LEON A. WEISBERG, M.D.

Department of Psychiatry and Neurology
Tulane Medical Center
New Orleans, Louisiana

CHARLES NICE, M.D.

Department of Radiology
Tulane Medical Center
New Orleans, Louisiana

MYRON KATZ, Ph.D.

Department of Mathematics
Arizona State University
Tempe, Arizona

CEREBRAL COMPUTED TOMOGRAPHY
A Text-Atlas

W. B. SAUNDERS COMPANY
Philadelphia London Toronto

W. B. Saunders Company: West Washington Square
Philadelphia, PA 19105

1 St. Anne's Road
Eastbourne, East Sussex BN21 3UN, England

1 Goldthorne Avenue
Toronto, Ontario M8Z 5T9, Canada

Cerebral Computed Tomography   ISBN   0-7216-9167-6

Last digit is the print number: 9   8   7   6   5   4   3

To Dr. Robert Heath, who had the wisdom to appreciate the value of the collaboration of neurologists and radiologists in the study of cerebral computed tomography, and who has worked continuously toward this joint approach, and to my family, whose inspiration and encouragement made the completion of this book possible.

L.A.W.

Preface

The introduction of cerebral computed tomography (CT) in the investigation of suspected intracranial pathological processes has revolutionized the approach to clinical neurological practice. Since the initial description of the practical scanning apparatus by Hounsfield and the results of the early clinical studies reported by Paxton and Ambrose less than five years ago, CT has been demonstrated to be an extremely sensitive, accurate and safe technique to investigate many neurological disorders. In addition, acceptance of CT by the medical community has occurred much more rapidly than the acceptance of isotope scan, angiography and air study. Such early acceptance is a result of low patient discomfort, minimal radiation exposure comparable to that of routine skull radiogram, and the highly developed technological capability of the first generation of CT scanners, which had diagnostic sensitivity and accuracy greater than other noninvasive imaging techniques and, in some cases, equal to that of the invasive contrast procedures — air study and angiography.

The initial published studies of CT emphasized the technical aspects, including description of the apparatus, physical principles of operation and image reconstruction, computer system, specific normal anatomical details of the transverse brain tissue sections and abnormal scan findings in pathological conditions. The initial clinical and radiographic studies were retrospective analyses of findings in patients whose diagnoses had been confirmed by complementary neurodiagnostic studies and operative and necropsy examination. These studies emphasized the radiological and pathological correlation which was necessary to assess the sensitivity, validity and reliability of CT in neurological diagnosis, and also confirmed that the technique of image reconstructive tomography was a significant and dramatic advance in neurological diagnosis with possible application for the entire field of diagnostic medicine.

These early CT studies investigated the diagnostic accuracy in many specific pathological conditions, including neoplasms, intracerebral hematoma, cerebral infarction, hydrocephalus and cerebral atrophy. However, no attempt was made to undertake prospective studies of the value of this new imaging technique in the investigation of specific neurological symptoms so as to place CT scanning in appropriate diagnostic perspective relative to other currently available diagnostic studies, both noninvasive and invasive. At present, CT is accepted as a highly accurate technique, but some health care planners have suggested that over-utilization is occurring and that the technology is expanding so rapidly that it is becoming an extremely expensive procedure. In addition, in certain clinical diagnostic situations it may not be superior to less expensive conventional diagnostic studies. Rapid technological advances have been achieved, including a matrix system of finer resolution, more rapid scanning time, thinner section scans, higher contrast resolution, and multiplane scans to include coronal and sagittal sections. These improvements have required continual upgrading of the existing models to achieve greater diagnostic detail and more precise anatomical localization, but at increasing cost. Studies have not addressed the questions of how these advances have affected diagnostic accuracy, utilization of other studies and total medical costs. Furthermore, initially CT was labeled as a noninvasive study but recent changes, including widespread utilization of contrast infusion studies with material which has known neurotoxicity and has been administered intravenously, intra-arterially or intrathecally, have modified this technique so that it is becoming an increasingly invasive study.

This book has been conceived and developed to serve as an introduction to the utilization of the CT scanner in evaluating neurological disorders, and is directed toward the neurologist, neurosurgeon, psychiatrist, internist, pediatrician and other physicians who will be ordering this study in the course of their investigation of a patient with neurological symptoms. It is hoped that this book will familiarize the physician with an approach to utilization of this diagnostic technique which is based upon a knowledge of its sensitivity and accuracy but also upon its limitations and an awareness of conditions in which alternative more readily available diagnostic tests will provide equivalent information. Because of limited access and high cost, there are frequently one- to five-week waiting periods for CT scans; the physician must choose those patients in whom the diagnostic yield is greatest. This can best be achieved by awareness of the CT scan's potential yield and accuracy as compared with other diagnostic procedures. The clinical neurological problems which are reported in this book are based upon over two years of clinical experience by neurologists and radiologists working together to determine the potential yield of CT scanning in specific neurological symptomatology. The organization of this book emphasizes the role of CT in specific clinical situations as they initially present to the physician, as well as the appropriate role of CT in the broad field of diagnostic evaluation.

LEON A. WEISBERG

Acknowledgments

I would like to thank Dr. Robert Heath for directly involving me in cerebral computed tomography and for providing support and encouragement. Almost all scans included in this book were performed at the Tulane Medical Center utilizing the Mark I EMI head scanner with the 160×160 matrix and $4^1/_2$ minute scan time. Mr. John Ariatti of EMItronics was most helpful in providing information and keeping us up to date about technical developments in CT. Our radiology technicians were responsible for the high quality of the scans and we owe special thanks to Mr. David Falterman and Ms. Norma Binns for their assistance in obtaining many of the scans. Thanks to Dr. Roger Tutton, Dr. Allen Roses and Dr. Albert Goree, who kindly lent several valuable scans, and to the American Journal of Medicine and the Radiological Society of North America, who permitted reprint of scans previously published in their journals. Dr. David Dunn and Dr. Jeff Ellison were especially helpful in collecting the clinical data on many patients. Dr. Donald Richardson and Dr. Rich Palmer carefully reviewed the chapter on the theory and computer aspects of CT. My wife Laurie provided invaluable secretarial and editorial assistance. And the publishers, especially Mr. George Vilk, were most helpful and supportive in seeing this book to completion.

L.A.W.

Contents

xi

PART ONE

OVERVIEW OF COMPUTED TOMOGRAPHIC (CT) SCANNING

The impact of the CT scanner upon the traditional and conventional concepts of management of patients with neurological symptoms can best be appreciated by an analysis of the increased early diagnostic sensitivity and accuracy in many neuropathological conditions with excellent clinical pathological correlation, decrease in utilization of other invasive diagnostic procedures, and assessment of its cost effectiveness in neurological diagnosis. At the Tulane Medical Center, 5500 scans have been performed on 5000 patients with 9 percent of scans representing repeat studies. For purposes of this analysis, the scans have been divided into two groups, each representing one-half of the total number (2750 CT studies), and comparison of diagnostic trends in these two groups demonstrates several interesting patterns (Table 1–1). In the initial series, the frequency of contrast infusion was 20 percent but, with reports of increasing pathological information which may be obtained with contrast infusion, this is now being performed in 53 percent; this compares to other series in which 50 to 70 percent of scans are subject to contrast enhancement. In patients with certain neurological disorders, including neoplasms, the necessity of a prior "routine" or noncontrast infusion study has been questioned. Elimination of the plain scan would increase the number of patients who could be studied per working day.[1] This dependence upon

TABLE 1–1. Reason for CT Scan Referral in 5500 Patients

Referral	Initial Series (per cent)	Current Series (per cent)
Specific Disorders	76	65
cerebrovascular disease	15	12
seizures	10	8
dementia	8	7
head trauma	7	9
suspected primary tumor	12	11
supratentorial	10.5	10
infratentorial	1.5	1
suspected metastases	6	5
visual or endocrine disorder and sella abnormality	1	1
disturbed consciousness	2	1
evaluation of previously documented lesion	2	1
post surgery or irradiation	6	4
orbital lesion	2	2
increased intracranial pressure	1	1
pediatric		
increasing head size	1	1
poor development	1	1
hearing loss	1	1
Nonspecific Disorders	24	35
headache	10	16
dizziness	8	10
syncope	2	4
vague psychiatric symptoms	1	2
weakness	3	3

contrast infusion may alter the nature of CT scanning to that of an invasive contrast study, and attempts are therefore being made to limit its use to cases in which postinfusion information may help establish specific pathological diagnoses or to cases in which the initial scan is negative but other reported studies have indicated a high probability of positive results with infusion study of a suspected lesion. Initially, low dosage (20 cc) contrast material infusion was associated with only infrequent enhancement pattern in non-neoplastic conditions as compared with a much higher incidence of enhancement in neoplasms, but by utilizing a higher dose (50 to 100 cc) or a rapidly administered drip infusion (300 cc administered over five minutes), the frequency with which enhancement has been detected in non-neoplastic conditions has increased to the extent that differentiation now is best established by the pattern, intensity and location of enhancement rather than simply by the presence of enhancement (Table 1–2). One consequence of this higher dose infusion study was that there was an immediate

and dramatic increment in the number of angiograms performed in cerebrovascular disease to differentiate infarction from neoplasm, vascular malformation or abscess, but this trend has decreased as greater clinical experience has been achieved and the temporal evolution of the enhancement pattern in non-neoplastic conditions has been documented. This trend toward increasing frequency of enhancement in non-neoplastic conditions brought with it certain associated problems in differential diagnosis, but this was later balanced by greater diagnostic accuracy, especially in the diagnosis of cerebral inflammatory disease, infarctions, and hematomas.

Of all scans performed, 44 percent were abnormal, 51 percent were normal, 4 percent were technically unsatisfactory, and 1 percent were indeterminant — that is, no specific diagnostic conclusion was possible based upon scan pattern. These indeterminant scans included studies that were technically adequate for interpretation but that showed an unusual ventricular asymmetry without accompanying distortion or displace-

TABLE 1–2.   Enhancement in Differential Diagnosis

	Frequency of Enhancement		
Pathological Condition	50 cc BOLUS (PER CENT)	100 cc BOLUS (PER CENT)	300 cc DRIP INFUSION (PER CENT)
cerebral infarction			
non-hemorrhagic	5	10	60
hemorrhagic	0	0	40
intracerebral hematoma	0	0	15
extradural hematoma	0	0	15
neoplasm			
meningioma	90	90	100
glioma	85	85	95
pituitary adenoma	100	100	100
craniopharyngioma	60	50	50
acoustic neurinoma	100	100	100
pinealoma	100	100	100
aneurysm	0	0	40
angioma	10	10	100
abscess	33	50	100

ment, an abnormal density pattern contiguous to bone or ventricles an unexplained region of abnormal density visualized on only one section, nonvisualization or an asymmetrical basal cisternal space. In these cases subsequent contrast infusion is indicated, and if this is negative, no further studies are usually indicated, although occasionally angiography or air study has been performed, confirming the lack of pathological findings indicated by CT.

If the CT scan showed an abnormality, it was necessary to correlate the finding with the clinical disorder to determine if the reported abnormality could explain the clinical symptoms or if it was perhaps an incidental findng. In 300 consecutive abnormal scans, analysis of clinical data and results of other neurodiagnostic studies indicated that in 10 to 15 percent of cases it was highly likely that the abnormality did not explain the clinical symptoms that were the indicated reason for the scan referral. This was most frequent in cases reported as cerebral atrophy, in which there were no concomitant intellectual or psychiatric symptoms. In another 1 to 2 percent the scan showed either infarction, subdural hematoma, cystic lesion or neoplasm in patients with vague nonspecific symptoms and without focal signs, seizures or a history of sudden or progressive clinical worsening, and in whom the symptoms persisted without change following treatment of certain conditions deemed surgically remediable. In these cases, further diagnostic and therapeutic procedures after detection by CT may have been initiated by the fact that the physician is provided with more information about brain structure than ever previously available; if an abnormality is suggested by the CT scan report, there is an obligation to evaluate this finding despite a paucity of clinical symptomatology. This is the case because of the physician's training, which is directed toward com-

pleteness of evaluation and because of a defensive tendency of the physician aimed at avoiding future malpractice litigation. In addition, there have been an increasing number of recent referrals for CT scan in cases involved in litigation, such as those involving possible cerebral concussion in which the medical indication for the scan is quite limited.

In March, 1975, it required an initial two- to three-month period to familiarize physicians with the potential capabilities of CT scanning, but after this time our scheduling was completely saturated, with a waiting period of two days for inpatients and four to 16 days for outpatients. With increasing awareness within the medical community about the capability of the CT scanner, the opening of new installations has usually produced a saturated schedule from the onset. As the clinical demand for CT increased, the scanner was made operational for up to 15 hours per day on a five-day schedule with additional use for four to seven hours on a sixth day. This has permitted us to perform 50 to 70 scans per week, a rate which compares to the average of 58 reported by Evens and Jost.[2] With a scanning time of four minutes, this required an appointment schedule with 20 to 45 minutes allocated for each patient, depending on the need for contrast study and sedation. There may be occasional delays of one to four hours, which are usually due to technical factors or the sedation of restless and uncooperative patients, but much of this problem will be obviated with more rapid scanning time. With increasing awareness of the availability of the scanner, the scheduling delay has increased, but this has recently been balanced by an increasing number of scan installations throughout the region. Furthermore, since CT is especially valuable in head trauma, it should be available on 24-hour emergency basis; this is not presently feasible in many installations, although angiography is usually performed on an emergency basis. Careful studies will be necessary to compare the diagnostic sensitivity and accuracy of the dedicated head model with the body scanner, but with the present generation of scanners it is generally agreed that the dedicated head unit is superior in studying suspected neurological disorders. Despite this fact, one-half of referring physicians were not aware of any differences or limitations and in ordering the study opted for the facility with the shortest scheduling delay, regardless of the specific disorder to be investigated.

Our clinical data has been derived from referrals generated from multiple sources, including the Charity Hospital of New Orleans, which is a large state-run hospital, Veterans Administration Hospital and other private hospitals in the greater New Orleans regions. Of the patients studied, two-thirds were inpatients and one-third were outpatients referred either by private physicians or from multiple clinics of the Charity Hospital or Veterans Administration Hospital system. Fifty-two percent of patients studied were ambulatory, 22 percent were in wheelchairs and 26 percent were on stretchers. Following the introduction of CT scanning the number of neurological and neurosurgical inpatients at the Charity Hospital increased by 25 percent over the number in the preceding years without any possible alternative explanation, and the number of neurosurgical operations performed also increased. The number of ambulatory inpatients who were studied by CT was greater than the number of ambulatory inpatients who had EEG, skull radiogram or isotope scan, and this may reflect the need to hospitalize patients for CT. Due to certain well-conceived carefully monitored economic restraints imposed upon the physicians of the Charity Hospital and Veterans Administration Hospital, all scan requests had to be approved by a neurology or neurosurgical attending physician. In the first year of operation more than 58 percent of studies were abnormal; this was higher than in all other neurodiagnostic procedures performed during this period. With somewhat greater flexibility in the availability of the scan, the incidence of abnormal studies has decreased, but this may reflect either of two trends. Firstly, the obvious conclusion was that less care and discrimination were being employed in the selection of patients for scanning, but this was not reflected in the analysis of the clinical data available with each patient, which confirmed that there was no increase in the number of scans performed for vague and nonspecific symptoms. Secondly, the more likely explanation was that there had been a change in the approach to the selection process such that patients in whom other contrast studies had been contemplated but in whom the indications were questioned initially had CT scans and if they were normal it obviated the need for further contrast studies. If the clinical situation indicated that a preoperative angiogram would still be needed, CT was frequently not performed. In support of this approach, several angiomas, aneurysms and neoplasms were directly studied with angiography; although CT may have been valuable in their detection, subsequent preoperative contrast study was still necessary. Viewed in this perspective, a negative result of CT serves as a "positive" study, since it reduces the indication for other invasive time-consuming procedures and reduces hospital stay. This lowered incidence of positive studies reflects a change in the position of CT from that of a "revolutionary and special" procedure in which indications for its use were unsettled to one with which the clinician felt increasingly comfortable and knowledgeable about its value in the diagnosis of specific clinical problems.

Of the initial 2750 scans performed, approximately 90 percent were referred by neurologists and neurosurgeons; of these 54 percent were abnormal. In the most recent studies, the frequency of physicians who request the CT scan but have not received specific training in neurological diagnosis has increased to 30 percent, and the incidence of abnormal studies has decreased to 38 percent. This trend appears to reflect utilization of the CT scan as an expensive triage procedure that may be used to replace the performance of a complete neurological history and examination. Analysis of the reason for referral has demonstrated an increasing number of patients who have been referred because of vague, nonspecific and poorly defined neurological symptoms. In some instances referral was directly related to an abnormality of EEG or skull radiograph which may not have always warranted further study if reviewed by a neurologist prior to availability of the CT scan. The physician may have followed the patient's clinical status, but now these patients are frequently referred for CT study to exclude any "structural" pathology, even in the absence of definite symptoms. Because of this trend, it may be prudent to have a physician who has received formal training in neurological diagnosis evaluate the patient prior to CT scan.

Initial experience in the CT era derived from the Mayo Clinic showed that, following the installation of their first scanner, the number of neurological and neurosurgical patients increased by 15 to 20 percent. Because of this, the number of EEG studies also increased, but utilization of isotope scan, echoencephalogram, and air study significantly decreased, while angiography remained at a relatively constant level.[3] At the Mallinckrodt Institute, there was a 66 percent reduction for air study, 34 percent for angiography, and 29 per-

cent for isotope scan.[2] At Mayo, the number of negative angiograms decreased from 30 percent in 1972 to 22 percent in 1975; this 25 percent drop reflects the high sensitivity and accuracy of CT, utilized as a screening procedure. In addition, there was a marked change in the type of pathological process studied by angiography, including a 50 percent decrease in the diagnoses related to traumatic hematoma and edema; tumors increased by 50 percent and vascular lesions by 25 percent. Several other results in the diagnosis of tumors by CT are worth emphasizing. Prior to CT, the incidence of Grade I and II astrocytoma, documented by operative findings, was only 5 to 7 percent, whereas in 1975 those low-grade gliomas comprised 30 percent of all histologically proven cases, although earlier diagnosis does not appear to be associated with an improvement in prognosis.[3] Furthermore, grossly visible incidental meningiomas are not infrequently detected at the necropsy examination, but these lesions are not usually detected by isotope scan, EEG or skull radiogram. With CT, asymptomatic meningiomas have been visualized, whereas other studies were negative. Although initial studies indicated difficulties in studying posterior fossa lesions, our experience has reflected a marked increase in the early diagnosis of posterior fossa lesions prior to the development of signs and symptoms of increased intracranial pressure. There has been a marked increase in the frequency of the diagnosis of acoustic neurinoma, tentorial meningioma, and brain stem tumors; such diagnosis was quite difficult prior to CT; and the frequency of the diagnosis of porencephalic, epidermoid and arachnoid cysts in the last 18 months at several institutions is greater than that of the previous five years.

Wortzman and Holgate analyzed the cost effectiveness of a neurological evaluation utilizing the CT scan, specifically in regard to the need for contrast procedures and subsequent hospitalization.[4] They evaluated the importance of the CT findings in 203 patients in influencing the decision to perform or avoid angiography or air study; in 61 instances angiography was prevented, and air study was obviated in 89, whereas in 11 instances angiography or air study was deemed necessary because of CT findings. An additional 241 patients were analyzed in reference to the value of CT in deciding the need for subsequent hospitalization. This showed that CT prevented hospitalization in 140, prompted admission in 28, and was 'not a crucial factor in 73 cases. This is in agreement with the experience of other centers with CT, as it has become possible to evaluate patients with common complaints such as seizure, headache, dizziness and syncope on an outpatient basis if the CT scan is negative.

In our experience in our large ambulatory neurology clinic where patients are usually seen on a referral basis, the most common problems related to possible CNS lesions include headache, dizziness, syncope, seizures, mental change, and gait or visual disturbances. Of those patients in whom the neurological history and examination raised suspicion of specific organic neurological lesions, further neurodiagnostic studies were performed in 60 percent. Ten percent of patients had abnormal neurological signs, abnormal EEG or abnormal skull radiograph that required further investigation, and in some instances may have required delineation with contrast studies. In these patients CT confirms the presence or absence of an underlying lesion and it was on this basis that the decision for admission was then made. In the 30 percent who had negative CT, no lesion was subsequently diagnosed. Of 200 patients who were evaluated with headache only, 20 had an abnormality defined by EEG or skull radiograph;

and of these 20, CT confirmed the presence of a lesion in only three, which then required inpatient hospitalization for contrast studies, whereas in 17 CT was negative. Of those 17 CT-negative patients, subsequent isotope scan, angiography or air study confirmed the negative results of CT with follow-up of 12 months or longer.

In the decade 1962–72, there was a tenfold increase in the number of isotope scans performed at the Johns Hopkins Hospital. Despite this, there was no increase in the number of brain tumors operated upon or in the mortality rate, although the interval between the onset of neurological symptoms and the time of tumor diagnosis was decreased by the use of radionuclide scanning. For example, 93 percent of meningiomas, 67 percent of astrocytomas and metastases had positive scans at onset of symptoms, whereas 100 percent of meningiomas and 87 percent of astrocytomas had positive scans by 28 months, and 100 percent of metastatic lesions had positive scans by eight months.[5] Furthermore, isotope brain scan was the most sensitive screening procedure to detect the presence of potentially operable and remediable neurosurgical lesions, and negative studies frequently obviated the need for hospitalization and invasive contrast procedures, but it was recognized that low-grade and small-sized lesions were not always detected by isotope scan. In one study comparing the results of isotope and CT scan in 297 patients it was shown that they were frequently in agreement but CT was more sensitive; they provided similar results in 185 (both positive in 52 and negative in 133), whereas in 87 cases CT was positive but isotope scan was negative; in only nine cases was isotope scan positive but CT negative.[6] Of 25 patients who had CT scan performed primarily because of positive isotope scan, CT demonstrated single or multiple lesions in 10 but was negative in 15 cases. The impression of a falsely positive isotope scan was confirmed by subsequent angiography or air study. In the study of patients with suspected cerebrovascular disease, isotope and CT scan were complementary, as isotope scan is more sensitive in detecting abnormalities of cerebral blood flow but less sensitive than CT in differentiating uptake in normal and infarcted tissue. In the diagnosis of suspected neoplasms, isotope scan is much less effective as a sensitive screening procedure because contrast discrimination between normal parenchyma and neoplastic tissue must be quite pronounced before it can be detected, but more subtle differences may be defined by CT. In the evaluation of cerebral atrophic and hydrocephalic conditions, intravenous use of gamma-emitting radionuclide has little place; although isotope cisternography may demonstrate abnormalities of CSF flow patterns, CT directly visualizes enlarged ventricular and subarachnoid spaces. The value of the combined negative results of these two studies is that there have been no cases in which both isotope scan and CT are negative and subsequent studies have detected a pathological lesion, with a follow-up of 12 to 18 months.

REFERENCES

1. Butler AR, Kricheff I: Non-contrast computed tomography in brain tumor suspects: is it necessary? Abstract presented at American Society of Neuroradiology, Atlanta, May 1976. Neuroradiology 12:48, 1976.
2. Evens RG, Jost G: Economic analysis of computed tomography units. Am J Roentgenol 127:191, 1976
3. Baker HL: CT and neuroradiology: a fortunate primary union. Am J Roentgenol 127:101, 1976.
4. Wortzman G, Holgate RC, Morgan PP: Cranial computed tomography: An evaluation of cost effectiveness. Radiology 117:75, 1975.
5. George RD, Wagner HN: Ten years of brain tumor scanning at Johns Hopkins. In: Noninvasive Brain Imaging HJ DeBlanc, JA Sorenson (eds). Society of Nuclear Medicine, New York, 1975, pp 3–16.
6. Clifford JR, Connolly ES, Voorhies RM: Comparison of radionuclide scans with CT in diagnosis of intracranial disease. Neurology 26:1119, 1976.

Chapter 2 Principles and Technique of Image Reconstruction with CT

Myron Katz, Ph.D.

Tomography is a radiographic diagnostic technique which attempts to improve visualization of certain regions by increasing our ability to localize areas of the body. Conventional or geometric tomography commonly refers to the original techniques in which the x-ray source and photographic plate are moved in opposite directions within parallel planes in a coordinated manner. If the source is moved at the same speed as that of the film, then a planar section of the patient one half the distance from the film to the source will have a projection which moves with the film. The planar section remains in focus on the tomogram while the rest of the intervening tissues are blurred. Conventionally, the coordinated motion of the source and the x-ray plate is along a line. The region of the body which stays in focus and has a particular *section thickness* diminishes as the magnitude of the angular displacement *(tomographic angle)* increases. Although a tomogram usually provides quite good spatial resolution, with increasing tomographic angle the image contrast diminishes owing to blurring. Spurious or *phantom images* have been described and are caused by this blurring. Such imaging and localization problems have en-

couraged the use of other planar paths, including circular, elliptical, spiral or hypocycloidal. In conventional tomography contrast has remained poor, but its good spatial resolution maintains the usefulness of conventional tomography in high-contrast (bone, airways or contrast media) studies.[1, 2]

To improve image contrast, it has been necessary to inject air or iodide substances to create artificial differences in x-ray attenuation so as to visualize accurately the ventricles, subarachnoid spaces and blood vessels. Other methods to improve imaging were explored by D. E. Kuhl, who used a computer to process data collected by a gamma detector at various axial angles after injected radionuclides localized a tumor.[3] The output image, actually a reconstruction, was of a cross-sectional plane parallel to the paths of the detected gamma rays. Since no overlying structures were sampled by radiation, they could not blur the image, but with this technique only passable resolution was obtained. This exploration into the use of computer processed, axially collected data had an earlier proponent in W. H. Oldendorf. He added a collimated scintillation counter, and recognized the potential to the study of biological systems —

especially the brain.[4] It was not until G. N. Hounsfield and EMI Ltd. utilized these ideas with x-rays that computed tomography became firmly established as a medical diagnostic technique.[5, 6]

The most effective use of computed tomography requires an understanding of the theory of the technique — *reconstruction from projections*. In most examples a transverse planar section is sampled by a beam narrowed to intersect only that particular section. Projection data collected by a collimated detector or an array of detectors is processed by a computer according to an algorithm. The digital output displayed on a cathode ray tube is an approximation of the distribution of the x-ray attenuation coefficients in the transverse section. Computed tomography is basically noninvasive, low in radiation and provides excellent contrast at modest spatial resolution.

CT is subject to misinterpretations arising from almost every aspect of its various designs. Currently available devices apply the theory of reconstruction from projections in a way that is open to mathematical criticism. Data collection methods are under the conflicting stresses of image contrast, spatial resolution, scan speed and dosage requirements; accuracy is further hampered by the nonhomogeneity of the physical phenomena involved. Algorithms are also evolving to handle these changing constraints; speed and stability in the presence of erroneous data are among the critical issues. Even when the output is virtually error free, interpretation of the image may be difficult.

RECONSTRUCTION FROM PROJECTIONS

In 1917, an Austrian mathematician, J. Radon, proved that all of the inner structure of an object can be determined from the information available in the infinite set of all of its projections.[7] More recently, it has been recognized that any infinite subset of the set of all projections will suffice. Therefore, it was established that the idea of reconstruction from projections makes sense theoretically, but no one had shown that any finite number of projections contains sufficient information. With this theoretical background alone, physical implementation was attempted.

Scientists recognize that there is a limit, referred to as the spatial resolution, which determines how closely projection data can be examined for additional information. *Resolution* is generally defined as the size of the smallest part of the observation or image that can be reliably discriminated. High resolution means finer or smaller values for resolution. For this reason, scientists view projections as discrete functions. To a scientist a projection is a function which takes a different value only on small (nonoverlapping) subregions of the film, where these regions have a diameter no smaller than the resolution of the projection data.

An *algorithm* is a rule of procedure for solving a problem (like the long division algorithm) that frequently involves repetition of an operation. Scientists present their descriptions of the theory of reconstruction from projections via the justification of algorithms. The mathematicians prove that conclusions are determined by assumptions; in many cases, these proofs do not explain how to perform that deduction. In the context of computed tomography, an algorithm uses the projection data to choose a particular reconstruction from a predetermined class of feasible reconstructions—called the *reconstruction space*. The reconstruction space for some algorithms which were considered for the EMI head scanner is the set of all 160×160 arrays of real numbers. This was done since that device represents a cross-section of a head on a 160 × 160 array of small squares. The number for each square, or *pixel*, indicates the average x-ray attenuation within a 1.5 × 1.5 × 13 mm rectangular parallelopiped of brain matter.

More than a year after the initial work of Hounsfield, a mathematician, Kennan T. Smith, proved that, without some *a priori* information about the sampled object, that object cannot even be estimated from a finite number of projections.[8] This result cast quite a shadow over the application of the theory of reconstruction from projections for the following reasons: Firstly, there is only a finite number of projections (and these are discrete, not continuous), and secondly, no one had found reasonable *a priori* assumptions that together with a finite set of projection data allow for a mathematically sound theoretical treatment.

The currently employed methods of data collection followed by computed choice of a reconstruction have not overcome the hurdle illuminated by Kennan Smith. No rigorous argument has been presented to date which expresses the reliability of such a reconstruction. The meaning of a particular CT scan can at present only be inferred from past performance. With certain alterations in the existing equipment, a new algorithm could be applied which uses special projection angles and sets standards for the resolution of the projection data. This method lets the physician know that the reconstruction obtained is the unique reconstruction that best fits the empirically obtained projection data. Furthermore, this algorithm provides an upper limit on the error in the reconstruction, and it is now possible to determine the reliability of a reconstruction obtained with this algorithm. In this case error could only result from errors in the original projection data. When this occurs the inconsistency of the projection data

can be used to depress the reliability indicator to permit warning about the degree of uncertainty in the reconstruction.[9]

DATA COLLECTION

When a monochromatic x-ray beam, of intensity I, passes through an object, the attenuation, ΔI, causes fewer x rays to pass through to the detector. The linear x-ray attenuation coefficient, μ, expresses the instantaneous ratio $\dfrac{\Delta I/I}{\Delta x}$ at any point along the path of the beam. For a homogeneous object, μ is a constant and the penetrating intensity, I, can be related to the incident intensity, I_0, by $I = I_0 e^{-\mu x}$ where x expresses the thickness of the transmitting object and e = 2.718. The result is that intensity of the transmitted beam decreases exponentially as the thickness of the attenuator increases.[10, 11]

Attenuation is defined as reduction in intensity. Only two processes significantly diminish the number of x-ray photons which penetrate the object under the conditions prevalent in computed tomography. More important at lower x-ray energies is the photoelectric effect. On the other hand, Compton scattering of x-rays by water is more than nine times as likely as the photoelectric effect if the energy of the incident photon exceeds 57 keV.

True absorption of x-rays is called the photoelectric effect. An impinging *photon* can be absorbed via the excitation (increase in energy) of an electron of an atom—thereby causing that electron to jump to a higher energy level or even escape from the atom. The photoelectric effect is more probable with the inner shell electrons since they can more easily accept the incident energy at x-ray frequencies. The "potential well" is deeper (the energy required for escape is greater) the larger the atomic number (Z). The probability of a photoelectric absorption per gram, that is per unit mass, varies as Z^3. For example, since oxygen has $Z = 8$ and calcium has $Z = 20$, an electron of calcium is almost 16 times as likely to photoelectrically absorb an impinging photon as is an electron of oxygen.

Like the photoelectric effect, Compton scattering can occur as an interaction between a photon and an electron. This process is most probable when a photon interacts with an outer, loosely bound atomic electron. Similarly, a transfer of energy occurs but the overriding concern is the change in direction of the altered photon. It is the density of the matter or, more precisely, the number of electrons per cubic centimeter which most accurately predicts the probability of Compton scattering. This may partially explain the significantly lower x-ray attenuation of fat than that of protein.

Attenuation of the x-ray beam is generally proportional to the number of electrons encountered, since electrons are responsible for both effects, but the atomic number of the atoms in the tissue greatly affects the probability of photoelectric absorption. A scale of attenuation has been named after the inventor of CT, Hounsfield. One Hounsfield or EMI unit represents a 0.1 percent change in attenuation relative to that of water.

Another aspect of the passage of the x-ray beam through living tissue results in a change in the nature of the spectrum of the incident beam, since the x-ray source is not monochromatic. Lower energy photons are more likely to be absorbed, as photoelectric absorption varies inversely as the cube of the energy of the incident photon. This results in a change in the spectrum of the penetrating x-ray beam toward the higher energies. Such high-energy photons are characteristically more penetrat-

ing, or harder. This beam hardening alters the probability of an average x-ray photon from the beam to undergo Compton scattering or photoelectric absorption and favors the former effect.[12]

The attenuation coefficient expresses the amount of scattering plus absorption per unit length of a particular kind of living tissue. It is generally assumed that the attenuation coefficient observed for any part of the body will be the same for each projection, but beam hardening invalidates this assumption mildly. To minimize this error, 4 to 5 mm of aluminum is used to preharden the beam.

Another important aspect of attenuation results from the distribution of scattering angles accompanying the Compton effect. With an x-ray energy of 73 keV and an accelerating potential of 120 kVp (used by the EMI Scanner) more than half of the scattered photons are deflected through an angle of less than 45°. This means that the geometry of data collection plays a major role in the contrast and noise in the data. Some authors report that in conventional radiology over 90 percent of the photons incident on the film are forwardly scattered through an angle less than 90°.

The Meaning of a Projection

Imagine that an object is composed of various thicknesses of materials, each with its characteristic attenuation coefficient (μ_1, μ_2, μ_3, ..., μ_n) and particular thicknesses (x_1, x_2, x_3, ..., x_n). The observed transmitted intensity I of an incident beam with an intensity I_0 would be given by:

$$I = I_0 e^{-\mu_1 x_1} e^{-\mu_2 x_2} e^{-\mu_3 x_3} \ldots e^{-\mu_n x_n}$$
$$= I_0 e^{-(\mu_1 x_1 + \mu_2 x_2 + \mu_3 x_3 + \ldots + \mu_n x_n)}$$

or equivalently

$$\ln (I_0/I) = \mu_1 x_1 + \mu_2 x_2 + \ldots + \mu_n x_n.$$

The idea of computed tomography is to treat the x_i's as knowns and try to determine the μ_i's. This is plausible if the problem is viewed as a linear system where the unknowns can be remotely sampled via a sufficient set of simultaneous equations. To get the required set of linear equations an object is assumed to have constant attenuation on (usually square) uniform subregions — each subregion having a known position and shape. Then a planar object can be represented by an array of attenuation coefficients:

$$
\begin{array}{cccc}
\mu_{11} & \mu_{12} & \mu_{12}...\mu_{1n} \\
\mu_{21} & \mu_{22} & \mu_{23}...\mu_{2n} \\
\vdots & \vdots & \vdots \\
\mu_{n1} & \mu_{n2} & \mu_{n3} & \mu_{nn}
\end{array}
$$

Similarly, a three-dimensional object could be represented by a three-dimensional array of attenuation coefficients. The simultaneous equations can be obtained by taking projections along the rows, giving n equations, along the columns, giving n more equations, along the diagonal directions, upper left to lower right and upper right to lower left, giving $4n - 2$ more equations. Similarly, projections can be taken in other directions. Clearly, at least n^2 equations would be needed to determine the n^2 unknowns which specify a planar object — therefore the need of a large number of projections to get the required data. The decision to allow n^2 numbers to specify the distribution of the attenuation coefficients in an arbitrary object is choosing a reconstruction space. The problem is to make measurements which will allow the determination of the best reconstruction of the x-ray attenuation distribution among the class of reconstructions that can be specified by such an array. A three-dimensional object can be imaged by independently imaging each two-dimensional cross-section. The engineer concerned with data collection will endeavor to provide, with a minimum of error, the required values of $\ln(I_0/I)$ for those equations.

When a three-dimensional object is considered to be a stacked array of two-dimensional planar arrays, rectangular parallelopipeds are usually specified as the uniformly shaped subregions. There are clear advantages to having the thickness of the slice or equivalently the height of each of these parallelopipeds as small as possible. This would provide good spatial resolution in the vertical direction and minimize the partial volume phenomenon (discussed later). Unfortunately, the available methods for collecting data about a thin region necessarily diminish the number of photons which reach the detectors. The x-ray beam can be collimated before entering the patient so that only the particular slice is irradiated. In actual practice, a larger wedge-shaped region is sampled by the beam. To avoid counting the only slightly scattered x-rays by collimating the beam at the exit face further decreases the number of photons reaching the detector.

Another difficulty associated with the use of thinner slices is time. If thinner slices are used, more slices may have to be studied. In most cases, thinning the slice only increases the amount of time needed to collect the data for that slice. Therefore, thinning the slice dramatically increases the amount of time necessary for adequate examination of the patient.

Types of Detectors

There are two types of detectors in use: scintillation crystals, frequently composed of sodium iodide, and multiwire gas chambers, frequently filled with xenon. The scintillation detectors produce a signal by allowing x-rays to excite electrons in the crystal.

When an electron returns to an empty orbital of the lattice, light is produced. This signal is amplified via an optically coupled photomultiplier which produces the electronic impulse. Since the time required for the crystal to reach an unexcited state can be comparable to the time between adjacent data collections, this "afterglow" effect can produce distortions near transitions between bone and air. Multiwire gas chambers act like Geiger counters. When a photon knocks out an orbital electron of xenon, the resulting ions carry an electric current between wires that are kept at a constant potential. This current provides the signal for the data collection. Scintillation counters provide high amplification of the input x-ray intensity; however, they are large in size and relatively costly. The cheaper gas chambers are smaller and can be packed closely together. Currently, scintillation detectors are used in systems that require a small number of detectors, whereas the gas chambers are incorporated when the design calls for a large number of detectors packed closely together. An important advantage of these photon-electronic detector systems over photographic film is that the spectrum of response available more than matches the variations in the output intensities of the x-ray beam.

Parallel and Fan Beam Techniques

The gantry is the structure which holds the x-ray source, the detector system and various collimators; the motion of these components is provided by the gantry. The first generation machines employ the parallel technique of data collection, and require both translational and rotational motions. Each projection is a series of data collections in which the beam is made to pass through a single row of attenuation values. If we call the projection angle in the direction of rows $0°$, then n data would be collected: I_1, I_2, I_3, $\ldots$, I_n. These data would then be considered the projection data for the $0°$ direction. The ith datum, I_i, provides $\ln (I_0/I_i) = \mu_{i1}x_1 + \mu_{i2}x_2 + \ldots + \mu_{in}x_n$. Therefore, the data are collected via the transmission of parallel beams. The motion of the x-ray source and the detector is a translation perpendicular to the direction of the paths of the x-rays. After the data for this direction have been collected, the gantry rotates to a new projection angle and collects another set of data, which becomes the projection data for this angle.

Following the first generation machines, various types of fan beam geometry have been used. The key to the use of fan beams is a linear or circular array of detectors. The only collimation applied in such a system restricts the x-rays to the particular slice of interest. Within that slice the x-rays from a small source are allowed to diverge into a fan beam. The array of detectors can simultaneously record the intensities over large portions of the slice — thereby receiving the data for many equations at the same time.

The second-generation machines employ the fan beam geometry and utilize the same translational and rotational motions of the x-ray source and the rigidly connected detector array that were used by the first machines. This form of data collection can be viewed as a parallel beam geometry in the sense that the information collected by a particular detector in the array collects only parallel beams of photons within a single translational pass. If the linear array had five detectors, the projection data collected would be virtually equivalent to the information available in five repetitions of "translate then rotate" in a first-generation machine. Such a device would have shorter scanning times, as this changes inversely with the number of detectors.

New scanners do not employ translational motions at all; they use fan beam geometries and gas chamber detectors so that rotation of the gantry collects large amounts of data in very short periods. The realization of the data for each projection requires the computer to sort out data collected at many different angular positions. In one case, the x-ray source and a relatively large number of detectors are rigidly connected. Because each detector is involved in the sampling only of an annular region and since calibration in this system is very difficult, circular or onion-shaped inaccuracies frequently show up in the reconstructions. Finally, the resolution of the projection data is limited by the size of the detectors and their distance from the x-ray source. The newest data collection method requires an entire circle of detectors. In this case, only the x-ray source moves; the detector circle is motionless. The shortcomings of this system are (1) the cost of such an extensive detector array, (2) difficulty in collimation of scattered radiation and (3) inefficient use of radiation passing through the patient.

Resolution of the Data

Since the data must be discrete to be measured experimentally, it is necessary to separate the x-ray photons into compartments so that the intensity within each compartment can be measured independently. In the fan beam model, this is accomplished spatially by the use of an array of detectors. The separation of the compartments chronologically can be done by an internal clock within the computer or by pulsing the x-ray source as the x-ray gantry is rotated. It is a different matter in the devices which employ translational and rotational motions. In this case a glass plate, on which is placed a series of parallel thin strips of lead, is put between the patient's head and the detector. This grid, called the graticule, provides the spatial and chronological separation required for the collection of the photons.

Although each system has a clearly defined distance for the resolution of the collected projection data, the utility of that data depends as well on the expected accuracy. This accuracy can be expressed as *contrast*. Here the reference is made to the precision of the measurement. If σ is the standard deviation of the error in the measurement of the intensity of the emerging x-ray beam when, for example, 150 photons originally entered the patient, then the standard deviation of the measurement when N times 150 photons enter the patient will be $\sigma/\sqrt{N}$. Therefore, if N = 10^4 then the standard deviation of the error in the measurement will decrease by a factor of 10^2. This would suggest that if a finer graticule were used, say twice as fine, and everything else remained the same, then the resolution of the data will improve by a factor of two but the contrast of the data will degrade by a factor of $\sqrt{2}$. The situation regarding the trade-off between the contrast and spatial resolution of the fan beam systems is important. Owing to the size of the detectors within the array, resolution is hard to improve, and because of the effects of forward scattering, the standard deviation of the error in the measurements would also be high. On the other hand, time is not critical, since there is no need for translational motion, so longer exposure time can allow some improvement in the contrast.

Maximum exposure to the patient has been estimated from 2.5 rads to 4 rads per scan for a series of three to four scans; this is comparable to a plain skull series. These exposure rates are consistent with the asymmetric nature of x-ray attenuation — as explained in the discussion of beam hardening. For example, 2.8 rads has been quoted as the maximum dosage to the right eye (the one closer to the x-ray tube) in an orbital scan, but the left eye may have only one fifth the exposure.

In those CT scanners which incorporate rotational and translational motions, the number of projection angles, as well as the specification of the particular angles themselves, has been a moderate design problem. Led by some theoretical studies and experimentation, Hounsfield and EMI decided upon the use of equally spaced projection angles and chose 180 for the number of these angles. Recently, EMI has decided to utilize one third this number of angles for certain optional modes of operation. This would reduce scanning time, but only further experimentation can recommend the quality of the produced reconstruction under these conditions.

Scanning time is often a consideration given much importance. The advantages of brief scanning include improved versatility, if motion is a problem, and more efficient use of the scanner. The EMI head scanner yields two images through the use of two detectors which collect photons in adjacent slices in a total scanning time of about 270 seconds. The use of fan beam geometry allows much improved scanning time. Such scanners have succeeded in cutting scan time to between 150 and 20 seconds and recently marketed scanners have scanning times under ten seconds, but with faster scanning comes loss of accuracy in calculating attenuation coefficients.

Calibration of the source-detector system is of fundamental importance. Since the observed attenuation must allow for the distinction between various tissues, even the slightest insta-

bility in the output of the x-ray source or the sensitivity of the detector system can lead to important misinterpretations. The EMI Scanner literally recalibrates itself during each projection through the use of a plastic rod. By assuming that the NaI crystal and the coupled photomultiplier as well as the x-ray source are operating consistently during the data acquisition for a single projection, and given that the x-ray attenuation of the plastic rod is known, the computer can rescale the projection data for that projection angle so that it is consistent with the known information. Similar rescaling procedures are available for the second generation, fan beam machines. But frequent rescaling of the source-detector system is difficult and time-consuming for the newer models, and this may result in the production of artifacts.

A problem receiving recent attention involves the hardware device which converts the analog electronic signal generated by the detector to a form which is (digital) computer-readable. The problem is one of accuracy of conversion. The resulting error can be around 0.5 percent — a value that exceeds manufacturers' estimated requirements of about 0.1 percent error in the projection data.

The EMI Scanner employs another mechanism to facilitate accurate data collection. The patient's head is inserted into a cavity fitted with a water bag so that air near the head can be forced away by water pressure. This water arrangement serves at least three purposes. (1) The water tends to preharden the beam. (2) Since water instead of air is adjacent to bone, the detectors are not required to measure very great differences in attenuation over short time intervals during the translational sweep required for each projection — a problem that tests the accuracy of response of the detection instruments. (3) The outer container for the water allows the beam to traverse a fixed length (27 cm) of waterlike attenuating matter—this further diminishes the stress on accurate response of the detector system.

The gantry of the EMI Scanner uses a conventional x-ray tube energized to about 120 to 140 kVp with a current of 30 mA. The beam produced is collimated to a rectangle 26 mm tall and a few millimeters wide. At the receiving end is a pair of NaI scintillation detectors coupled to photomultipliers, each responding to half the beam. A graticule placed right before the detectors collates the photons so that 240 transmission readings are stored by each detector during each translational sweep. The entire gantry rotates 1° and repeats the process in the same plane. This is repeated for 180° taking about 4.5 minutes and produces two CT scans: 13 mm thick adjacent cuts.

ALGORITHMS

Although fundamentally different algorithmic processes have been explored, the basic idea behind the prominent methods for passing from radiological projection data to a reconstruction is described in the *back-projection* or *summation* method.[13, 14] This technique produces a reconstruction by overlaying a series of spread-out or back-projected images which can be obtained from the data in each projection; the value at each point in the reconstruction is the sum of the densities of each ray passing through that point. If a test object consists of a single disk in a homogeneous background and four projections of it were made, the reconstruction would be similar to an eight-pointed star (Fig. 2–1). The back-projection method is not accurate since the original disk has been spread out in eight directions. In the example of the reconstruction of the disk, the simple nature of the original object is reflected in the single star pattern created, but when more general objects are imaged with this technique, spurious details may be hard to recognize and discount. In addition, the reconstruction does not have projection data which agree with the original data provided.

To improve the back-projected image, spurious details can be avoided by a process which removes the star-shaped or point-spread effects; such an algorithm is named *convolution* or *filtered back-projection*. Alternatively, it is possible to concentrate on the production of a reconstruction whose projection data agree with the original data; algebraic reconstruction technique (ART) is the best known algorithm based on this idea. Both kinds of algorithms utilize the back-projection process, but only after they employ rules to alter the projection data. The key difference lies in the way the data are transformed. ART proceeds iteratively by altering the data for each projection angle in a way which depends on the present guess for the reconstructed image, so that when this data is then back-projected, the new image agrees with the original data at that projection angle. Convolution uses a simple rule to change or filter all of the projection data uniformly before any back-projection proceeds.

Originally, the EMI Scanner programmed its computer to calculate a reconstruction using the ART algorithm because of the following: (1) when the data is error-free, ART tends to pick the reconstruction (from the reconstruction space of 160 × 160 arrays of real numbers) which agrees with the projection data and is closest (in the least sum of squared deviation sense) to the zero array, i.e., the 160 × 160 array of zeros. It is not in the nature of ART to introduce spurious

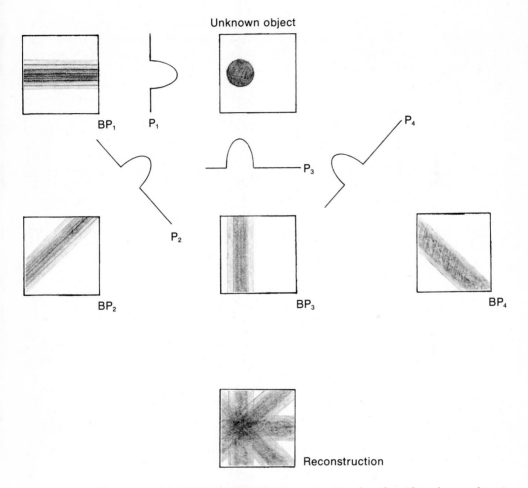

Figure 2–1.   Illustration of the BACK-PROJECTION reconstruction algorithm. The unknown object is top central. Given information is the set of projection data: P_1, P_2, P_3, P_4. The back-projected images, BP_1, BP_2, BP_3, and BP_4, are the spread out values of the corresponding projections. The reconstruction is obtained by adding together or overlaying the back-projected images.

images when good data are available. Nothing so clear-cut has been deduced about the convolution algorithm; the reconstruction produced by convolution may not even tend to agree with the provided projection data. (2) Compared to convolution ART is less affected by noisy data in its choice of reconstruction as long as the noise level exceeds a modest figure. (3) ART's mathematical description is flexible enough to accept the introduction of additional information (called constraints); this flexibility has allowed the creation of various other algorithms in the same family. (4) ART allows the use of projection data which do not span a full semicircular arc; this is definitely not the case for convolution. (5) Generally, ART has the capability to more accurately depict large local fluctuations in attenuations without a concomitant amplification of the effects of noise in the data than its rival, convolution.

With the demand for faster scanning and the rise in confidence in data collection, EMI switched to convolution; they may have considered the following reasons: (1) ART is significantly more time-consuming than convolution. Convolution utilizes only one third the amount of computer time; this was not an issue when the gantry motions required 4.5 minutes but newer machines operate in one third to one twentieth of these times. (2) Because of the iterative nature of ART — it proceeds by utilizing the projection data at each angle in isolation and then continues to the next angle, continuing for a number of cycles — and the fact that real projection data will not match any feasible reconstruction (with probability 1.0), the current guess will tend to wander among virtually equivalent reconstructions after a few cycles of iterations. Convolution's two-step nature (first filter all of the data, then backproject) does not present this difficulty. (3) Since ART tends to wander,

some criterion must be used to end its execution; this stopping criterion affects the accuracy of the reconstruction but has not been logically linked to that accuracy. Convolution requires no such arbitrary condition.

Other results further suggest the implementation of convolution including: (1) Convolution has been shown to be equivalent to another technique called Fourier filtering under various ideal conditions; this near equivalence has lent more credence to the algorithm and provided insights into and guidelines for its improvement. (2) Under conditions generally available in current practice, convolution has been shown to be statistically reliable; in particular, with current limits on computer time, convolution performs better than ART in the representation of small fluctuations of brain matter (when such matter is at least a small distance from the skull), when the projection data has low error content.

The current emphasis is on speed since fan beam geometries have greatly reduced scanning times. "Real time" computational speed refers to the amount of time required to complete the computation of a reconstruction on a computer when the speed of data acquisition is recognized as a limiting factor. It is difficult to surpass convolution's time of execution since it is almost "real time constrained." Since the eventual effect of the projection data at any angle on the reconstruction is independent of the data collected at other angles, this effect can be calculated while the data is collected at the next projection angles. Some scanners utilize this fact in their display system. New algorithms will probably have to demonstrate improved reliability or require less data acquisition in order to replace convolution; in particular, the speed of execution of the algorithm will not be a controlling issue.

REPRESENTATION OF A RECONSTRUCTION

A reconstruction is a (finite dimensional) approximation of the x-ray attenuation distribution in a transverse section of the patient. The quality of such an approximation is characterized by two parameters: resolution and accuracy. These terms are applied in the same way as in a description of the information in a photographic record. There is a significant difference between the interpretation of these two kinds of images with respect to the derivation of information at the limits of resolution and accuracy. When a photograph is enlarged so much that the grain size is apparent, the photograph still contains all of the information available in the negative; in particular, if one observes such an image at a greater than normal distance, the high-resolution spurious details are blurred out and only coarser but informative aspects remain. By making choices which are analogous to choosing the enlarging parameters, a reconstruction is created to depict information at a particular resolution. If the choice of that resolution is inappropriately fine, the reconstruction will be unpredictably inaccurate in its representation of details about that size. Rigorous theories place a strict limit on the resolution available from a particular machine design. If an attempt is made to synthesize an image beyond this resolution, misleading image features may appear. These features will not be removed by viewing the image subsequently at lower resolution. Figure 2–2 clarifies this point. This means that careful consideration must go into the choice of the (mathematical) resolution of the reconstruction.

An important aspect of the presentation of a reconstruction is the use of algorithms to post-process the original reconstruction. These image-enhancing techniques may involve the presentation of the reconstruction on a finer grid than the one used for its original synthesis. These methods remove graininess, smooth curves, take out "inaccuracies" or may even sometimes add "missing" features. The problem with these post-processing schemes is their dubious validity, in that they imply an improvement in accuracy and resolution.

The interpretation of a reconstruction is also confused by the nonisotropic resolution presented; for example, a single pixel represents 1.5 x 1.5 x 13 mm of brain matter in an EMI reconstruction. Some authors have described this aspect of computed tomography as the major technological shortcoming of present devices. So often has this problem caused confusion that it has acquired a special name — the *partial volume phenomenon*. The typical situation that has caused this type of misinterpretation involves a pixel near the boundary between brain and skull in a cut near the top of the head. If the rectangular parallelopiped intersects both brain and bone tissues, the value for that pixel represents the average attenuation and therefore will be a number intermediate between the normal attenuation values for bone and brain matter. This means that careful interpretation is required in regions where the kind of tissue varies significantly with small changes in depth. Unlike other effects responsible for misinterpretation, the partial volume phenomenon is not responsible for inaccuracies of the image. The problem here is simply one of interpretation of the reconstruction. When this situation is suspected of hiding a pathological process, contrast can be enhanced by injection of a radiopaque dye followed by collection of another set of projection data.

The manufacturers of these scanning devices recognize that there are difficulties inherent in interpretation; various viewing techniques have

-50	-50	-50	-50	-50	-50	-50	-50	-50	-50	-50	-50
-50	-50	-50	-40	20	30	30	28	14	-50	-50	-50
-50	-50	-20	30	13	3	3	13	30	15	-50	-50
-50	-40	30	8	3	3	3	3	3	30	-40	-50
-50	15	15	3	3	3	3	3	3	18	15	-50
-50	30	3	3	3	3	3	3	3	5	30	-50
-50	30	3	3	3	3	3	3	3	3	30	-50
-50	15	13	3	3	3	3	3	3	13	20	-50
-50	5	30	6	3	3	3	3	6	30	-40	-50
-50	-50	10	30	6	3	3	7	30	-20	-50	-50
-50	-50	-50	10	30	30	**30**	**30**	**-20**	**-50**	**-50**	**-50**
-50	-50	-50	-50	-50	-50	-50	-50	-50	-50	-50	-50

-50	-50	-50	-50	-50	-50	-50	-50	-50	-50	-50	-50
-50	-50	-50	-40	20	31	29	28	14	-50	-50	-50
-50	-50	-20	29	13	3	3	13	31	15	-50	-50
-50	-40	31	8	3	4	2	3	3	29	-40	-50
-50	15	15	3	3	3	3	3	3	18	15	-50
-50	29	3	2	3	3	3	3	4	5	31	-50
-50	31	3	4	3	3	3	3	2	3	29	-50
-50	15	13	3	3	3	3	3	3	13	20	-50
-50	5	29	6	3	4	2	3	6	31	-40	-50
-50	-50	10	31	6	3	3	7	29	-20	-50	-50
-50	-50	-50	10	30	29	31	30	-20	-50	-50	-50
-50	-50	-50	-50	-50	-50	-50	-50	-50	-50	-50	-50

Figure 2–2.   Although these two images are diagnostically different, they could not be distinguished from their projection data. This is an example of insufficient design. The two simulated reconstructions are displayed on a 12 by 12 array. (This represents an array of uniform squares, each over a centimeter on a side.) Each number is chosen to be approximately one tenth of the appropriate EMI number for slices taken through a patient's head. If projections of these two images are taken at exactly eight equally spaced projection angles, then the corresponding projection data will not disagree more than one part in one thousand at any datum. Notice that the lower image shows diagnostically significant fluctuations that are not present in the upper image; in particular, consider the 4's in the intracranial portion of the array.

been provided. The window width control allows the viewer to distort the normal contrast of the image in such a way that small differences in brain matter can be accentuated while setting irrelevant values to either white or black. This is particularly important since the variations of greatest interest occupy only 5 to 5.5 percent of the total range of attenuations. Some companies also provide the viewer with a control which allows him to explore small regions of the reconstruction. Practical experience with those controls can be very useful in the diagnosis of subdural hematomas. This author's experience suggests using a smaller window width than for normal viewing and varying the "center" control until the two regions to be distinguished show a marked contrast.

To provide a measure of accuracy to reconstructions, experiments have been performed using inanimate objects in the place of patients; these objects are usually called *phantoms*. Phantom experiments indicate that reconstructions are statistically likely to accurately represent attenuations within 0.5 percent of the difference between air and water. Such experiments indicate that accuracy may not be the same everywhere within a particular reconstruction.

To provide a measure of experimentally established resolution, abnormal regions which are 1.0 cm in diameter and exhibit 4 EMI units of contrast are close to the smallest details that can be reliably discriminated. In special cases, objects as small as 6 mm have been observed.

Part of the strength of the viewing system is the accessibility of the reconstruction in many forms. It can be stored on magnetic tape, floppy disk, or in printed form. Perhaps the most valuable aspect of the memory feature is the retrospective examination of a reconstruction, which is again available for viewing with the "center" and "window width" controls.

ARTIFACTS

In order for a physician to draw accurate conclusions about data obtained from any experimental test, he should understand both its meaning and reliability, and it would be nice if these two subjects could be separated in computed tomography. Since even the best images produced by CT scanners are at least mildly inaccurate, a physician should decipher the informative from the misleading details in each reconstruction. This skill must be developed from experience, but a guide through the reasons for artifacts (inaccuracies) in a reconstruction should be helpful.

Despite the statistical unlikeliness of their occurrence, as demonstrated by phantom experiments, mathematical proof has established the existence of grossly inaccurate reconstructions that exactly match error-free projection data. Manufacturers claim that attenuation coefficients exhibited in a reconstruction are most often accurate to within 0.5 percent of the difference between air and water; this represents about 2.5 EMI units of expected error. Mathematicians, on the other hand, have shown that by choosing to represent a reconstruction at a resolution which exceeds the validity of any particular set of projection data, both a healthy-looking and a pathological image have that same projection data. Statistical tests notwithstanding, mathematical justification of the resolution used in existing scanning equipment has not been presented. That is, consistent and error-free data are not always sufficient to (uniquely) determine a reconstruction at high resolution.

Projection data are not completely consistent or error-free, but the magnitude of such discrepancies is small. As previously mentioned, the convolution algorithm performs well in such cases. It is important to understand that the convolution algorithm represents inconsistencies in the error in a characteristic way. To clarify this point, the reader should realize that the total error is a sum of consistent and inconsistent components. No reconstruction algorithm can distinguish the accurate (and consistent) data from the inaccurate consistent data — so it will tend to present an image derived from their sum. However, the inconsistent part of the data is also exhibited in a reconstruction produced by the convolution algorithm. When the convolution algorithm presents inconsistent information, the back-projection patterns or streaked patterns that are generated are not damped out by compensating streaks from other directions. Since the convolution algorithm imposes an oscillating character to projection data just before back-projection occurs, uncompensated streak artifacts will tend to have an oscillating or ringing nature. This means that the presence of a ringing or alternating anomaly in the reconstruction should be suspected of being associated with inconsistencies in the data. Fortunately, if an object within a patient is involved with erroneous data collection that object is usually near the presented ringing artifact in the reconstruction. Experience indicates that if a detail within a reconstruction is spatially removed from all suspiciously oscillating features, that detail is likely to be more reliably depicted. This last comment refers to reconstructions which have not been post-processed to remove such oscillations. Also keep in mind that the consistent component of the error in projection data will produce artifacts which are not flagged by a ringing feature in their vicinity.

The filter function (which is another name for the rule to change the projection data just before back-projection) used by a particular convolution algorithm represents a compromise between two goals. It would be desirable to be able to represent large local fluctuations in x-ray attenuation coefficients. It is also important that high-frequency error in the data not be amplified to a point which distorts the reconstruction. These goals are contradictory for the convolution algorithm. The effect is that a filter function is chosen which removes the worst part of the high-frequency error while living with the less common medium-frequency kind. In particular, the reconstruction algorithm is chosen to best match the expected error and the expected relief in the data. This means that either an unusual extreme of x-ray attenuation in the patient or a significant increase in moderate frequency error will overwhelm the filter function — thereby causing a streaked, ringing artifact in the former case or a grainy image in the latter.

The kinds of artifacts associated with data collection can be presented starting from the obvious artifacts associated with the most inconsistent kinds of data to the least discernable artifacts that are associated with more consistent erroneous data. For reconstructions produced by the convolution algorithm, the more inconsistent the data, the more streaked and oscillating will be the reconstruction.

Grossly inconsistent data can be collected because of hardware malfunctions. A brief drop in the x-ray source output or a faulty detector connection can produce extremely pronounced black and white bands. A herringbone pattern imposed on a reconstruction can be caused by inaccurate rotation of the scanner. Misalignment of the center of rotation of the scan literally shifts correct data to inappropriate equations and can cause gross inconsistencies. In the third-generation devices calibration of the sensitivity of each detector during a scan is not feasible; this means that a drift in sensitivity cannot be easily determined. When this happens, one or more concentric circles of artifacts are produced; this is called the "onion" artifact.

The most common form of artifact is associated with patient motions. In most cases small patient motions do not cause significant inconsistencies; this is not the case, however, when a bone structure is greatly displaced. Motion artifacts are usually quite visible and distinctive. When an in-and-out motion, i.e., along the axis perpendicular to the scans, occurs, streaks are most visible in the reconstruction near areas where there was the greatest change in attenuation. In a basal section a slight in-and-out motion can reveal or hide the petrous pyramids. Side-to-side or rotary motions are frequently displayed by vertically oriented bands, often exterior to the skull. Similarly, up-and-down motions are indicated by horizontal streaks of oscillating gray levels. When a water bag is used, air trapped near the temporal hollow (or other places) can shift significantly even with slight motions of the patient — this creates streaks which emanate from the offending region. Even the motion of fluid within the body can cause serious artifacts; the paranasal sinuses have been so implicated. At least two remedies to the patient motion problem have been employed in addition to the use of more stable support for the patient's head. One company provides the operator of the scanner with a "patient motion correction" option. This allows the collection of data at 225° instead of the normal 180°, and an auxiliary program discards up to 45 projections before convolution is applied. Another device performs the convolution reconstruction process on the display console as the data is collected, so that the experienced operator can recognize a forming motion artifact and stop the scan sequence in midstream. It should be clear, however, that in a reconstruction marred by a motion artifact, the resolution will be degraded everywhere and probably not in a homogeneous manner.

Probably the most pervasive and difficult to remedy defect in data collection is associated with the beam-hardening problem. Also called the *spectral shift* artifact, this error in a reconstruction is associated with the polychromatic nature of the x-ray beam and the fact that different tissues have different percentages of attenuation resulting from the photoelectric and Compton effects at each photon energy. In particular, this difference is quite pronounced between brain matter and bone and is completely out of hand if metal objects are also present. Judging from the nature of the artifact produced in a head scan, the erroneous part of the data seems to have a large consistent component; this means that the reconstruction algorithm, per se, would not be expected to remove the artifact. The characteristic spectral shift artifact seems to make the skull thicker (by about 2 to 5 mm). The error in the reconstruction represents areas nearer to the skull with progressively larger attenuation values. The artifact, which depends on the hardness of the penetrating beam, can be grossly described as a cusped discrepancy ranging from a factitious increase of 12 EMI units about 30 mm from the skull to a rise of 50 EMI units at about 5 mm from the skull. Other bony regions present their own kinds of artifacts. The region between the petrous pyramids is frequently exhibited with depressed attenuation values. The first procedure that is used to remove the spectral shift artifact is the employment of a preprocessing algorithm that is designed to adjust the collected data to a kind that would result from more homogeneous attenuation phenomena. This type of preprocessing is quite successful in removing a large percentage of the artifact, but it necessarily creates one of its own since it must be based on fixed percentages of brain matter to bone at each observed intensity level.

High-density regions or regions with a large local fluctuation in attenuation cause both data collection problems and difficulties for the convolution reconstruction algorithm. This effect is generated to some extent in every scan, since bone-to-air and bone-to-brain interfaces are universal. Previous diagnostic tests can leave residual matter which display great local fluctuations in attenuation; residual Pantopaque or intraventricular gas left over from pneumoencephalography can detract from the clarity of a reconstruction. Metallic clips left by previous surgical procedures, metal casings of a valve or a tantalum plate can cause quite significant artifacts, the extent and severity of which vary with the size and proximity of the objects. An important error in data collection (apart from the effects of beam hardening) lies in the detector crystal which must accurately register intensity values, however abruptly these decrease during the scan. Because of afterglow in NaI, such a detector may not be able to provide the proper signal to the computer memory. Afterglow in CaF_2 is shorter-lived, so it is used in some scanners. As previously mentioned, even slight motion can be a significant source of inconsistent data if large changes in attenuation result; therefore, high-density regions make data collection much more sensitive to movement. It was previously explained that too large a local fluctuation in attenuation values cannot be reconstructed with the convolution algorithm. Note that even when motion is not present, the reconstructions produced when high local fluctuations or extremes of attenuation are present are characterized by streaks (overshoots and undershoots) that pass through the unusual region.

The prominent and most typical example of this kind of artifact is the ringing artifact, which appears as a thin line of relatively low attenuation values located about 5 mm from the skull. Such a streak does not result from inconsistent or even inaccurate data but from the choice of the filter function, which is inappropriate for this particular kind of error-free projection data.

FUTURE DEVELOPMENTS

During the last few years, the emphasis for improvement of computed tomography has been on reduction of the time required to go from data collection to presentation of the image. One suggestion is the recording of more than two slices simultaneously; this is important since many physicians routinely order a large set of adjacent cuts. Another improvement may be the use of hard-wired computers which can perform the reconstruction algorithm in much less time than a general purpose digital computer can. The trend may change, however, to a greater emphasis on accuracy and resolution, both of which require longer data acquisition times.

Data collection will probably involve more optional modes of operation. Theoretical evidence suggests that projections at other than equally spaced angles may be advantageous. Collecting multiple projections at the same projection angle has already been used to provide data for high-resolution images. By collecting data in thinner slices (already 4 mm in some devices) the partial volume phenomenon can be further alleviated. More and more machines are employing variable tilting gantries; this is particularly important for viewing the head of a patient who has limited flexibility in the spine. The most radical departure in data collection may be the use of a pulse-height analyzer at the x-ray detectors. Research has demonstrated that by recording the x-ray photon intensities above and below some medium-energy value, the available information will allow the creation of a photoelectric absorption as well as an independent Compton scattering reconstruction. This information would be free of the spectral shift artifact and even provide improved diagnostic clarity.

The programs which control the computer will also become more flexible in the future. It should be possible to adjust the filter function at will so that unusual projection data can be more accurately depicted. This is just one of many ways in which various reconstruction algorithms can be optionally retailored to a particular need. There are many proven and largely unimplemented possibilities in computation. It is possible to perform tests on the projection data so that the closeness of the reconstruction provided can be mathematically estimated; this estimate can be given to a physician along with the image. Such a system would probably close the gap in the meanings of the three types of resolution discussed in the section on representation of a reconstruction. It is also possible to create reconstructions of thinner slices than were physically sampled, by processing two or more overlapping slices. A recent development in computing involves a relatively sound postprocessing technique for removal of the spectral shift artifact. Although it presently takes hours to run on digital computers (only minutes are required on hard-wired computers), it suggests that the artifact can be removed in large measure if the need for great accuracy persists.

REFERENCES

1. Gordon RR, Herman GT, Johnson S: Image reconstruction from projections. Sci Am 133:56, 1975.
2. McCullough EC, Baker HL, Houser DW: Evaluation of the quantitative and radiation features of a scanning x-ray transverse axial tomograph: the EMI scanner. Radiology 111:709, 1974.
3. Kuhl DE, Edwards RQ: Reorganizing data from the transverse section scans of the brain using digital processing. Radiology 91:975, 1968.
4. Oldendorf WH: Isolated flying spot detection of radiodensity discontinuities displaying the internal structural pattern of a complex object. IRE Trans Bio-Med Elect BME 8:68, 1961.
5. Hounsfield G: Computerized transverse axial scanning. Part I: Description of the system. Br J Radiol 46:1016, 1973.
6. Ambrose J: Computerized transverse axial scanning (tomography). Part II: Clinical application. Br J Radiol 46:1023, 1973.
7. Radon J: Uber die Bestimmung von Funktionen durch ihre Integralwerte langs gewisser mannigfaltigkeiten. Ber Verh Sachs Akad 69:262, 1917.
8. Smith KT, Solomon DC, Wagner SL: Practical and mathematical aspects of the problem of reconstructing objects from radiographs. Bull Am Math Soc 83(6):1227, 1977.
9. Katz MB: Questions of Uniqueness and Resolution in Reconstruction of 2-D and 3-D Objects from their Projections. Lecture Notes in Biomathematics, Springer-Verlag, New York. (In press.)
10. Ter-Pogossian MM: Computerized cranial tomography: equipment and physics. Semin Roentgenol 12:13, 1977.
11. Rao PS, Gregg EC: Attenuation of monoenergetic gamma rays in tissues. Am J Roentgenol 123:631, 1975.
12. Brooks RA, Di Chiro G: Beam hardening in x-ray reconstructive tomography. Physiol Med Biol 21:390, 1976.
13. Edholm P: Image construction in transverse computer tomography. Acta Radiol (Supple) 346:21, 1975.
14. Herman GT, Rowland SW: Three methods for reconstructing objects from x-rays: a comparative study. Computer Graphics and Image Processing 2:151, 1973.

Chapter 3 Normal Tomographic Anatomy

To understand the alterations in tissue density and associated displacement and distortion caused by pathological lesions visualized by CT, it is necessary to have a clear understanding of the normal anatomical landmarks that may be visualized by plain scan and of the vascular anatomy that may be defined following infusion of contrast media.[1-4] The exact orientation of the scan is determined by the specific anatomical region that is to be visualized. For routine scans the head is positioned 15 or 20° relative to the orbitomeatal line. To focus more clearly on specific regions, certain modifications in angulation are necessary. To visualize the posterior fossa, 25° angulation is necessary to avoid bone structures at the skull base, which may be a source of confusing artifacts. This steeper angulation requires an increasing degree of neck flexion; this may be difficult in patients with headache, nausea and vomiting, commonly present in patients suspected of having posterior fossa lesions. Because of the small size of the posterior fossa, 8 mm collimators may be necessary; the decrease in section thickness may require extra scans to study this region completely. To visualize the orbits, zero degree angulation, with 3 to 5 mm sections, is used. To visualize the sellar region and temporal horn, zero degree angulation is optimal, although the suprasellar region may be visualized with 15° angulation. Because of variability of individual skull shape and positioning of head, differences in structures may be seen on

identical CT sections in different individuals; for example, in patients with elongated dolichocephalic skulls an extra scan sequence may be required to reach the vertex.

The lowest scan, which was obtained with 15 to 20° angulation, includes the orbital-inferior surface of the frontal lobe, temporal lobe, cerebellum, brain stem and basilar cisterns (Fig. 3–1, A). Anteriorly, if the cut is slightly lower it may include the orbital roof, crista galli, sphenoid and frontal sinus, and posteriorly may include the region of the foramen magnum. The middle fossa is bounded anteriorly by the sphenoid bone, posteriorly by petrous bone and medially by the lateral margin of the suprasellar cistern; and it contains the inferior and medial gyri of the temporal cortex. The narrow slitlike or comma-shaped low-density structures in the middle fossa represent the temporal horns; they are usually not visualized because of partial volume effect except if they are dilated (Fig. 3–1, B).

Located directly posterior to the sphenoid bone and lateral to the suprasellar cistern is the sylvian cistern, which is oriented horizontally. In this section the most inferior portion of the fourth ventricle may be visualized in 50 percent of normal cases. In normal subjects the height of the fourth ventricle is 6 to 15 mm, and it is frequently necessary to use 8 mm collimation to visualize this structure. The fourth ventricle has a triangular shape. It may be indented and distorted in posterior aspect by the nodulus of the cerebellum, which

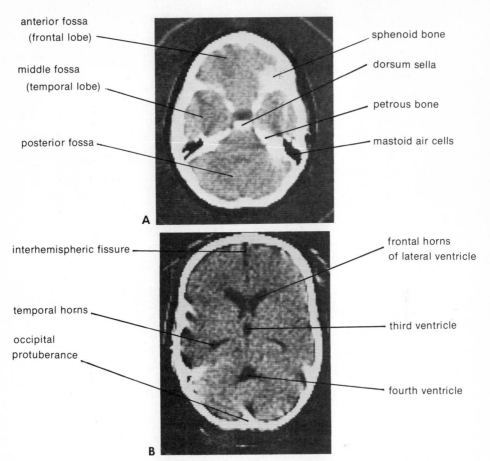

anterior fossa
(frontal lobe)

sphenoid bone

middle fossa
(temporal lobe)

dorsum sella

petrous bone

posterior fossa

mastoid air cells

A

interhemispheric fissure

frontal horns
of lateral ventricle

temporal horns

occipital
protuberance

third ventricle

fourth ventricle

B

Figure 3–1.   *A*, Scan section passes through the inferior portion of the anterior middle and posterior fossae, with good definition of the sphenoid bone, dorsum sella, petrous bone, and mastoid air cells. *B*, This section includes the frontal and temporal horns of the lateral ventricle, the anterior portion of the third ventricle and the fourth ventricle. Note the comma shape of the temporal horn, which may be confused with the retrothalamic cistern.

appears as a round high-density structure. Also included is the cisterna magna; this has a triangular shape, with its base directed posteriorly toward the occipital bone, and has the density of CSF. The vallecula passes from the cisterna magna anteriorly to the fourth ventricle and is medial to the high-density round cerebellar tonsils (Fig. 3–2, *A*). Directly underneath the petrous pyramids are the low-density cisterns of the cerebellopontine angle, which continue anteriorly, and the pontine cistern, located directly posterior to the dorsum sella. The horizontal fissures which separate the cerebellar folia are visualized only if there is a pathological atrophic disorder. Because of its small size and orientation relative to scanning angulation, the aqueduct is not visualized unless it is markedly dilated and zero degree angulation is used.

Because of the many prominent bony structures in the basal region, slight head motion may cause significant artifacts simulating abnormalities. These artifacts may be minimized by decreasing effective contrast by altering the window width control. On this section artifacts include linear high-density streaking originating from the frontal

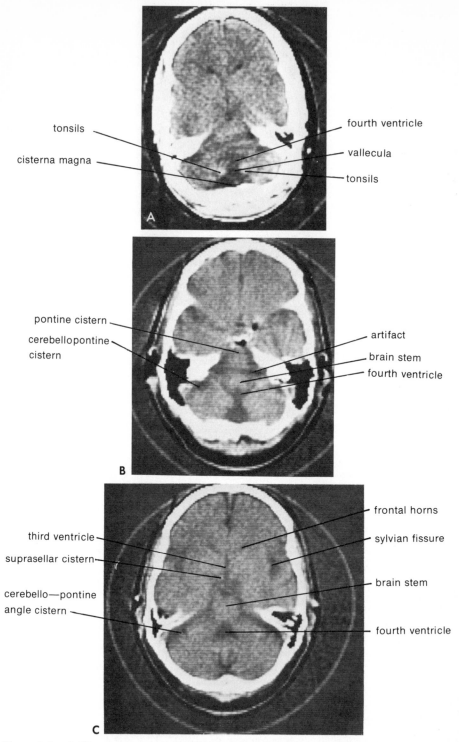

Figure 3–2.   A, The cisterna magna continues anteriorly as the vallecula and is bounded by paired cerebellar tonsils. B, Section includes pontine cistern and cerebellopontine angle cistern. The transverse low-density line in the posterior fossa is a frequent artifact. C, Section includes frontal horns of the lateral ventricle, third ventricle and sylvian fissures. The suprasellar cistern is faintly outlined, and posterior to this the pontine cistern surrounds the brain stem.

and occipital protuberance. Another frequent finding is a low-density horizontal band traversing the posterior fossa (Fig. 3–2, *B*). The anatomy of the ethmoid and sphenoid sinuses, internal auditory canal, dorsum sella, anterior and posterior clinoid processes, foramen magnum and other foramina at the base of the skull may be demonstrated, but the bony details are not as well visualized as with conventional tomography. The anterior clinoids are visualized as paired high-density structures medial to sphenoid, and the dorsum sella is located in the midline. These normal structures may be confused with high-density lesions in the sellar region, but they are not associated with displacement or contrast enhancement, although the pituitary gland may show slight enhancement. Superimposed upon the sellar region are the very low-density air cells of the sphenoid sinus, which may be averaged with higher-density structures, including pituitary tissue and CSF in the suprasellar cistern. Complete evaluation of this region requires thinner sections and coronal orientation.

On a higher section, the lateral wings of the sphenoid and petrous bones are still included but are less prominent (Fig. 3–2, *C*). Anteriorly, the section passes through the orbitofrontal cortex, and the two hemispheres are separated by a low-density longitudinal fissure. At this level a vague impression of the anterior horns of the lateral ventricles is obtained, but they are better defined if enlarged. In the middle fossa the sylvian fissure is visualized as a comma- or Y-shaped structure. In only 5 percent of scans in which there are no clinical symptoms referable to the temporal region and no abnormality subsequently demonstrated by other diagnostic studies, the anterior tip of the temporal horn is demonstrated. This structure is visualized by CT only when the lateral cleft is 6 to 8 mm or more in height.

It has a hockey stick, slitlike or comma-shaped appearance, with the concavity directed posteriorly. The temporal cortex occupies the middle fossa and the medial temporal region (uncus) abuts into the lateral edge of the suprasellar cistern; alterations in its shape may define transtentorial herniation. This cistern is located directly above the sella turcica.

Also, on this section the suprasellar cistern has the configuration of a 5- or 6-pointed structure, depending upon the angulation (Fig. 3–3, *A* and *B*). Its anterior boundary is the inferior portion of the frontal lobes, and extending from the midline is the cistern of the lamina terminalis, which appears to reach the posterior-inferior portion of the frontal longitudinal fissure. The anterolateral portion is made up of the sylvian cistern (middle cerebral artery cistern) as it diverges to reach the sylvian fissure, and the posterior boundaries consist of the brain stem. The interpeduncular cistern is oriented horizontally and outlines the rounded cerebral peduncles. The convergence point of the peduncles forms the posteromedial sixth point of the star. If angulation is less steep the plane of the scan intersects the pons rather than the interpeduncular fossa, so that the posterior edge is flat due to the configuration of the vertical edge of the pons and in this instance the suprasellar cistern, and it has a pentagonal (crown) shape. The superior-inferior boundaries of this cistern are not well delineated by the transverse axial section.

Within the anterior portion of the suprasellar cistern, it is frequently possible to visualize the optic chiasm and paired optic nerves. The chiasm appears as a V-shaped high-density area, and the optic nerves appear as symmetrical, paramedian, round, high-density masses located anteriorly in the chiasm; CT does not allow the detailed anatomical delineation of this region that is obtained with polytomoencephalography.

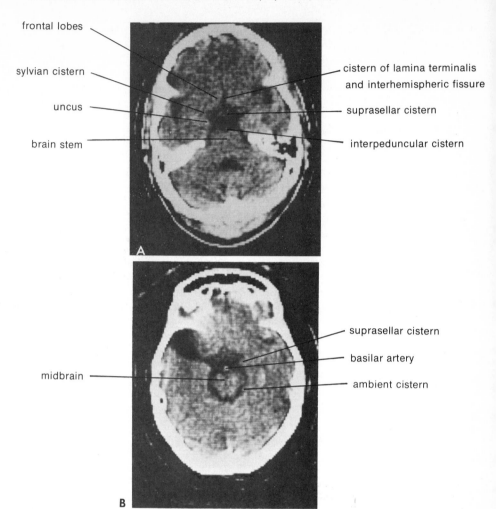

frontal lobes

sylvian cistern

uncus

brain stem

cistern of lamina terminalis and interhemispheric fissure

suprasellar cistern

interpeduncular cistern

midbrain

suprasellar cistern

basilar artery

ambient cistern

Figure 3–3. *A* and *B*, The suprasellar cistern has either a pentagonal or hexagonal shape, depending on whether it intersects the pons *(A)* or cerebral peduncles posteriorly *(B)*. The anterior border includes the frontal lobe; the lateral border is the uncus. The basilar artery is located in the interpeduncular fossa, and the interpeduncular and crural cisterns surround the brain stem.

The blood vessels composing the circle of Willis form the outer perimeter of the suprasellar cistern: the internal carotid arteries are located at anterolateral points, with the middle cerebral artery extending into the sylvian cistern; the anterior cerebral artery extends along the anterior portion, directed toward the midline, and the posterior cerebral artery extends posteriorly to surround the brain stem. The basilar artery is a round, irregularly shaped, high-density structure located in the interpeduncular cistern. In routine scan sequences the outline of the suprasellar cistern is adequately visualized in 60 percent of cases. If a juxtasellar lesion is suspected, this region may be outlined by utilizing zero degree angulation to obtain four 8 mm tissue sections at 1.6 cm intervals, or scanning at 25° angulation to obtain three overlapping 13 mm tissue sections at 10 mm intervals. In those cases in which complete visualization cannot be obtained, contrast enhancement is performed to exclude an abnormality.

BUSINESS REPLY MAIL

FIRST CLASS   PERMIT NO. 101   PHILADELPHIA, PA

Postage will be paid by addressee

W. B. Saunders Company

West Washington Square
Philadelphia, PA 19105

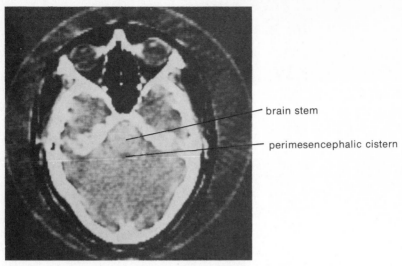

brain stem

perimesencephalic cistern

Figure 3–4. Scan obtained at zero degree angulation shows a round midline high-density area, which represents the brain stem, surrounded by a low-density cistern.

In the majority of tomograms the configuration of the cistern is symmetrical but in 5 percent of cases a mild asymmetry is detected; no lesion or evidence of transtentorial herniation is subsequently demonstrated by other diagnostic studies. The suprasellar cistern is visualized in only 50 percent of patients with supratentorial lesions, an incidence significantly lower than the 90 percent visualization with routine studies; this is believed to be due to uncal herniation.[5]

In the posterior fossa the triangularly shaped fourth ventricle is usually visualized. In 5 percent of normal cases no visualization is obtained despite utilization of 8 mm collimators and steeper angulation. Nonvisualization of this structure raises the suspicion of a posterior fossa lesion. Directly anterior to the fourth ventricle is the brain stem, which appears as a round high-density mass surrounded by the cisterns. The high-density round appearance of the brain stem surrounded by cisternal spaces is best visualized with zero degree angulation (Fig. 3–4). Directly posterior to the fourth ventricle is the vallecula,

which extends to the cisterna magna. This cistern is a relatively free space with a wide separation of the pia and arachnoid and few intervening arachnoid trabeculations. It may reach the undersurface of the tentorium and occasionally extends supratentorially if there is a small defect in the tentorium. There may be wide variation in the CT scan size, extent and shape of this cistern. Rarely, it may be confused with a posterior fossa cyst. Visualization of this cistern is obtained in 40 percent of scans, and in 10 percent of those cases it extends supratentorially. The cerebellopontine angle cisterns are visualized in 50 to 84 percent of cases and in two-thirds of cases are symmetrical. The frequency of other cisternal structures includes vallecula (47 percent), superior cerebellar cistern (37 percent), crural (63 percent), ambient (63 percent), prepontine (90 percent) and quadrigeminal cistern (90 percent).[6]

The next section best visualizes the lateral and third ventricular region. Anteriorly, the frontal lobes are separated by the interhemispheric fissure (Fig. 3–5, A). In the middle fossa the sylvian cistern may still be seen. In

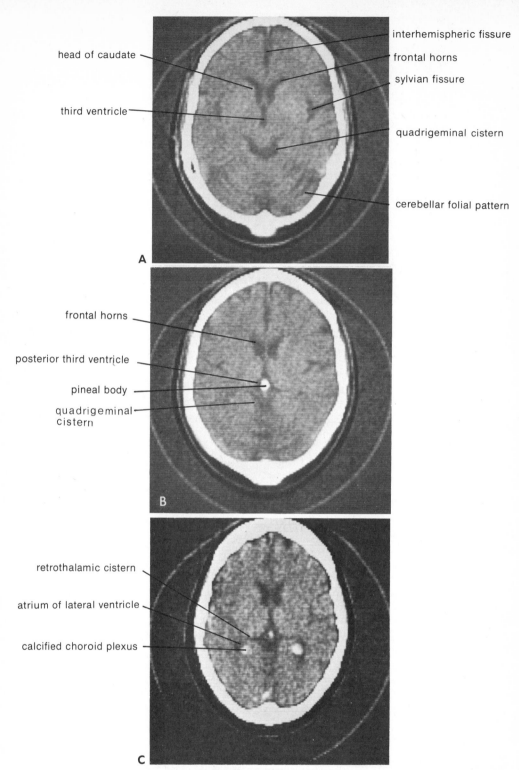

Figure 3–5. *A*, This demonstrates the quadrigeminal cistern, which is indented by the colliculi. The cerebellar folial pattern is well outlined, as there is cerebellar atrophy. The head of the caudate nucleus abuts into the wall of the lateral ventricle. *B*, The pineal body is located within the posterior third ventricle and the quadrigeminal cistern is located posteriorly, forming a diamond-shaped low-density area. *C*, The retrothalamic cisterns extend laterally from the quadrigeminal cistern, and the atrium of the lateral ventricle is visualized.

the posterior region angulation may be such that the most superior portion of the cerebellum and the superior cerebellar cistern are included. This is midline in location and forms a roughly triangular or wedge-shaped region of relatively lower density than the supratentorial cortex, and occasionally the folial pattern of the cerebellum is demonstrated. The most constant landmarks on this section are the frontal horns of the lateral ventricle, third ventricle, and quadrigeminal. The frontal horns are seen at this level; the maximal width of the lateral extremities ranges from 21 to 36 mm. The anterior portion of the corpus callosum is not directly delineated. The lateral ventricles are separated by the septum pellucidum, and at its lower edge the rounded masses consisting of the anterior columns of the fornices may be outlined. The ventricles are usually symmetrical but occasionally are asymmetrical, with the right frontal region wider than the left. Directly adjacent to the frontal horn is the caudate nucleus, which indents its lateral wall to produce a concave shape in the wall. This nuclear mass is bounded laterally by the white matter of the internal capsule. Because of the higher concentration of high-density substance (calcium, iron) and more abundant circulation of the nuclear mass, it appears more opaque compared to the lateral ventricle and internal capsule. The caudate nucleus is clearly seen in only 35 percent of scans; this finding is inconstant because certain scans will average the nuclear mass with larger sections of white matter to produce lower attenuation value. The putamen and thalamus are less frequently seen than is the caudate nucleus but all have similar density. The degree of anatomical detail may be increased by increasing the radiation exposure, and certain scanners permit this variation if this detail is required.

The region of the intraventricular foramina is seen at the level of the anterior-superior portion of the third ventricle. The anterior portion of the third ventricle appears as an elongated tubular structure that is 3 to 8 mm in width. It becomes more bulbous at its lowest portion, which represents middle and posterior expansion, and it is most clearly defined when angulation is parallel to its lumen. The massa intermedia is a commissural or gray-matter bundle, which connects the two halves of the thalamus; it is seen as a high-density mass separating the anterior and posterior portions of the third ventricle. The lateral walls of the third ventricle are formed by the thalamus, which may indent the walls to produce lateral concavity, and immediately posterior to the third ventricle the quadrigeminal cistern may be identified. This cistern is usually symmetrical, although the lateral portion may be asymmetrical. The shape of the cistern is determined by the colliculi that indent its floor. At this level a round low-density area is located posterior to the quadrigeminal cistern and this represents the superior cerebellar cistern. It is best seen in atrophic pathological processes and if prominent may be misinterpreted for a cystic lesion. The superior cerebellar cistern may appear continuous with the quadrigeminal cistern and posterior third ventricle, although there is a definite anatomical separation.

The next scan section 2B outlines the lateral and third ventricular regions (Fig. 3–5, *B*). The walls of the third ventricle diverge with increasing width and posteriorly it has a roughly triangular shape. The shape of the quadrigeminal cistern shifts to triangular and the combined posterior third ventricular quadrigeminal cistern forms a diamond shape containing the pineal body (Fig 3–5, *C*). In those cases in which it is visualized it is not necessarily calcified because it has a higher density compared to low-density CSF. The presence of a shift of the pineal body is best detected at this level. The retrothalamic cistern extends laterally from the diamond-shaped confluence and may appear to be contiguous with the trigonal area of the lateral ventricle. Located within the lateral ventricle, calcified glomeruli of the choroid plexus appear as round high-density masses. They are usually symmetrical in position and shape, but slight rotation of the head or normal anatomical variation may create an impression of asymmetry. The calcified choroid plexus in the left lateral ventricle is more frequently located posterior to the structure on the right side.[7]

Because of the difference in density between that of the caudate, putamen and thalamus and the lower density of the white matter, the linear low-density anterior and posterior limb of the internal capsule may be outlined. At this level the section passes through the frontal horns, thalamus and third ventricle, then re-enters the lateral ventricle at the level of the trigone, and the cortex represents the frontal and temporal region. Posteriorly, in the midline a small amount of cerebellar hemisphere or superior cerebellar cistern may be visualized. With contrast infusion, enhancement of the lateral edge of the tentorium and the incisura is identified; it delineates the lateral extent of the infratentorial region. The vein of Galen, straight sinus, lateral sinuses draining into the torcular (confluence of sinuses) region may also be visualized.

This section includes the bodies of the lateral ventricles and also the superior portion of the frontal and occipital horns (Fig. 3–6, A). This level, (3A) is used to measure the maximal width between the lateral aspects of the cella media, which has a range of 24 to 39 mm. The calcified portion of the choroid plexus is seen on noncontrast scan, and following contrast infusion the well-vascularized noncalcified glomeruli become more dense. The posterior portion of the corpus callosum produces divergence of the lateral ventricle but cannot be visualized directly. The occipital horns may also be visualized but are best defined on a higher section. The cortex included in this section cannot be identified or separated by any specific anatomical landmark, but the following may be inferred: the frontal lobe is anterior to the frontal horn; the parietal lobe extends from posterior to frontal horn to body of lateral ventricle, the temporal region from body to lateral extent of occipital horn; the occipital cortex is located medial to the occipital horn.

The appearance of the occipital horns by CT has confirmed air-study findings which emphasize marked asymmetry, even in the absence of disease (Fig. 3–6, B). The occipital horns may vary from a small tentlike structure that projects backward from the atrium to a well-developed fingerlike projection that extends posteriorly to within 1 to 2 cm of the occipital bone. The tips of the occipital horn may be rounded, bulbous or flared or may taper to a point. In some sections, the calcar avis is seen as a relatively high density which projects into the medial aspects of the occipital horn (Fig. 3–6, C), and the left occipital horn is usually wider than the right. The cortical boundaries are poorly defined unless the sulcal markings are prominent.

The highest scan sequences include the most superior portion of the body of the lateral ventricle. The anterior or posterior portion will be most prominent, depending upon angulation — the steeper the angulation, the more posterior portion is seen. In addition, the steeper the angulation, the more anteriorly located will be the position of the central sulcus. It is frequently possible to identify the longitudinal, precentral, central and postcentral fissures because of relatively constant position. Above the ventricular system the centrum ovale may be visualized; it is located medially as a low-density area with jagged irregular margins, or occasionally as a more regular ovoid region. At this level the brain has homogeneous density except for the central low-density white matter. The two hemispheres are separated by the

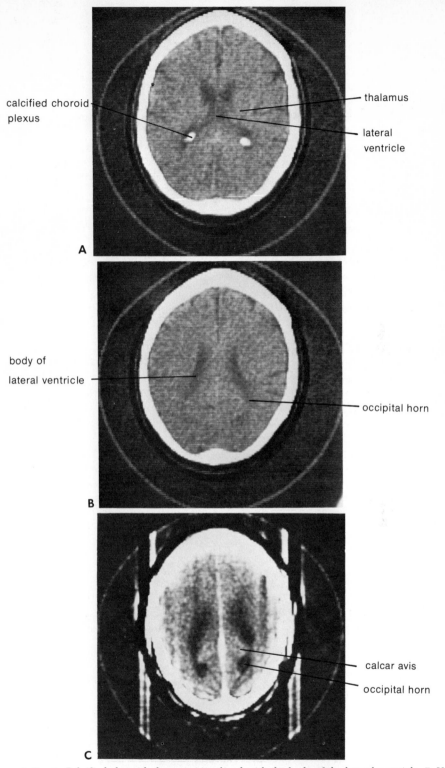

Figure 3–6.   *A*, Calcified choroid plexus is visualized with the body of the lateral ventricle. *B*, Usual appearance of body and occipital horns. *C*, Calcar avis abuts into occipital horn.

falx, which may contain high-density calcified plaques, not visualized by plain skull radiographs. The falx is best visualized in the postinfusion study. Posteriorly in the midline the triangularly shaped superior sagittal sinus is visualized. This is an important landmark because, if there is swelling of one hemisphere, the falx may be bowed and stretched.

CONTRAST ENHANCEMENT ANATOMY

Following intravenous injection of iodinated contrast material, there is an increase in the density and the computed attenuation coefficient great enough to visualize intravascular blood and to outline certain larger vascular structures.[8] The circle of Willis forms the perimeter of the suprasellar cistern, with the anterior cerebral artery extending forward and directed medially, the middle cerebral artery extending laterally into the sylvian cistern and the posterior cerebral artery directed posteriorly around the brain stem (Fig. 3–7). The basilar artery is located in the center of the interpeduncular cistern. There is extensive enhancement in the vascular portion of the choroid plexus.

Following infusion, the falx and tentorium may enhance, as may occur with angiography.[8] The outline of the falx may provide an important diagnostic key to the presence of hemispheric swelling even if no mass is clearly visualized, as it may be bowed and stretched. Posteriorly, the tentorial incisural region and straight sinus may be visualized (Fig. 3–8, A and B).

Normal venous structures frequently visualized include the round-shaped vein of Galen, which drains posteriorly into the straight sinus. The torcular Herophili is visualized in the midline posteriorly as a triangular high-density region that receives contribution from the straight and transverse sinuses (Fig. 3–8, C). Frequently, the vascular anatomy of the larger vascular structures may be well defined, but this does not provide the spatial resolution or evidence of vascular development that is possible with angiography. In addition, the average density measurements made on the computer printout in identical areas on pre- and postinfusion scan in both the basal ganglia and parietal convexity region show a definite increment if the scan is performed immediately after infusion.

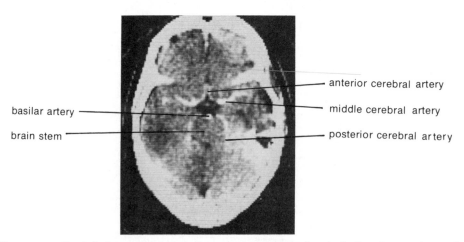

basilar artery

brain stem

anterior cerebral artery

middle cerebral artery

posterior cerebral artery

Figure 3–7.   Postinfusion study outlines the major arterial branches, including the anterior cerebral artery continuing into the interhemispheric fissure, the middle cerebral artery, extending laterally into the sylvian cistern, and the posterior cerebral artery, extending posteriorly around the brain stem.

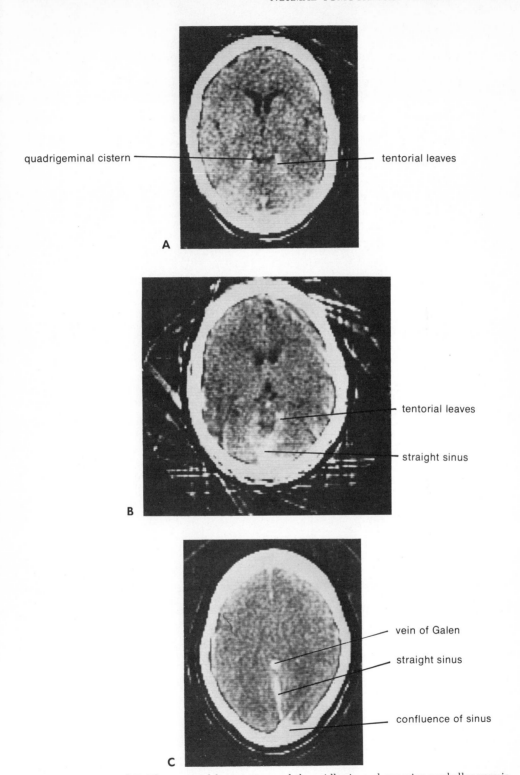

Figure 3–8. *A* and *B*, The tentorial leaves surround the midbrain and superior cerebellar vermis, and the tentorium extends posteriorly to the straight sinus. *C*, The vein of Galen, straight sinus and confluence of the sinus are visualized.

REFERENCES

1. New PFJ, Scott WR: Computed Tomography of the Brain and Orbit. Williams and Wilkins, Baltimore, 1975. pp 54–115.
2. Schoultz TW, Morrison JR, Calhoun JD: Atlas of the human brain for use in diagnosis by CT. Surg Neurol 5:255, 1976.
3. Muller HR, Wuthrich R: A graphical reporting system for CT. Eur Neurol 11:197, 1974.
4. Huckman MS, Grainer LS, Clasen RC: The normal computed tomogram. Semin Roentgenol 12:27, 1977.
5. Naidich TP, Pinto RS, Kushner MJ, et al: Evaluation of sellar and parasellar masses by CT. Radiology 120:91, 1976.
6. Naidich TP, Lin JP, Leeds NE, et al: CT in the diagnosis of posterior fossa masses. Radiology 120:333, 1976.
7. Messina AV, Potts DG, Sigel RM, et al: CT: evaluation of the posterior third ventricle. Radiology 119:581, 1976.
8. Naidich TP, Pudlowski RM, Leeds NE, et al: The normal contrast-enhanced CT of the brain. J Comput Assist Tomog 1:16, 1977.
9. Naidich TP, Leeds NE, Kricheff I, et al: The tentorium in axial section. 1. Normal CT appearance and non-neoplastic pathology. Radiology 123:631, 1977.

Chapter 4 Performance and Interpretation of the CT Scan

There is no special preparation that is necessary for the scan, but the patient must remain motionless during the scan sequence. Even a small amount of movement may significantly degrade the scan quality. This was a major problem when scanning time required several minutes, as 3 to 5 percent of studies were technically unsatisfactory, but recent advances, including the utilization of the fan-shaped x-ray beam with a series of multiple detectors, have reduced scanning time to 5 to 20 seconds.[1] Head movement occurs because the patient may be uncomfortable owing to neck flexion or extension or more frequently relates to altered mentation, adventitious movements, coughing or hiccoughs.

If sedation is required and the risk of cardiopulmonary complication is considered low and is justified for the amount of diagnostic information gained, 10 mg of intravenously administered diazepam (Valium) has been effective in 60 percent of adult patients, whereas 30 percent require an additional 10 mg after 10 minutes. In 10 percent of cases adequate sedation is not achieved with this drug; further increments increase the risk of oversedation significantly so that the procedure should then be terminated and rescheduled. An alternative sedative drug is amobarbital (Amytal) administered intravenously at 50 mg per minute to a maximum of 500 mg, and this has been effective in all cases without any untoward effects. This drug should not be used immediately following diazepam because of the potential synergistic cardiorespiratory toxicity. In only rare instances has general anesthesia been required in adults. Children represent a significant problem and sedation is required in almost all children less than four years old. Chloral hydrate has been the most efficacious and safest when used in dosage of 50 to 75 mg per kilogram of body weight 20 minutes prior to the scan and then repeated 40 minutes later if adequate sedation has not been achieved. No untoward effects have occurred with this drug, and technically satisfactory studies have been achieved in 95 percent of children. In 1 to 5 percent of cases other agents, including secobarbital, meperidine, atropine, chlorpromazine or hydroxyzine pamoate or anesthesia utilizing intramuscularly administered ketamine, have been employed, and in these cases hospitalization is required.[2, 3]

A question regarding advisability of sedation is most frequent in the head-injured patient, since negative CT scan almost always obviates the need for angiography; but prior cervical spine x-ray is necessary before neck manipulation to position in the scanner is attempted, and oropharyngeal airway or endotracheal intubation with careful monitoring of ventilatory status is mandatory to avoid airway obstruction.[4] Head movement may

41

cause linear, vertically orientally, alternating high- and low-density streaking; this artifact is most severe if air and bone overlap but may be minimized by the Patient Movement Correction option.

For the CT scan, the patient is positioned supine on a standard x-ray table and the head is fitted into the head cone, which contains a rubber water bag. With the newer generation of scanners, the need for the water-bag has been eliminated, and this advance has facilitated the range of head positioning which is necessary for direct biplane coronal and sagittal scanning. As the head is positioned into the head cone, the radiology technician draws a line from the superior rim of the orbit to the external auditory meatus, and a second line is then made to correspond to the desired degree of angulation (0, 10, 15, 20, 25) relative to the orbito-meatal line. The patient's head is then positioned so that this line is parallel with the outer margin of the head cone, and the scanning sequence begins with this lowest section. After each sequence the head is moved 25 mm in or out of the scanner to obtain sequences from the skull base to the vertex. The routine sections are 13 mm in thickness, but thinner collimation and overlapping sections may be necessary for specific regions.

It must be remembered that as thinner sections are obtained, it is usually necessary to increase the dosage of radiation exposure. The x-ray source consists of a stationary anode tube energized at 120 kv with 0.6 mm focal spot diameter, although several models now use a rotating tube. The beam is thinly collimated to minimize radiation scatter, and after the beam passes through the head it is detected by sodium iodide or calcium fluoride scintillation detectors coupled to a photomultiplier tube for signal amplification or alternatively utilized multiple xenon gas detectors; these record a series of x-ray transmission data at a finite number of angles. The computer analyzes this data and reconstructs a two-dimensional image in a matrix consisting of 160 × 160 pixels (picture elements) in which each pixel represents a 1.5 mm × 1.5 mm area with a thickness of 13 mm, and this resolution has now been increased in certain models for finer details. The images reconstructed represent a two-dimensional image of the transverse axial projection, and this is adequate to detect the presence of pathological lesions, enlargement of ventricles and subarachnoid spaces; but in certain cases a three-dimensional display, including coronal and sagittal planes, is

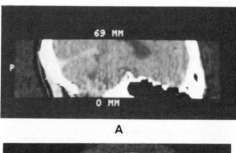

A

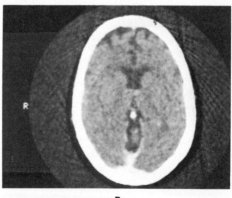

B

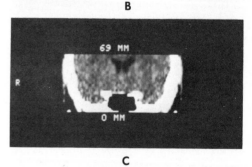

C

Figure 4–1. Transverse section (B) and the accompanying coronal (C) and sagittal reconstruction (A). (Courtesy of Artronix Company, St. Louis.)

necessary to define the relationship of the lesion to normal anatomical landmarks in order to determine its intra- or extra-axial location. This may be especially important in defining the extension of a pituitary tumor inferiorly into the sphenoid sinus, in detecting the point of origin of an aneurysm from the parent vessel and in establishing intra- or extracerebral origin and extension of mass lesions.

To obtain these coronal or sagittal sections, the patient must be rescanned and multiple overlapping sections obtained, but this increases radiation exposure significantly. Recently, a technique has been developed in the computer circuitry which provides thin transverse axial tissue sections, and the projection data are stored in such a manner that it is later possible to reprogram the computer for coronal and sagittal reconstruction of the specific area desired without the necessity of rescanning the patient[5] (Fig. 4–1). The computer provides a reconstruction as a numerical display of the attenuation values of all the individual pixels in the matrix, but this is difficult to work with on a routine basis. It is easier to work with a cathode ray oscilloscope display in which these numerical values are displayed on a gray scale in which lower values appear blacker and higher attenuation values appear white, and a permanent record is obtained with a Polaroid camera picture.

SCAN REPORT

A complete study consists of three or four sequences, each containing two scans. If contrast infusion study is also included, this doubles the time and radiation exposure. A careful review of the clinical and laboratory data may reduce the number of sections needed and focus directly on the most likely involved area. In suspected juxtasellar lesions, plain scan to visualize the suprasellar cistern should initially be performed and then contrast infusion initiated and complete study performed. This shortens the scanning procedure and decreases unnecessary radiation exposure without eliminating diagnostically useful sections. A similar format should be utilized for suspected posterior fossa lesions in which infusion is started after the fourth ventricle and basal cisterns are visualized. In the majority of cases, only one section above the ventricular cast is necessary, but if metastasis, subdural hematoma, convexity neoplasm or cortical atrophic process is suspected, an extra section extending to the vertex is needed. The scan report should describe the technical quality of the scan and include description and identification of the source of any artifacts that may degrade the scan quality and interfere with the ability to visualize normal or pathologic structures.

The report should include a description of the following anatomical structures:

1. Size, shape and symmetry of the ventricular system, including the presence of certain common anomalies (common ventricle, cavum septum pellucidum, cavum vergae). Twenty-five percent of scans show an asymmetry of the choroid plexus or occipital horn region and 5 percent have an asymmetry of the anterior frontal region, but this finding does not usually suggest an obstructing lesion unless there is accompanying distortion or displacement.

2. The fourth ventricle should always be visualized, but this may require 8 mm collimation and steep (25°) angulation; nonvisualization of this structure is a definite indication for postcontrast study.

3. With routine 15° angulation the posterior portion of the third ventricle is better visualized than the anterior region which is frequently poorly visualized.

4. Midline indicators, including the pineal body, falx cerebri, suprasellar cistern and tentorial leaves.

5. Presence and symmetry of cis-

ternal and cortical sulcal spaces. The sulci are not seen until they are at least 3 mm in size, and this is suggestive of an atrophic process, although they are visualized in 10 to 15 percent of normal subjects. The suprasellar, quadrigeminal and sylvian cisterns are usually visualized, but other cisterns are more variable in their appearance.

6. If an abnormality of either high or low attenuation value is detected, it must be carefully described as to its size, shape, location, associated mass effect and its complete density characteristics. The actual size of the lesion may be determined by multiplying the measured value by a factor of three. The shape of the lesion is frequently an important clue to the location of the lesion, as round or wedge-shaped lesions are usually intra-axial, whereas concave or convex lesions are usually extra-axial in position. If the lesion is contiguous with bone it is usually extra-axial, whereas the presence of significant ventricular displacement and distortion is more indicative of intra-axial location. The most characteristic sign of extra-axial location is widening or obliteration of cisternal spaces ipsilateral to the lesion. The density characteristics of the lesion may help to predict certain pathological features and the exact attenuation value may be determined by a simple mechanical manipulation.

The "window width" control may be adjusted to different attenuation values. By increasing the width the sharp black and white contrast is lost and this is helpful in reducing an artifact due to moving from high to low attenuation value in a small area. This is the case in visualizing the orbital contents, and a window width of 200 is frequently used. To detect differences of 2 to 4 attenuation units in the intracranial compartment, high-contrast resolution is necessary and a window width of 75 is used. In addition, there is an "M" or measure setting such that with the window width set at measure all values above this designated level appear white. By utilizing this control it can be determined if a low-density lesion is homogeneous, usually consisting of fluid or air, or nonhomogeneous (speckled or mottled), usually consisting of necrosis, petechial hemorrhages or neoplasia. If the lesion is of high density it may be dense or consolidated. This usually suggests a homogeneous appearance and may indicate hemorrhage or calcification, whereas malignant neoplasms usually show a mixed high-density appearance. By utilizing computer histographic analysis, it is possible to determine if a lesion is homogeneous, in which case a frequency profile of the attenuation values for the central portion of the lesion should have a smooth, narrow, symmetrical curve, whereas with nonhomogeneous lesions the curve will be spread out and quite uneven.[6]

The density pattern following contrast infusion should be described and includes the following:

1. No enhancement, characteristic of poorly vascularized neoplasms and old chronic infarctions, hemorrhage or contusion.

2. Patchy nonhomogeneous enhancement, most indicative of malignant neoplasm.

3. Linear nonhomogeneous enhancement, consistent with recent infarction, contusion or angioma.

4. Dense homogeneous enhancement, most often seen with meningioma.

5. Peripheral rim of enhancement, which may have several patterns, including complex rings of a malignant neoplasm, a smooth regular rim seen in abscesses, or metastases with a necrotic central core, and a thin regularly shaped rim of enhancement, which is due to peripheral neovascularity and does not represent capsule formation. This latter pattern may be seen in hematoma or infarction but is not specific as other conditions, including abscesses, postsurgical change and rarely, malignant neoplasm, show a similar pattern.

6. A thick rim of enhancement with no enhancement of the central region, as contrast does not reach the central portion with certain neoplasms.

7. Enhancement in the medial wall of extracerebral lesions, including subdural hematoma, empyema or effusion; this is due to neovascularity.

8. Homogeneous sharply-margined enhancement, most characteristic of non-invasive lesions, including meningioma, pituitary adenoma and acoustic neurinoma.

Scan interpretation may be influenced by the prior knowledge of the clinical history and the results of other diagnostic studies. The incidence of false positive scan findings — which imply that a pathological lesion exists at a certain location when in fact it does not — is greater if the scan is initially interpreted with this information available; this occurs most frequently when the scan is not completely satisfactory technically.

The problem of this bias is obviated by an initial interpretation without any clinical or diagnostic studies available, and a second review of the scan after study of the entire clinical picture. These "false positives" result from misinterpretation of normal parenchymal and vascular structures, which may appear to be sufficiently different in attenuation values so as to suggest a pathological process. In addition, the image reconstruction produced by the computer algorithm is an approximation and not an ideal reconstruction; therefore, if the discrepancy is great enough, a false image may be produced. If these are constant and their exact source understood, it may be possible to reprocess the image to correct or eliminate these false images without any reduction in the sensitivity of the study.

On the other hand, the incidence of false negative studies — in which the scan findings imply normality in an area in which a pathologic condition exists — is higher if the scan is initially interpreted without knowledge of the clinical history, but it is not influenced in this direction if the EEG, skull radiogram or isotope scan results are not known. Currently, the incidence of false negative studies is less than 1 percent but is a definite problem in identifying lesions contiguous with bone; this includes tumors at the base of the skull, such as acoustic neurinomas and sella lesions, as well as extracerebral hematoma. In addition, lesions of insufficient size or having attenuation values too close to surrounding brain are more likely not to be detected, and the anatomy of normal and abnormal vascular structures are much better outlined by angiography.

In some cases CT may identify the presence of a lesion; but the density pattern, morphological and enhancement characteristics are not sufficiently unique to permit differentiation of a neoplastic from a non-neoplastic process and complementary procedures are still required. If the patient's clinical condition permits serial studies to be obtained with specific attention to mass effect and enhancement, it is possible to differentiate neoplasm from an inflammatory process, infarction or hematoma without angiography or surgical biopsy. The CT pattern of certain neoplasms may be so similar that preoperative angiography is still required, as CT frequently provides insufficient information relative to tumor extension or pathological features to determine the appropriate treatment modality. Following medical, irradiation or surgical therapy, the image reconstructed by CT is more valuable in evaluating the results than other neurodiagnostic studies.

CONTRAST ENHANCEMENT STUDIES

Early experience indicated the value of intravenous administration of iodinated contrast material to increase resolution of structures in both tumorous and nontumorous conditions. Ambrose attributed this tumor blush to the passage of iodine through the basement membrane of the capillary endothelial cells of abnormal tumor vascularity.[7] Other studies confirmed that enhancement was due primarily to extravascular diffusion because the absorption attenuation increment was too large in proportion to the regionally small cerebral blood volume.[8] Additional support for extravascular diffusion was derived from the demonstration of enhancement in angiographically avascular lesions, and correlation of contrast CT enhancement with positive isotope scan, in which concentration of radioisotope in the lesion is believed related to the passage of isotope into the tumor cells and the extracellular fluid.[9] Furthermore, in cystic avascular tumors contrast infusion study shows persistence of iodide in the cyst for as long as 18 to 24 hours.[10] In normal subjects contrast material may diffuse into the dura; this diffusion may be related to the effect of the hyperosmolar substance's causing disruption of the blood-brain barrier by opening tight endothelial cell junctions of the capillary walls. Alternatively, it has also been postulated that contrast enhancement may be related to intravascular iodide concentration, which would explain the visualization of larger cerebral arteries and veins in both normal and pathological conditions.[11] Large aneurysms may be well visualized only immediately after contrast infusion, whereas in angioma there may be an initial increase up to 15 minutes after contrast infusion due to the intravascular phase, and there may also be a high residual attenuation value at three hours due to the extravascular phase.

Recent studies of the mortality rate of intravenous contrast infusion revealed one death in 50,000 examinations and an incidence of 5 percent for all untoward effects. Utilizing contrast in CT, the incidence of complications has been 3.8 percent and these have included nausea, vomiting, throat discomfort, hives, rhinorrhea, and other skin reactions. Most reactions have occurred in the first few minutes after starting the infusion and they are rarely severe enough to terminate the infusion.[12, 13] If the contrast material is infused too rapidly, nausea and vomiting may occur; this will disappear if the rate of infusion is slowed. All symptoms respond to treatment with 50 mg of Benadryl or 0.2 ml epinephrine. In rare instances a superficial phlebitis has developed several hours following infusion, and this has responded to elevation and warm soaks of the involved arm. The incidence of complications is not different from that in the early studies when a bolus of 20 to 60 ml of 60 percent sodium meglumine iothalamate was used (Conray); more recently with rapid drip infusion over five minutes of 300 ml of 25 percent sodium meglumine diatrizoate (Hypaque) or Conray is used.

With the introduction of contrast injection as an important complementary part of CT, the nature of the examination has been changed from an almost completely noninvasive procedure, which did not require prior patient consent or a more complete explanation than that required for plain skull radiogram, to a procedure that now requires prior informed consent by a physician, venipuncture and infusion of a pharmaceutical agent which is usually safe but carries a small but definite risk of toxic effect. Initial CT studies without contrast infusion had a diagnostic accuracy of 82 percent, and this was increased to 92 percent if scanning with 20 ml of contrast infusion was also performed.[7] After the introduction of the 160 × 160 matrix system, enhancement was detected in 73 percent of tumors, and when the contrast dose was increased to 60 ml, enhancement was detected in 90 percent of tumors. Several studies have investigated the criteria for contrast infusion. These include:

1. The presence of a pathological lesion which has previously been demonstrated by other diagnostic studies, including isotope scan, air study, angiography, biopsy and skull radiogram.

2. Any patient with evidence of an extracerebral neoplasm in whom there was suspicion of intracerebral metastases.

3. The suspicion of a cerebellopontine, posterior fossa or parasellar lesion.

4. Suspicion of aneurysm or angioma.

5. Finding of an abnormality on the neurological examination or a history of seizures.

6. Symptoms suggestive of occlusive or hemorrhagic cerebrovascular disease.

7. Evidence in preinfusion study of a possible space-occupying lesion, as manifested by an unexplained shift of midline structures, asymmetry or nonvisualization of ventricles or abnormal tissue density.[11, 12]

As greater experience with contrast infusion is obtained, the indications for it appear to be increasing, but it should not be considered as a "routine" procedure. From our experience, contrast infusion is indicated in the following clinical situations:

1. Since the majority of parasellar lesions show evidence of enhancement with contrast infusion, it should always be performed in patients with radiographic evidence of abnormal sella, endocrine symptoms of hypothalamic pituitary disturbance and visual symptoms suggestive of optic pathway involvement. In 5 percent of parasellar lesions, preinfusion study showed no abnormal tissue density but the lesion was readily detected with infusion.

2. In patients who have evidence of sensorineural hearing loss, vertigo or unsteadiness of gait with radiographic evidence of abnormality of the internal acoustic canal the suspicion is raised of cerebellopontine angle tumor. In 15 to 20 percent of tumors, the tumor was visualized only following contrast infusion, with no detectable abnormality of the cisterns or fourth ventricle. In 200 patients who had only "dizziness" without accompanying neurological signs or radiographic abnormalities, infusion study detected no abnormalities.

3. In patients with suspected posterior fossa tumor, especially if plain scan does not clearly visualize the fourth ventricle as a normal-sized midline structure. Two percent of these posterior fossa neoplasms showed abnormal density with infusion only. In several cases the tumor was not detected by initial CT scan, as the significance of nonvisualization of the fourth ventricle was not initially appreciated and a contrast medium was not always administered.

4. In patients who have a known intracranial lesion and have had surgery, radiotherapy or chemotherapy, as it is not possible to differentiate the effect of surgery from tumor recurrence without contrast enhancement. In addition, the intensity and extent of enhancement may correlate with the clinical course and may be used as a most reliable monitor of therapy.

5. The previous finding of a positive isotope scan or angiography.

6. If a patient has evidence of visceral carcinoma and treatment and the modality of therapy will be altered by the presence of intracerebral deposit, contrast CT should be performed even if there are no symptoms referable to CNS, as 5 percent of asymptomatic lesions are detected by CT even in the presence of a normal EEG and isotope scan.

7. In patients with clinical symptoms of increased intracranial pressure, contrast study should be performed if there is evidence of dilatation, distortion, displacement or compression of

the ventricular system, but infusion study may be avoided if the ventricles are normal in size and position.

8. In patients with suspected occlusive cerebrovascular disease 10 to 25 percent will show a striking enhancement pattern only. Failure to perform infusion study with a high dose of contrast medium may partially explain why some early studies showed only 55 percent of infarctions. With hemorrhagic disorders enhancement may establish the temporal profile and the etiology of the hematoma, including neoplasm, angioma and aneurysm.

9. If angioma or aneurysm is suspected, contrast enhancement may demonstrate a marked intravascular component.

10. Patients with generalized seizures alone have routinely had infusion studies, but in a study of 200 patients with a negative plain scan only 1 percent had a positive postinfusion study, and in these cases EEG and isotope scan were also positive.

11. If the plain scan shows ventricular dilatation consistent with an obstructive process, infusion is indicated, but if there is ventricular dilatation and sulcal widening consistent with an atrophic process, this is unnecessary. If the ventricles are displaced or compressed without evidence of an abnormal lesion, infusion is necessary to identify an isodense lesion.

12. In cases of craniocerebral trauma, infusion may be necessary to define enhancement in a contusion. In isodense extradural hematoma, the only finding may be enhancement in the medial membrane. In patients with a clinical history consistent with diagnosis of concussion but without neurological signs, both plain and postinfusion studies were negative.

Metrizamide Cisternography

Metrizamide (Amipaque) is a water-soluble iodine-containing contrast material that is a non-ionic substituted amide and not a salt. It results in high iodide content with lower osmolarity.[14, 15, 16] The combination of high iodide concentration with lower toxicity increases its contrast resolution and decreases its systemic toxicity and neurotoxicity. Because of the risk of seizures, premedication with phenobarbital (130 mg) has been routinely employed, and this is repeated immediately before the study and up to 24 hours after the study. Following lumbar puncture performed under fluoroscopic control on a standard myelographic table, metrizamide is instilled so as to fill the basilar cisterns, fourth ventricle, and, rarely, the third and lateral ventricle. This outlines the cisterns surrounding the brain stem and may therefore detect brain-stem neoplasms and may also be of value in detecting smaller suprasellar tumors. In addition, by utilizing metrizamide the dynamics of CSF in hydrocephalus may be evaluated and the findings correlated with those of isotope cisternography. The results obtained with this technique have not been sufficiently superior to those obtained with conventional contrast-enhancement CT to warrant the risk of its neurotoxicity and patient discomfort.

REFERENCES

1. New PFJ, Scott WR: Computed Tomography of the Brain and Orbit. Williams and Wilkins, Baltimore, 1975. pp. 30–34.
2. Welborn SG: Anesthesia for EMI scanning in infants and small children. South Med J 69:1294, 1976.
3. Gomez MR, Reese DF: CT of the head in infants and children. Pediat Clin N Amer 23:473, 1976.
4. French BN, Dublin AB: The value of CT in the management of 1000 consecutive head injuries. Surg Neurol 7:171, 1977.

5. Rosenbaum HE: Three dimensional computerized tomographic scans of brain. Arch Neurol 34:381, 1977.
6. Reese DF, O'Brien PC, Beeler GW, et al: An investigation for extracting more information from CT scan. Am J Roentgenol 124:177, 1975.
7. Ambrose J, Gooding MR, Richardson AE: Sodium iothalamate as aid to diagnosis of intracranial lesions by CT scanning. Lancet 2:669, 1975.
8. Gado MH, Phelps ME, Coleman RE: Extravascular component of contrast enhancement in cranial CT. Part I: The tissue blood ratio of contrast enhancement. Part II: Contrast enhancement and blood tissue barrier. Radiology 117:589, 1975.
9. Messina AV: CT: contrast media within subdural hematoma. Radiology 119:725, 1976.
10. Messina AV, Potts DG, Rottenberg D, Patterson RH: CT: Demonstration of contrast medium within cystic tumors. Radiology 120:345, 1976.
11. Huckman MS: Clinical experience with intravenous infusion of iodinated contrast material as an adjunct to CT. Surg Neurol 4:297, 1975.
12. Kramer RA, Janetos GP, Perlstein G: Approach to contrast enhancement in CT of the brain. Radiology 116:641, 1975.
13. Fischer HW, Doust VL: Evaluation of pretesting of serious and fatal reactions to excretory urography. Radiology 103:497, 1972.
14. Roberson GH, Brismar J, Weiss A: CSF enhancement for CT. Surg Neurol 6:235, 1976.
15. Drayer BP, Rosenbaum AE, Kigman HB: CSF imaging using serial Metrizamide CT cisternography. Neuroradiol 13:7, 1977.
16. Greitz T, Hindmarsh T: CT of intracranial and CSF circulation using a water soluble contrast medium. Acta Radiol (Diagn) 15:497, 1974.

PART TWO

EVALUATION OF SPECIFIC NEUROLOGICAL SYMPTOMS AND SIGNS

Chapter 5 Neurological Deficit of Rapid Onset

The Stroke Syndrome: Cerebral Infarction and Intracerebral Hematoma

A stroke syndrome is defined as a relatively sudden or apoplectic onset of focal neurological deficit, which rapidly reaches a plateau. The subsequent course is varied. One third of patients die in the acute stage, whereas the remainder regain some degree of function and may recover completely.

The clinical classification is based upon the temporal evolution of the deficit and this has therapeutic and prognostic significance. In the majority of stroke syndromes, the neurological dysfunction develops rapidly, and this is contrasted with the slower progress characteristic of neoplastic disorders. Transient ischemic episodes (TIE) are characterized by brief episodes of focal neurological deficit which develop rapidly, persist for several minutes to 24 hours and resolve spontaneously and completely. They may be recurrent and the harbinger of a fixed or completed deficit in 50 to 80 percent of cases. A "completed stroke" is the prototype disorder in which deficit develops acutely over several minutes. The term "completed" is used in its temporal sense to define rapidly developing and persistent deficit, which is maximal at onset and has progressed no further, although the deficit may be less than expected for a hemorrhage or occlusion involving the entire distribution of the involved vessel. The spatial completeness depends on other factors. The temporal profile of patients with stroke-in-evolution (SIE) is more varied, and the deficit occurs more slowly, in a step-wise series of events, which may take up to 96 hours before maximal deficit is reached.

The most usual pathological process causing this clinical condition is a progressive stenosis and occlusive process leading to a more gradual interference with the blood supply; the collateral circulation is not adequate to prevent subsequent ischemia and infarction. Although the majority of SIE are caused by nonhemorrhagic cerebral infarction, several studies have found that in 10 to 18 percent of cases of necropsy-proven cerebral hemorrhages the onset was more gradual than apoplectic. Other causes include cerebral embolism and nonvascular mass lesions.[1]

Since cerebral infarction and hemorrhage occur in characteristic locations, the clinical pattern of the deficit may define the specific pathological process and vascular territory involved; and this clinical impression may be confirmed by the results of EEG, isotope scan, CSF examination or angiogram; but the underlying pathological process cannot always be accurately determined without necropsy study. The study of Dalsgaard-Nielsen demonstrated that necropsy evaluation in stroke syndromes was frequently at variance with the clinical presentation; the clinical diagnosis of cerebral hemorrhage was confirmed at necropsy in 65 percent of cases, whereas the diagnosis of cerebral infarction was confirmed in only 57 percent.[2]

Although the majority of clinically diagnosed stroke syndromes are due to cerebral vascular disorders, not infrequently the episode of rapid clinical neurological deterioration is due to the presence of neoplasm, abscess, subdural hematoma or demyelinating disorder.[3, 4, 5] This rapid clinical deterioration may be due to the effects of sudden shifts in intracranial pressure dynamic relationships, mechanical compression by the tumor causing venous infarction, hemorrhage within the neoplasm or sudden paroxysmal electrical discharges due to the irritative effect of the tumor. In these latter cases there is frequently an antecedent history of headache, nausea and vomiting; neurological examination indicates altered mentation and evidence of intracranial hypertension. An important differentiating point in the temporal evolution of cerebrovascular stroke syndrome is that there is usually no further progression after the deficit has become maximal unless there is continued hemorrhage, recurrent infarction or progressive cerebral edema. If hemorrhage has occurred within a neoplasm, there may be some initial clinical improvement for several days as the hemorrhage resolves. As the continued growth of the tumor occurs there is subsequent clinical worsening, but initial diagnostic confusion with primary intracerebral hemorrhage may occur.

Until the introduction of the CT scan, the error in the initial misdiag-

nosis of an acute stroke syndrome was 2 to 4 percent. In one report of 300 patients initially diagnosed on a clinical basis alone as having cerebral infarction, Groch identified four previously unsuspected cases of intracranial tumor or abscess, and Carter reported 10 neoplasms in 289 patients with clinically diagnosed cerebral infarction.[6, 7]

The identification of the underlying lesion frequently depended upon the utilization of angiography or air study. Bull assessed the accuracy of clinical diagnosis of "acute stroke" prospectively by performing angiography on 80 consecutive patients, and a glioma and metastatic neoplasm were visualized. In both patients initial clinical improvement of six weeks' and three months' duration occurred and was followed by subsequent deterioration. In 40 cases angiography defined the exact location of the vascular occlusive process, and in 20 cases showed evidence of an avascular mass presumed to be an intracerebral hematoma; however, in 18 cases angiography did not identify an underlying lesion.[8] In patients with clinical signs of an acute stroke syndrome, the indications for cerebral angiography include: (1) suspicion of a potentially surgically accessible extracranial carotid lesion; (2) suspicion of the presence of an intracerebral hematoma; (3) clinical uncertainty as to the exact nature of the underlying lesion, including possible nonvascular mass, angioma or aneurysm. In certain cases of clinically suspected cerebellar infarction or hemorrhage and lateral ganglionic hematoma, angiography is frequently performed, as these cases may require neurosurgical intervention, but angiography in patients with atherosclerotic and hypertensive vascular disease is associated with a morbidity and mortality of 5 to 10 percent. If angiography is not performed the diagnosis is based on clinical analysis and is confirmed by more indirect studies, including CSF examination, EEG and isotope scan with both static and dynamic flow studies, but this pathological diagnosis is frequently incorrect.[9]

Utilizing CT, the most accurate anatomical localization and definition of the pathological sequelae to occlusive or hemorrhagic disorders is obtained, although angiography is required to define the specific underlying vascular etiology. Serial scanning also now enables the clinician to determine the evolution of the pathological changes in nonfatal cases and to achieve a high degree of pathological correlation. Based on plain and post-contrast infusion scan findings, it is usually possible to differentiate primary intracerebral hemorrhage and hemorrhagic and nonhemorrhagic infarction, and with serial studies to exclude other nonvascular causes. Clinical and necropsy studies prior to CT classified the incidence of stroke syndromes in the following order: cerebral embolism, 2 to 5 percent; primary hemorrhage, 7 to 23 percent; subarachnoid hemorrhage, 5 to 10 percent; nonembolic cerebral infarction, 52 to 70 percent; uncertain diagnosis, 7 to 9 percent; clinically unsuspected space-occupying lesion, 3 percent; and transient ischemic attacks without infarction, 6 percent.[10, 11] Utilizing CT, early studies of stroke patients have shown a much higher incidence of intracerebral hemorrhage with a wider clinical spectrum, as well as higher incidence of nonvascular conditions, than indicated by other studies.

Of 111 patients with cerebrovascular syndromes studied by CT, Kinkel reported that 90 had nonhemorrhagic and 21 had hemorrhagic disorder. Of these patients 32 were believed clinically to have transient ischemic episodes, but in 9 cases an area consistent with nonhemorrhagic infarction was detected by CT; this finding may alter the need for anticoagulation, angiography and surgery. In 58 cases nonhemorrhagic infarction was suspected clinically on the basis of sudden or rapidly progressive deficit be-lieved to be due to supratentorial vascular occlusion; CSF was negative for presence of red blood cells or xanthochromia and no meningeal signs were present. CT scan confirmed this diagnosis in 42 cases; in 11 others an intracerebral hematoma (ICH) or neoplasm was present, and in 5 the CT scan was negative or showed only generalized atrophy. In one unusual case angiography showed branch occlusion of the middle cerebral artery, and immediate and serial studies up to 12 months later were entirely normal. The diagnosis of an ICH was clinically established in patients who presented with sudden neurological deficit associated with nuchal rigidity, bloody or xanthochromic CSF and angiographic analysis showing shift of midline vessels by an avascular mass, and the CT scan confirmed the presence of an ICH in 12 cases, but nonhemorrhagic infarction was demonstrated in 9 others. In those cases in which CT scan demonstrated ICH, CSF was bloody or xanthochromic in 52 percent, a lower rate than the 74 to 80 percent previously reported from other studies.[12]

In early studies of sensitivity of the CT scan in cerebral infarction, Paxton and Ambrose reported positive findings in 27 of 55 cases; scan was positive in 8 of 15 studies in the initial 7 days, 8 of 17 studied at 7 to 21 days, but positive in only 4 of 23 scanned after three weeks.[13] This was consistent with other studies which reported positive findings in 50 percent. With nonhemorrhagic cerebral infarction the initial finding was the appearance of a nonhomogeneous low-density region (+3 to 13) which had regular and sharply defined margins, although frequently the edges were slightly irregular.[14, 15] This change may be visualized within 24 hours, and our earliest detectable lesion was present 12 hours after the ictus. Conversely, the longest interval after the onset of the clinical ictus until the scan showed a low-density area consistent with infarction was 72 hours, and in this case the scan had been negative at 48 hours.

In patients whose only abnormality is contrast enhancement without a low-density area, the scan may be normal up to 10 days after ictus. It is believed that the low absorption area represents cerebral edema, which correlates with the experimental evidence that significant tissue swelling begins 12 to 24 hours after the ictus and becomes maximal at 72 to 96 hours. Approximately 20 percent of infarctions show significant mass effect; this correlates directly with the clinical observation that those patients with scan evidence of a large area of edema have altered mentation due to mass effect (Fig. 5–1). In addition to edema, the earliest detectable pathological changes include slight tissue hyperemia due to dilatation and congestion of the subpial vessels, which is not demonstrated by CT. Within the first 72 hours, the CT scan shows a speckled nonhomogeneous low-density lesion resulting from a mixture of edema, vascular congestion and early tissue necrosis. Serial scans obtained in the first week may show progressive enlargement of the low-density region, which may be due to increasing edema or necrosis. The lesion usually attains maximal size by 96 hours, although in several cases substantial enlargement of the infarction occurred 7 to 10 days later. With significant cerebral edema there is pathological evidence of loss of gyral pattern, and the edema spreads to involve the deep white matter. In the CT scan the edema fluid may be isodense, and this may be visualized only as loss of sulcal pattern over the involved hemisphere. The low-density area has a rounded wedge shape which extends to the periphery and its apex is directed deeply.

By the end of the first week, the mass effect begins to diminish, the margins of low- and normal-density tissue become more clearly defined, and the lesion may appear more homogeneous in density pattern. Pathologically, the phagocytic macrophages migrate to the infarcted region and liquefaction necrosis begins. At this stage the necrotic area becomes replaced by cystic spaces, which have a uniform homogeneous density pattern consistent with CSF. In small infarctions the process of necrosis is less extensive and after several months the scan may be entirely normal owing to reduction in size of the abnormal area and partial volume effect. Pathological studies have shown that a cavity one centimeter in diameter takes two months to form, and larger cavities may be complete by four months.

In some cases the lesion consists of a mixture of cystic fluid, granulation tissue and normal parenchyma, and the density may be indistinguishable from that of normal brain. In old more extensive cerebral infarctions, the density is that of CSF, and the shape is rounded rather than triangular, with well-defined margins. Pathologically there are bands of well-

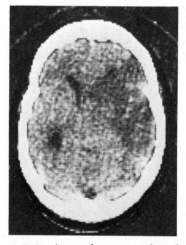

Figure 5–1. A very large area of nonhomogeneously decreased density, is confined to the territory of the middle cerebral artery and spares the region of the anterior and posterior cerebral arteries; it extends deeply, with compression and distortion of the left lateral ventricular system and no contrast enhancement. Necropsy examination confirmed the diagnosis of cerebral infarction due to occlusion of the middle cerebral artery.

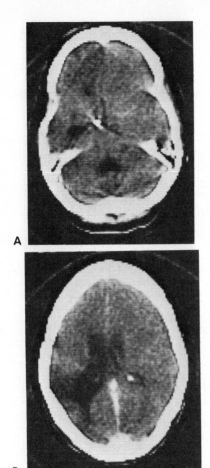

Figure 5-2. A low-density lesion in the left parietal–temporal region appears to be contiguous with the lateral ventricle. The left temporal horn is dilated and the lateral ventricle is shifted to the side of the lesion (A); there is no contrast enhancement (B). This is consistent with an old cerebral infarction.

with the ventricles. Several months later the infarction appears to be pathologically stable and remains visible by CT scan. By its location, shape and density characteristics it is not possible to determine if it was initially hemorrhagic or nonhemorrhagic in origin.[14]

Yock and Marshall concluded that establishing a timetable for evaluating the age of the cerebral infarction could only be roughly approximated.[15] They found that half the infarcts one to seven days old were visualized as well-defined low-density areas with no changes in margination or homogeneity from days one to three compared with days four to seven; in the second week the infarctions were equally divided between those nonhomogeneous irregularly marginated lesions and homogeneous well-marginated lesions. Therefore, definition of the visual appearance on precontrast infusion was not sufficient to determine its age, and this required contrast infusion. Twenty-five percent of patients showed a prominent increase in tissue absorption, and in one case the preinfusion study had been negative; this enhancement pattern was most prominent seven to 18 days after the ictus. The initial impression in those cases characterized by prominent enhancement without an initial low-density lesion was that they represented neoplasm or vascular malformation; angiography did not substantiate this impression, and the clinical course was most consistent with infarction. They concluded that, based on the visual appearance and actual density coefficients, it was not possible to approximate the age of the infarct. The presence of mass effect and enhancement were indicative of a lesion less than three weeks old. Serial studies may define the resolution of certain pathological changes which cannot be defined with a single study.

Early studies did not emphasize the importance and frequency of contrast infusion studies in the diagnosis

vascularized granulation tissue which extend across the cavity but are not detected by scan. Because of the loss of tissue parenchyma, there may be a shift of the ventricular system to the damaged region associated with ipsilateral ventricular dilatation (Fig. 5-2). From the scan appearance the low-density region may extend to the ventricular system and appear to communicate with the ventricles (porencephalic cyst); but based on the results of air studies and necropsy findings there is *no* communication

of cerebral infarction. Characteristically, the acute infarct is a low-density lesion without any evidence of contrast enhancement, although at this time there may be "luxury" or hyperfusion and leakage through an impaired vascular endothelium. Toward the end of the first week the enhancement pattern begins to become quite striking in 50 percent of cases, and this is seen from days seven to 17, after which time it becomes less striking (Fig. 5–3). The importance of performing both plain and contrast scans has been emphasized by Wing et al. who reported that 11 percent with contrast enhancement had a normal plain scan and the only abnormality was the enhancement pattern.[16] In 5 percent of cases contrast enhancement may obscure an initial low-density lesion — the abnormality may not be detected with only contrast infusion study. Yock and Marshall suggested the value of comparing numerical values on computer printout for pre- and postinfusion studies to detect a loca-

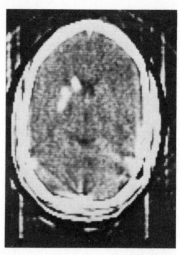

Figure 5–4. A 15-year-old boy developed sudden onset of headache and then became unresponsive for several minutes. When he became conscious he had a right hemiparesis, hemianesthesia and field defect and was aphasic. Initial isotope scan was negative but scan became positive by end of the second week, and angiogram showed occlusion of the distal intracranial portion of the internal carotid artery with faint blush, compatible with diagnosis of "Moyamoya disease." CT showed normal plain scan, but, following contrast infusion, there was dense enhancement in the left caudate and putamen, with no enhancement crossing the internal capsule or superficially in the gyrus.

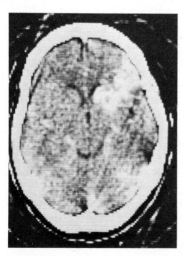

Figure 5–3. A 60-year-old woman had three episodes of transient left-sided numbness and weakness followed by sudden development of left hemiparesis–sensory syndrome. Isotope scan and EEG were normal. CT findings: a dense consolidated enhancement pattern in the right frontal parietal region extending to the paraventricular region, consistent with cerebral infarction.

lized increment of sufficient magnitude to be indicative of a pathological lesion.[15]

In other cases of nonhemorrhagic cerebrovascular disease due to carotid occlusion, the most striking feature is the enhancement pattern in the basal ganglion, parasylvian region and cortical regions. In addition to defining the presence of cerebral infarction with CT, it may be possible to predict certain angiographic findings. If total occlusion of the internal carotid artery occurs rapidly, there may be massive hemispheric infarction. In these cases CT findings include a low-density lesion in the distribution of the middle cerebral artery (MCA) and the anterior cerebral artery (ACA) with significant mass effect and no contrast enhancement. An unusual variant of stenosis or occlusion of the supraclinoid portion of one or both internal carotid arteries (ICA) is associated with an unusual vascular stain pattern in the ganglionic region; this occurs most frequently in young patients without a known underlying vascular disorder (Moyamoya syndrome).[17] There is a fine vascular stain in the ganglionic region and this corresponds with the CT finding of enhancement in the caudate and putaminal region (Fig. 5–4).

In most cerebral infarctions the enhancement is most prominent in the gray matter and skips the white matter; this is consistent with the higher blood flow to the gray matter. In rare instances there are strands of enhancement traversing the white matter of the internal capsule, but these are less dense and thinner than the enhancement seen in the nuclear masses and cortex (Fig. 5–5). This CT enhancement pattern frequently correlates with the finding of angiographic stain or presence of early draining vein; it is usually found seven to 30 days after the clinical ictus, even if angiography was negative and is negative two months later. The presence of enhancement with CT was associated with a higher incidence of positive static scan (65 percent) than in those CT scans characterized by only low-density abnormality (40 percent). In no case of a CT pattern of enhancing infarction did a dynamic scan show hyperfusion, whereas one third had evidence of decreased flow pattern. The enhancement pattern may be homogeneous, ringlike and speckled or may be linear, conforming to a more superficial gyral location (Fig. 5–6).

In patients with clinical and angiographic documentation of nonhemorrhagic infarction, this enhancement is not uniformly dense, and it is usually possible to detect low-density regions that correspond to the intervening cortical sulci. The enhancement in infarction is restricted to specific vascular territories and has intervening low-density areas. This latter finding is not visualized with neoplasms because the sulci are obliterated by tumor and edema. In neoplasms enhancement does not respect vascular borders and extends deeply into the white matter, whereas the finding of

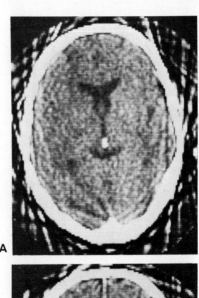

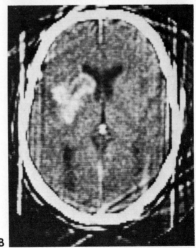

Figure 5–5. A 50-year-old physician became dizzy and then unable to express himself. Neurological findings included right hemiparesis, hemianesthesia and motor aphasia. CT scan performed eight hours after the deficit developed was entirely normal (A). Repeat study 14 days later showed a dense enhancement pattern in the paraventricular, caudate and putaminal region; linear strands of enhancement traversing the capsular region caused no mass effect (B). This pattern was consistent with cerebral infarction.

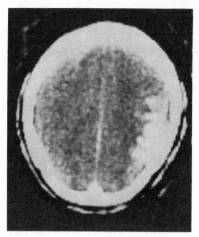

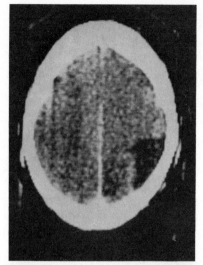

A

Figure 5–6. Patient developed severe temporal headache and left homonymous hemianopia with slight hemiparesis. Isotope scan was negative and EEG showed a mild slow-wave pattern over the right hemisphere. CT findings: plain scan was negative but following contrast infusion there were multiple enhancing gyri in the posterior frontal, parietal and temporal region, consistent with infarction of the middle cerebral artery. Angiography showed hyperperfusion in the right hemisphere with an enlarged early-draining vein in the right parieto-occipital region. Six months later there was no enhancement.

dense enhancement with minimal mass effect is quite characteristic of cerebral infarction.

If there is an occlusion of the mid-

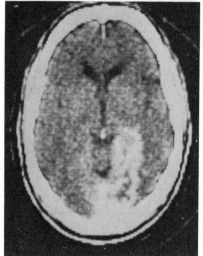

B

Figure 5–8. Patient developed left-sided weakness which worsened over a 72-hour interval. Neurological findings included left hemiparesis-sensory syndrome with left homonymous hemianopia. CT findings: a wedge-shaped area of low density in the right parieto-temporal region without mass effect (A), and dense enhancement in the thalamic superior temporal and right occipital region with several enhancing gyri in the right region (B), consistent with infarction in territory of the middle and posterior cerebral arteries.

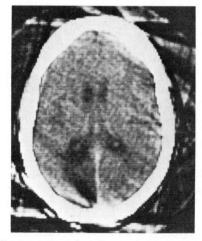

Figure 5–7. A low-density lesion in the left occipital region extends directly to the midline and appears contiguous with the occipital horn of the lateral ventricle. There was no enhancement, as is consistent with occipital infarction.

dle cerebral artery (MCA) branch, the enhancement may be located only in the paraventricular region (caudate), or more commonly in the cortical gyral pattern of the MCA territory. These patterns are quite specific for

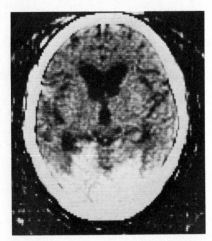

Figure 5–9. This patient presented with dizziness, blurring of vision, unsteadiness of gait and a confusional state. Neurological findings included broad-based gait, right homonymous hemianopia and inattention to the left visual field. Isotope scan was positive in the right occipital region. CT findings: a dense gyral portion of tortuous enhancement in both occipital regions consistent with occlusion of the distal portion of the basilar artery or bilateral posterior cerebral artery involvement.

infarction and should not be confused with the more serpentine enhancement of angioma, but serial scans and temporal profile provide the ultimate point of differentiation.

With posterior cerebral artery (PCA) occlusion the plain scan may visualize a low-density area in the occipital region medial in location, confluent with the tentorium, inferior sagittal and transverse sinuses, oval or crescent-shaped, and with minimal mass effect (Fig. 5–7). The enhancement pattern may be extensive, tortuous and serpentine, is usually confined to the occipital and temporal region and always respects the arterial boundaries of the PCA. In other cases, the plain scan is normal and enhancement is detected in these cortical regions, the thalamus and portions of the putamen (Fig. 5–8), because the PCA also supplies these deep nuclear masses. In rare instances of PCA occlusion there is a dense enhancement in both occipital regions (Fig. 5–9), consistent with an

occlusive process at a proximal portion of the PCA.

Infarctions involving the territory of the ACA usually demonstrate a low-density pattern in the anterior frontal region, which is sharply delineated from normal parenchyma. Following contrast infusion, there may be a linear enhancement pattern, most prominent at the periphery of the lesion. (See Figure 5–45).

Hemorrhagic infarction is usually caused by cerebral embolus and has a characteristic CT appearance. Pathologically, there are multiple petechial hemorrhages on the surface, which coalesce to form a larger hemorrhagic area, and this is surrounded by a more extensive necrotic and edematous region. As the embolus lodges in the cerebral vessel, it further occludes blood flow, but lysis occurs with dispersal of the clot and metabolic factors lead to local vasodilatation. This subjects the necrotic parenchyma to the full arterial force and leads to hemorrhage. With CT, the characteristic appearance of hemorrhagic in-

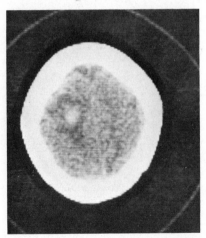

Figure 5–10. A patient who had chronic atrial fibrillation suddenly developed difficulty using her right hand, and this rapidly became hemiplegic. CSF examination showed evidence of red cells and xanthochromia. CT findings: a round high-density lesion surrounded by a low-density rim in the right parietal convexity. Lesion did not enhance, as is consistent with hemorrhagic infarction.

farction is that of high-density central areas, which are surrounded by a more extensive low-density region located in the peripheral distribution of the MCA; these lesions do not usually show an enhancement pattern (Fig. 5–10). Less commonly there may be dense central and peripheral gyral enhancement, and differentiation from nonhemorrhagic infarction is not always possible (Fig. 5–11). The presence of multiple lesions is consistent with cerebral embolism; but the scan appearance may be similar to that of several other pathological conditions, including metastases and abscesses. CT evidence of a hemorrhagic infarction pattern appears to be highly characteristic of cerebral embolus, and is an important finding in determining the risk of subsequent anticoagulation.

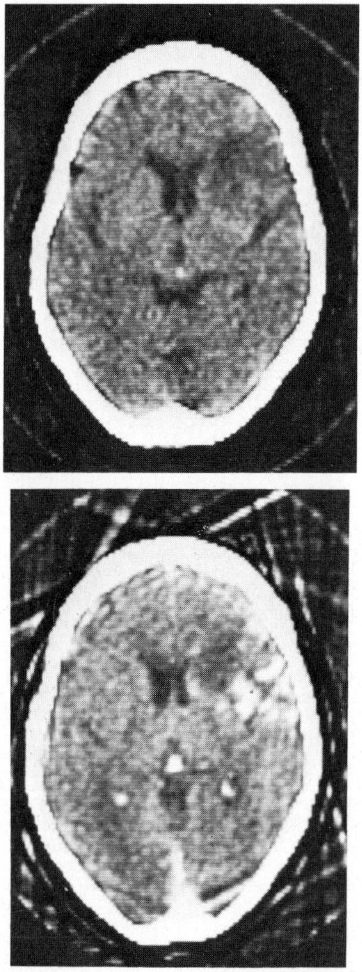

Primary intracerebral and intraventricular hematomas have a very distinctive appearance on the CT scan.[18] They are round or wedge-shaped, high-density (20 to 45 units) lesions having irregular borders. The central region is usually homogeneously dense, but the periphery may be less dense than the central region. These lesions are surrounded by low-density edema fluid; they usually cause significant mass effect, with compression, distortion and displacement of the ventricles and evidence of blood which has dissected into the ventricle (Fig. 5–12). Intraventricular blood conforms to the shape of the ventricular cast. With experience to date, there has been no report of an intracerebral hematoma (ICH) which was clinically symptomatic and not detected by CT, although partial volume effect may interfere with the diagnosis of hematomas less than 5 mm in diameter. Because of the relative density differences of white and gray matter, it would be theoretically more likely to fail to detect a small hematoma in the gray matter.

There is nothing characteristic about the CT appearance of a hypertensive ICH that permits distinction from those with other causes, but the localization of the hematoma is frequently helpful in predicting the results of angiography. If no further episodes of hemorrhage occur, as is usually the case with hypertensive ICH, there is a distinct change in the scan appearance of the hematoma. As there is phagocytosis of the blood pigment, necrotic tissue and xanth-

A

B

Figure 5–11. This patient initially developed left arm weakness and two days later noted that her left leg dragged. She was also in atrial fibrillation with rapid ventricular response. CT findings: a low density lesion in the right parietal region surrounded by a streak of high density, consistent with blood in the gyri (A); following contrast infusion there was prominent enhancement (B), and this was consistent with hemorrhagic infarction.

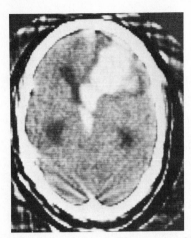

Figure 5–12.   A 40-year-old woman suddenly had a nongeneralized seizure. She regained consciousness but was confused and had a left hemiparesis. CSF examination was bloody and xanthochromic, and EEG showed a monorhythmic frontal delta pattern; isotope scan was negative. CT findings; a large irregular high-density lesion in the right frontal lobe, which extended into the anterior horn region of the lateral ventricle. In addition, blood filled the third ventricle, and the lateral and third ventricular system were dilated; there was no contrast enhancement. Angiography shows only an avascular mass in the right frontal region but no aneurysm or angioma.

ochromic fluid, the lesion may change from a high- to a low-density lesion. In this evolution the lesion may become isodense with brain parenchyma. This is usually associated with shrinkage in the size of the hematoma, but Messina reported necropsy evidence in two cases in which the CT density was normal or low but there has been minimal resolution in the size of the hematoma.[19]

As the ICH "ages," it may not be possible to differentiate it from a necrotic or cystic lesion. In other cases the high-density hematoma may resolve to normal density with no mass effect, so that it may not be possible to recognize the initial site of hemorrhage. In the first week after hemorrhage, the CT appearance is uniform, with a high-density region surrounded by a low-density rim, causing mass effect, and there is no enhancement. Between the second and sixth

week, a ring blush pattern following contrast infusion may be detected; this then decreases in intensity after that time. This pattern is not specific for hematoma, and if the initial scan is obtained during this time interval, diagnostic confusion with neoplasm or abscess may occur. If serial scans are available the entire sequence may be seen and this is diagnostic of an ICH. This ring blush pattern has

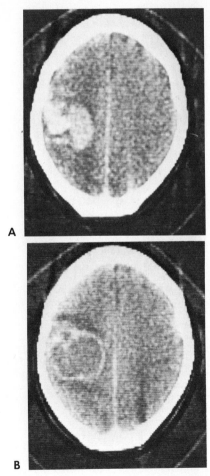

A

B

Figure 5–13.   A 44-year-old man developed a right hemiparesis without loss of consciousness or headache. Isotope scan and EEG localized a lesion in the left parietal region. CT findings: initial scan showed an irregularly shaped high-density lesion in the left parieto-temporal region that did not enhance (A). Two weeks later there was a peripherally enhancing ring surrounded by low-density edema and there was resolution of the core of the hematoma (B).

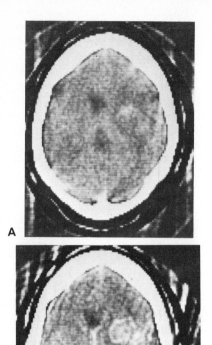

A

B

Figure 5–14. A hypertensive woman developed right-sided headache and left-sided weakness over 48 hours Neurological findings included a loud right carotid bruit and Horner's syndrome with left hemiparesis, constructional apraxia and hemianesthesia. EEG showed a right delta pattern: initial isotope scan was negative but repeat study ten days later was positive and CSF examination was negative, all consistent with a diagnosis of cerebral infarction. CT findings: plain study showed a small ganglionic high-density lesion surrounded by edema and causing ventricular displacement (A). Following contrast infusion there were definite areas of enhancement with a dense and complex ring pattern (B). Angiography demonstrated an avascular ganglionic mass consistent with hematoma. A clinical course of improvement for 12 months confirmed this impression.

tion of contrast material from intravascular space or hyperfusion. The ring is usually quite thin, consistent with the rim of neovascularity.[20] This pattern occurs in 5 percent of cases of ICH and is not related to specific etiology but is more frequently seen in lobar hemorrhage (Fig. 5–13).

Other enhancement patterns of ICH include the following: plain scan may show a small high-density area located in the ganglionic region surrounded by a low-density region with mass effect and striking irregular enhancement, suggesting a neoplasm (Fig. 5–14); or plain scan may show a mottled low-density area and contrast study show a peripheral ring and dense central enhancement. An identical scan pattern has been demonstrated in malignant glioma. This latter ring enhancement pattern may also be seen with cerebral infarction, and in these cases the enhancement

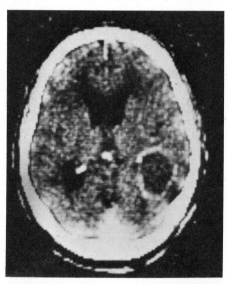

Figure 5–15. This patient developed left hemiparesis and hemisensory and homonymous hemianopic deficit, which cleared completely but then the patient developed left-sided focal seizures. Isotope scan was initially positive but became negative in two months. CT scan showed a round area of low density in the right parieto-occipital area with peripheral rim of enhancement. Angiography showed right MCA branch occlusion and the patient has remained asymptomatic except for infrequent seizures.

rarely been demonstrated with isotope scan and angiography. The mechanism is believed to be the hypervascularity of the collagen tissue surrounding the hematoma, extravasa-

is believed to represent neovascularity without capsule formation (Fig. 5–15).

CT AND ISOTOPE SCAN IN CEREBROVASCULAR DISEASE

Comparison of CT with isotope scan has demonstrated that CT is more accurate in detecting the presence of infarction or hemorrhage, but that isotope scan may detect certain lesions not detected by CT. Most investigators have reported a 20 to 30 percent incidence of abnormal isotope scan in patients with cerebral infarction studied within the first seven days after the ictal event, with a peak incidence of 60 to 80 percent for patients studied between seven and 28 days. Following this peak, the incidence of positive findings falls off sharply, so that it is unusual to detect cerebral infarction two months later; this differentiates infarction from ICH or other space-occupying lesions. Although the static scan is negative in the first week, the dynamic flow study may frequently show decreased perfusion in the territory of the involved vessel, although infrequently an increased flow due to hyperfusion may result. The use of serial scanning that shows an initial negative scan and then becomes positive between seven and 21 days is highly characteristic of cerebral infarction. In most cases, the scan then becomes negative one month after the clinical ictus. Several investigators have advocated the use of both immediate and delayed scans. In 10 percent of cerebral infarction the immediate scan is normal and the delayed scan is positive, but this technique has not been more widely utilized.[21, 22]

CT and isotope scan were comparable in the detection of the incidence of abmormalities in the early studies that utilized the 80 x 80 matrix system and a low dose of contrast infusion. In one study of cerebral infarction, CT was abnormal in 55 percent, whereas 69 percent had a positive isotope scan, but the results were not identical in 55 percent; this indicated that these were complementary and not alternative procedures.[23]

With the use of a higher-resolution matrix system and high-dose contrast infusion, the incidence of positive findings may approximate 85 to 95 percent for supratentorial vascular lesions, although the results are lower for infratentorial lesions and lacunar infarctions. During the first week following the ictus, the static isotope scan is negative, and this correlates with a CT low-density pattern without any contrast enhancement.

The highest incidence of positive findings with an isotope scan occurs between two and four weeks and this correlates with the maximal enhancement density with CT. After the fourth week the incidence of positive scan findings decreases and correlates with the decrease in frequency and intensity of enhancement; but enhancement persists longer than positive isotope scan finding. The mechanisms of contrast enhancement and uptake on isotope scan, therefore, appear to be similar and include the following: (1) abnormal vascular permeability of endothelial cells of capillary walls with extravascular diffusion, an occurrence that is unlikely since enhancement density rapidly declines by 30 minutes postinfusion; (2) increased vascularity due to development of neovascularity surrounding infarction, with later disappearance and subsequent replacement by cavity formation and hypovascularity; (3) luxury perfusion with focal hyperemia and early draining veins due to metabolic effects of the necrosis.

Chiu has compared the isotope scan patterns with the results of CT.[24] In MCA infarctions, 18 percent had an abnormal dynamic study with decreased flow but normal static study, 56 percent had linear or fan-shaped uptake along the Sylvian triangle, 21 percent had a crescent-shaped uptake, and 5 percent had multiple areas of uptake. Ten percent had entirely normal isotope study; this compared to 14 percent with normal CT scans. With occlusion of the PCA, the static scan was positive in 82 percent, and CT was positive in 93 percent. The radionuclide image of triangular uptake, with its base blending with the midline sinus

structure, correlates with the plain CT image of low density. Experience with occlusion of ACA was limited statistically but isotope scan shows uptake in the midline frontal region and CT shows a corresponding low-density region. With ICA occlusion there is usually extensive hemispheric infarction in the entire arterial supply of the MCA; in two thirds of cases this also includes the ACA and in 15 percent the PCA territory — this is more reliably detected by CT than isotope scan (Fig. 5–16).

The major diagnostic pitfalls in the diagnosis of cerebral infarction by CT and isotope scan include the following: (1) timing since isotope scan is negative in the first week and CT is negative in the initial 24 to 48 hours; (2) small size of lesion, with the isotope scan not detecting lesions smaller than 1.5 cm, and the resolving ability of CT dependent upon size plus density of surrounding structures.

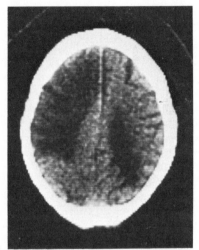

A

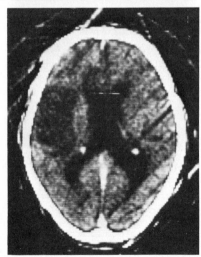

B

Figure 5–16. This elderly man suddenly became comatose with right hemiparesis. CT finding: a large low-density lesion encompassing the territory of the left middle (A) and anterior cerebral arteries (B), causing compression of the enlarged ventricular system. This was consistent with internal carotid artery occlusion, which was demonstrated by angiography.

CLINICAL STUDIES

Since the diagnostic and therapeutic procedures are dependent on the clinical pattern, the accuracy of these clinical diagnoses is crucial to further management. Since the risk that the patient with transient ischemic episodes (TIE) involving the carotid territory will develop stroke may be as high as 80 percent, angiography with subsequent vascular reconstructive surgery or anticoagulant therapy may be indicated. Complete neurodiagnostic studies should be done to exclude the presence of cerebral infarction or nonvascular cause of the symptoms. In one study of patients who presented with TIE, isotope scan was positive in 12 percent, and in another CT showed definite evidence of cerebral infarction in 27 percent.[12] The explanation of these diagnostic findings may be that an infarction occurred in which neurological deficit resolved in 24 hours or a silent infarction had occurred in the past and the transient cardiac arrhythmia decreased cerebral perfusion to cause a transient deficit in the previously infarcted area.

In patients with TIE due to carotid disease it is important to ascertain if there is any associated intracranial pathological process because in these patients a recent cerebral infarction alters the risk for carotid surgery. If a recent infarction is present the restoration of the cerebral blood flow may precipitate hemorrhage into the necrotic area. Of 40 patients with a clinical diagnosis of TIE, CT was abnormal in eight cases (20 percent). In four cases, the findings were consistent with recent cerebral infarction, and isotope scan was negative. All these patients had had multiple and frequent episodes of hemiparesis, occurring over a two- to three-week interval. In three instances angiography was performed and immediately following this study a completed stroke occurred. In two other patients who had a single transient ischemic episode lasting eight hours, CT showed a low-density lesion, whereas all patients with attacks lasting less than 30 minutes had normal scans. In one patient with multiple episodes of monoparesis, CT detected the presence of a glioma after EEG and isotope scan had been negative; the lesion appeared as an irregularly shaped, low-density area, which showed an irregular enhancement pattern, and the diagnosis was confirmed by surgical biopsy. In another case of clinically suspected TIE, CT showed a low-density lenticular extracerebral lesion consistent with chronic subdural hematoma. In this case the episodic neurological deficit may have been related to a transient reversible increase in intracranial pressure or to intermittent vascular compression.[3]

Stroke-in-evolution (SIE) refers to neurological deficit which evolves over several hours to days before reaching maximal dysfunction, and is usually due to nonhemorrhagic in-farction. In other cases the deficit occurs suddenly and then gradually increases over 48 hours, a course which suggests the presence of edema associated with infarction or, rarely, an ICH (Fig. 5–17). It has been the general impression that if the neurological deficit remains stable for 24 hours further progression is unlikely. If progressive and delayed neurological deterioration occurs after the patient's condition has stabilized, it is possible to document the underlying pathological process by CT. Of 30 patients in whom the diagnosis of SIE was initially made there were 10 patients in whom the underlying disorder was nonvascular, 7 with ICH and 17 who had nonhemorrhagic infarction defined by CT. In these cases the temporal evolution was the most critical determinant; in 8 cases the temporal evolution was stepwise and all had evidence of cerebral infarction, whereas in 22 patients in whom the deficit evolved more gradually over 96 hours, 10 had unsuspected neoplasm. If the deficit progressed to maximal dysfunction in less than 12 hours, CT showed evidence of infarction or hematoma in 90 percent, but if progression occurred over a longer interval, the incidence of nonvascular conditions was higher.

In patients with progressing stroke syndrome, appropriate therapy is dependent upon recognition of nonvascular conditions and awareness of the contribution of hemorrhage and edema formation. If the patient has a mild deficit which appears to be worsening, anticoagulation may be indicated but CT demonstration of an ICH or hemorrhagic infarction would interdict this. Since edema formation is maximal in the first 96 hours, it may be an important cause of progressive clinical deterioration, but it tends to resolve after this time. In several cases of SIE there has been progressive worsening for as long as one week after ictus, in which CT demonstrated only nonhemorrhagic infarction without mass effect or edema but with prominent enhancement, leading to the clinical suspicion of a neoplasm. In one case there was sufficient diagnostic confusion to require surgical biopsy prior to a more complete understanding of enhancement patterns (Fig. 5–17).

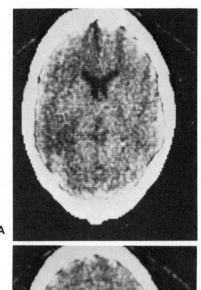

A

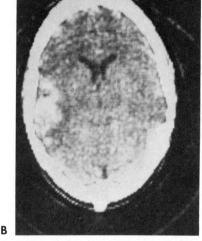

B

Figure 5–17. This young woman developed right hemiparesis progressively over one week without accompanying headache or altered mentation. EEG and isotope scan showed an abnormality in the left parietal region, and angiography showed a vascular stain with slight mass effect in this region. CT findings: preinfusion study showed no abnormality (A), but following contrast infusion there was dense irregular superficial contrast enhancement (B). Because the neurological deficit appeared to be worsening, craniotomy was performed. No tumor was found and a biopsy was consistent with cerebral infarction. (Courtesy of American Journal of Medicine.)

In patients with completed stroke the etiology may be either hemorrhage or infarction. Of 100 patients in whom the initial diagnosis was completed stroke, there were five nonvascular conditions. In only one of the five neoplasms was there evidence of hemorrhage into the tumor. Forty had nonhemorrhagic infarction, and several unexpected clinical findings were described, including the following: (1) One third of patients presented with severe unilateral headache at onset, a symptom that was only slightly less frequent than in those patients with ICH. (2) Generalized or focal seizures occurred as initial neurological manifestation in 25 percent. (3) One fourth of patients presented with impaired consciousness or a confusional state not believed to be related to a postseizure state. (4) One half of the patients were hypertensive; this rate is not statistically different than in those patients found by CT to have ICH. In 10 cases, CT defined the presence of hemorrhagic infarction, but the initial clinical picture was indicative of cerebral embolus in only two cases. Subsequent to the CT in which a pattern of hemorrhagic infarction raised the suspicion of embolus, careful evaluation detected previously unsuspected cardiac arrhythmias, valvular dysfunction and myocardial infarction and these conditions were the probable source of the embolus in these 8 patients.

CT is superior to CSF examination in showing evidence of hemorrhage, since in only 10 percent of cases of hemorrhagic infarction was there blood in the CSF. Since the risk of recurrence of embolus may be as high as 60 percent and subsequent mortality is quite high, anticoagulation should be considered to prevent recurrence. The recurrence role is highest in the first month, so the decision to anticoagulate must be made immediately. Hemorrhage may occur in 2 percent of patients treated with anticoagulants. Anticoagulation therapy should be avoided in patients with evidence of bleeding in the CSF or in whom severe neurological deficit is suggestive of hematoma rather than pale infarction.[25] In 3 patients heparin was started two to seven days before CT showed hemorrhagic infarction. It was continued and no clinical worsening developed.

In 45 cases of completed stroke, CT showed evidence of an ICH, and by its characteristic location the etiology of the hemorrhage could be determined without recourse to angiography. The majority of nontraumatic intracerebral hematomas in which angiography excludes other possible causes are related to hypertension, with bleeding occurring from small deeply located distal arterial aneurysms, most usually involving the lenticulostriate vessels. If the hematoma is located in a characteristic location, including the putamen, thalamus, brain or cerebellum, 90 percent of patients are found to have existing hypertension at the time of the stroke or to have manifestations of retinal changes, renal impairment or cardiac disease. With the diagnosis established definitively by CT, certain well-established clinical beliefs have been called into question. Firstly, the finding of evidence of hypertensive disease is not invariable and was presented in only 45 to 48 percent of cases. Secondly, the onset is apoplectic in only 70 percent and in 30 percent the development of deficit was more gradual, simulating other nonhemorrhagic disorders. Thirdly, in 20 percent of patients there were premonitory symptoms in the two weeks prior to the ictal event, a circumstance that suggested diagnosis of TIE and nonhemorrhagic infarction. Lastly, in one third of patients headache or alteration in consciousness were both absent, a finding at variance with the belief that patients with ICH present following a sudden episode of severe headache, nausea and vomiting followed by obtundation and focal deficit. The incidence of either generalized or focal seizures

was not different in ICH and infarction.

Previous studies have indicated that CSF examination shows evidence of blood or xanthochromia in 80 percent of cases of ICH but in CT-documented cases this was true in only 50 percent.[2] The mortality of ICH was only 30 percent, a figure significantly lower than in previous studies. The initial scan finding of severe ventricular compression, intraventricular hemorrhage and hydrocephalus was associated with mortality of 60 percent, which is lower than predicted from previous clinical studies.

CT was 100 percent accurate in detecting the presence of an ICH and is vastly superior to isotope scan and angiography. Previous studies have indicated that isotope scan is positive in only 50 to 60 percent of ICH; the uptake is usually round, crosses vascular boundaries, and is not associated with decreased flow; the scan is positive in the first week and then persists longer than uptake caused by infarction.[23] Angiography may not identify the source of apoplexy in 15 to 25 percent of cases of clinically suspected or necropsy proven ICH, and since clinical diagnosis is not always possible, the incidence of negative angiograms is probably much higher. The angiographic diagnosis of ganglionic hemorrhage is based on the following findings: (1) lateral displacement of the MCA; (2) characteristic displacement of lenticulostriate vessels medially or laterally, depending upon location of hemorrhage; (3) shift of the anterior cerebral artery and internal cerebral vein contralaterally; (4) ventricular dilatation with intraventricular hemorrhage. The hematoma may extend into the deep hemispheric white matter; if extension occurs into the temporal lobe, elevation of MCA is present; extension into the frontoparietal operculum causes stretching and spreading of these branches. Thalamic hematoma causes upward and medial bowing of the thalamostriate vein, with contralateral shift of the deep central vein. Gargano also reported that the lesion demonstrated by necropsy examination was larger than that estimated by angiography. If the hematoma originates in deep hemispheric white matter, there may be no angiographic signs of displacement and stretching of superficial arteries or shift of the internal cerebral vein, and a flattened spreading hematoma may not be detected by angiography.[26]

BASAL GANGLIONIC HEMORRHAGE

With direct visualization of the site, size and associated pathological effects of intracerebral hemorrhage by CT, we are becoming aware of an increasingly wide clinical spectrum of intracerebral hemorrhage. Previous studies have emphasized only two clinical syndromes of ganglionic hemorrhage: (1) lateral hematoma, following which the patient presents with symptoms developing over four to 12 hours, including mild impairment of mentation, development of an early spastic hemiparesis with mild sensory loss, but usually no hemianopia; (2) medially placed hematoma, in which the patient presents with more sudden and complete deficit and has pronounced alteration of mentation, flaccid hemiparesis with eyes deviated in either a downward position or conjugately and laterally to the side of the hematoma.

In the former group, the CSF examination is more likely to show evidence of a small number of red blood cells; the prognosis for recovery is better because the lesions tend to remain more localized with little tendency to extend into the ventricular system or hemispheric white matter. The prognosis for medial ganglionic lesions is worse because they are more likely to spread into the lobar white matter, rupture into the ventri-

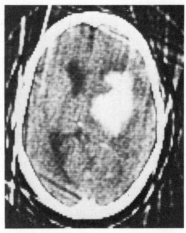

Figure 5–18. This hypertensive patient presented with generalized seizure and was found to be stuporous with left hemiplegia. CSF was bloody and isotope scan was negative. CT findings: a large consolidated high-density mass in the right ganglionic region, compressing and displacing the right lateral and third ventricle, with extension into the thalamic region.

cular system, and cause tentorial herniation with secondary brain stem hemorrhage.[27] Differentiation is important because if consciousness is normal but expected clinical improvement of the neurological deficit has not started to occur, this may be due to large volume and mass effect of the hematoma and may require neurosurgical intervention. Although angiography may show displacement of the lenticulostriate vessels due to laterally or medially placed hematoma, it may underestimate its size as determined by surgical or necropsy studies. This difference in size has been explained by continued progression of the lesion in the interval after angiography, but experimental studies have shown no evidence of continuing bleeding in ICH. With CT, there is excellent correlation between the size of the high-density lesion and pathological studies. The prognosis for recovery is best if CT localizes the hemorrhage to single tissue sections (two scans).

Based on the CT scan findings, it is possible to classify patients with putaminal hemorrhage in the following groups:[28] (1) patients who are initially comatose in whom CT scan shows large hemorrhage with wide extension, intraventricular blood and hydrocephalus (Fig. 5–18); (2) patients who are alert but have complete hemiplegia and with scan showing either laterally or medially extending hematoma, no intraventricular blood and less severe ventricular distortion;

(3) patients with hemiparesis-hemisensory syndrome without field defect, eye movement disorder, disorder of language or spatial relation or cortical sensory defect, with CT showing a small hematoma that may be medially or laterally located, with minimal ventricular distortion (Fig. 5–19). In 50 percent of the patients in the latter group, the initial diagnosis was nonhemorrhagic infarction, and in four cases isotope scan, angiography and CSF examination had been negative. In 10 percent of putaminal hematomas, the lesion extended to within one centimeter of the cortical surface, but the lesions usually extended along the pathway of the white matter tissue plane rather than dissecting laterally across the plane to the cortex. Initially, all hematomas are of high density with significant mass effect, but the hematoma may resolve to a low-density or isodense region within two weeks and then show a thin rim of enhancement.

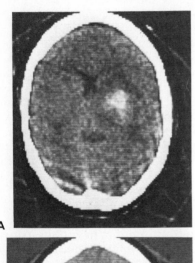

A

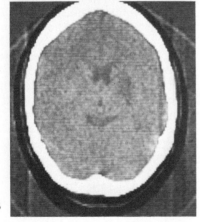

B

Figure 5–19. A 20-year-old woman developed left-sided numbness while driving her car. She had mild left pronator drift and persistent left-sided hypoanesthesia. CSF, EEG, isotope scan and four-vessel angiography were negative. CT findings: a high-density irregular lesion in the medial portion of the right putamen with surrounding edema and distortion of the ventricular system, consistent with putaminal hemorrhage (A). The patient recovered completely and three months later was asymptomatic. CT scan showed a slight residual low-density area in the right putamen (B).

THALAMIC HEMORRHAGE

This lesion accounts for 10 to 15 percent of all cases of ICH, and the clinical course is determined by the degree of mass effect and the tissue plane through which the hematoma dissects. Differentiation from medial ganglionic hemorrhage may not be possible based upon the clinical and angiographic findings, but is usually possible with CT. The characteristic clinical picture includes rapid impairment of consciousness, hemiplegia-sensory syndrome, impairment of vertical eye movement, usually with the eyes downwardly deviated, miotic and having poorly responsive pupils. If the hematoma extends laterally, the eyes are deviated laterally, usually away from the hemiplegic side as is characteristic of a supratentorial lesion, but occasionally toward the hemiplegic side as in an infratentorial lesion. The hematoma may rupture into the third ventricle and the occipital horns of the lateral ventricle. This usually causes obstructive hydrocephalus, and these patients present with increased tone in their legs and bilateral Babinski signs. This complication is associated with high mortality, and the CT finding of hydrocephalus and intraventricular extension of blood from a thalamic hematoma may be an indication for immediate shunting procedure. In only 60 percent of cases of thalamic hemorrhage did CSF contain blood or xanthochromia. EEG usually showed a bilateral slow wave pattern without lateralization in one half of cases, and isotope scan was positive in only 40 percent and did not localize the source of the blood.

CT visualized a nonhomogeneous, dense, consolidated round lesion, surrounded by a low-density region, which compressed and displaced the third ventricle; this was associated with hydrocephalus in two thirds of cases. The outcome was less favorable if blood was present in the ventricular system, but the prognosis did not correlate with a finding of ventricular dilatation (Fig. 5–20). In those patients who survived and were left with minimal neurological deficit, the ventricles returned to normal size and the high-density lesion was no longer present.[29] In certain patients clinical deterioration occurred over a 48-hour interval, and serial scan did not show any change to account for the observed clinical change. Since the introduction of CT, angiography has been performed less frequently in these cases; it was always positive in extensive lesions but was less accurate in smaller lesions and did not accurately define the entire extent of the hematoma.

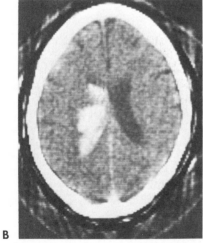

A

B

Figure 5–20. A 44-year-old hypertensive man developed headache and became unresponsive. Neurological findings included severe obtundation, right hemiplegia and hemianesthesia, with eyes deviated in downward position. CSF contained bloody fluid. CT findings: a high-density nonhomogeneous lesion in the left thalamic region with surrounding edema, impinging on the body of the lateral ventricle with intraventricular blood. In addition the ventricles are markedly dilated. This confirmed the clinical impression of thalamic hemorrhage with ventricular extension.

LOBAR HEMATOMA

In 25 percent of cases of nontraumatic ICH, the lesion is located in the deep white matter of the cerebral hemispheres. This was found most frequently in the frontal lobe but also occurred in other regions. These lobar hematomas are less likely to be related to hypertension than are striatal or thalamic hematomas; their occurrence should prompt a thorough investigation for angioma, aneurysm,

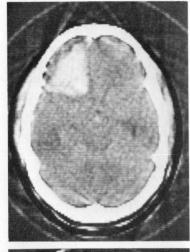

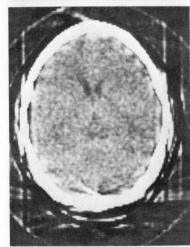

Figure 5–21. A 15-year-old boy developed obtundation following severe headache. CSF showed bloody fluid but an angiogram showed only an avascular mass in the left frontal region. CT findings: a wedge-shaped high-density lesion in the left frontal region, which did not enhance (A). Five months later the patient was asymptomatic and the hematoma not visualized; no residual mass effect is evident, as is consistent with complete resorption (B).

tomas did CT define the exact underlying pathological process. In all lobar hematomas visualized by CT, contrast studies should always be performed to define possible angioma. These lesions may extend deeply to rupture into the ventricular system and may also have a superficial portion. In those hematomas which extended to the cortex EEG showed a low-voltage slow wave pattern, and isotope scan showed a superficial crescentic uptake that simulated a subdural hematoma, but the intra-axial nature of the hematoma was visualized by CT. The frontal hematoma appeared as a wedge-shaped, high-density region, which frequently communicated with the ventricular system. Despite the large size of certain lesions with deep extension, 70 percent of patients recovered completely, with complete resolution of hematoma by CT study (Fig. 5–21). The presence of a temporal hematoma suggests a ruptured carotid aneurysm but it may occur spontaneously. If these lesions extend deeply, they may be confused with ganglionic or thalamic hemato-

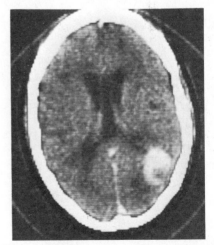

Figure 5–22. A 50-year-old normotensive male developed suboccipital headache and a confusional state. CSF was clear and EEG was diffusely symmetrically slow. CT scan showed a round high-density (30 to 40) hematoma in the right parietal-occipital area surrounded by edema with generalized ventricular dilatation.

neoplasm, blood dyscrasia, collagen vascular disease, cortical vein or dural sinus thrombosis. In McCormick's series, only 4 of 37 hypertensive patients had lobar hematoma. In two-thirds of all ICH a definite etiology was found and in 40 percent of presumed hypertensive ICH, one of the above listed etiologies was detected. In only 20 percent of our lobar hema-

mas, but primary temporal hematomas have a characteristic round or comma shape that is regular in form and displaces the uncal portion of the suprasellar cistern. The temporal, parietal and occipital hematomas appear as round high-density regions that usually extend to the superficial cortex but do not have the wedge shape of the frontal lesions (Fig. 5–22).

MULTIPLE INTRACEREBRAL HEMORRHAGE

Multiple hemorrhages are not usually seen in hypertensive patients but are most commonly associated with blood dyscrasias, coagulopathy,

septic emboli in infective endocarditis or multiple aneurysms. This diagnosis is usually established by necropsy and will not be detected if the condition is not fatal. In 3 percent of patients with ICH the lesions were multiple and, despite angiography and complete medical evaluation no underlying cause was found. In two patients who improved clinically CT showed reduction in size and density of the lesion (Fig. 5–23).

HEMORRHAGE CAUSED BY CEREBRAL NEOPLASM

Scott reported that 10 percent of cases of spontaneous ICH were

A   B

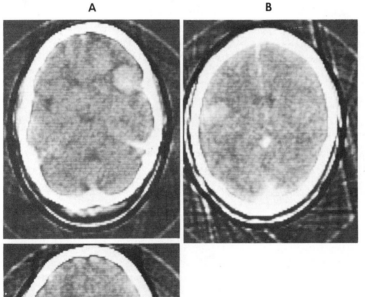

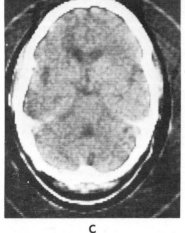

Figure 5–23. A 40-year-old man had episodes of subarachnoid hemorrhage. Four-vessel angiography was negative for angioma, aneurysm and mass effect. CT showed multiple high-density lesions (A, B), with surrounding edema and diffuse ventricular compression. Repeat study performed one month later showed definite evidence of resolution with no mass effect (C).

C

caused by either primary or metastatic neoplasms.[31] The patient may present with sudden onset of focal symptoms and intracranial hypertension, mimicking a "stroke syndrome" and this is most common in glioblastoma, metastasis, oligodendroglioma and pituitary adenoma. In glioblastoma there is tortuous and abundant neovascularity, which may explain the tendency to hemorrhage, but the mechanism with oligodendroglioma is less clear. Of the metastatic lesions, melanoma, choriocarcinoma and hypernephroma are the most likely to undergo hemorrhage. In the majority of cases, the tumor contains foci of hemorrhage, but the patient's course is that of progressive deterioration without an apoplectic onset. Conversely, in rare instances the onset of symptoms in glioblastoma is sudden but pathological study shows no evidence of hemorrhage.

POSTERIOR FOSSA VASCULAR DISORDER

Approximately 10 to 15 percent of cases of ICH are localized to the posterior fossa, and recognition of this disorder is important, as certain lesions require immediate neurosurgical intervention. Any patient who presents with headache, nausea, vomiting, vertigo and unsteadiness of gait, with or without altered consciousness, should be suspected of having cerebellar hemorrhage. Ott has reported that the triad of ipsilateral gaze palsy, appendicular ataxia and facial palsy is most suggestive of the diagnosis of cerebellar hemorrhage. In most instances this diagnosis cannot be made on a clinical basis alone, and differentiation from other conditions including cerebellar infarction, pontine hemorrhage, ruptured aneurysm and supratentorial mass lesions with brain stem compression is not possible.[32]

In one study of patients with proven cerebellar hemorrhage, the diagnosis was initially made in only 55 percent, and in several patients the clinical symptomatology was consistent with this diagnosis but they were proved to have other diagnoses.[33] On the basis of clinical findings alone, cerebellar hemorrhage and infarction may present an identical syndrome: differentiation is dependent upon results of CSF examination and radiographic studies (vertebral angiography and air study). Other conditions, including brain stem infarction, supratentorial mass lesion, ruptured aneurysm, brain stem encephalitis and multiple sclerosis, may occasionally present with a clinical picture simulating cerebellar hemorrhage, but results of diagnostic studies should enable diagnostic differentiation. Since cerebellar hematoma may cause brain stem compression, it may clinically present as primary pontine hemorrhage; and occasionally in pontine hematoma the onset is more gradual and gait disorder is more prominent, with some preservation of consciousness, causing confusion with primary cerebellar hemorrhage. Since the treatment and prognosis are quite different, diagnostic accuracy is essential, but there have been reported cases of negative angiography, ventriculography, and burr hole exploration in cerebellar hemorrhage with diagnosis established only by necropsy.

In cerebellar hemorrhage the onset may be acute or slowly progressive over several days. The hemorrhage frequently occurs in the region of the dentate nucleus, originating from the branch of the superior cerebellar artery and producing hematoma in the medial cerebellar hemisphere, with extension into the fourth ventricle — less frequently, into the occipital horn and third ventricle. Because of this the CSF is bloody or xanthochromic, but if hematoma is confined to the cerebellar hemisphere, the CSF may be clear. In two thirds of cases, ventricular dilatation with obstruction of the fourth ventricle is present. Fisher suggested that the diagnosis may be suspected on clinical grounds sufficiently to warrant posterior fossa exploration, but vertebral angiography is usually performed.[32]

Angiographic findings include demonstration of a posterior fossa avascular mass with characteristic vessel shifts to differentiate it from intrinsic

brain stem hemorrhage and to exclude an unsuspected angioma, aneurysm or neoplasm. Angiography was positive in 81 percent, but ventriculography is the definitive procedure.[33]

CT now appears to be the preferred initial study in patients suspected of having a posterior fossa hematoma or infarction.[34, 35] Cerebellar hematomas are visualized as high-density round masses located posterior to the fourth ventricle and may be midline or lateral in location. They usually compress and flatten the fourth ventricle with ventricular dilatation (Fig. 5–24). The lesion is usually well visualized on plain scan with no enhancement. With CT it may be possible to detect the dissection of blood into the ventricular system. Intrapontine hematomas appear as high-density masses on the plain scan; they are located posterior to the

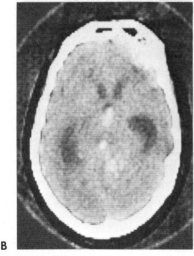

A

B

Figure 5–24. Patient developed sudden onset of inability to walk. CT findings: a large consolidated high-density region located to right of midline with surrounding low-density rim (A) and evidence of blood in the third ventricle (B). (Courtesy Dr. Roger Tutton, Ochsner Clinic.)

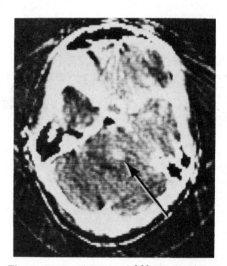

Figure 5–25. A 60-year-old hypertensive man developed right-sided weakness, blurring of vision and depressed consciousness. Neurological findings included right hemiplegia, bilateral Babinski sign, left sixth nerve paresis, left-sided cerebellar signs and conjugate eye deviation to the right side. CT findings: a high-density round lesion located posterior to the dorsum sella to right of midline, distorting the apex of the fourth ventricle, consistent with a small intrapontine hematoma.

dorsum sella and displace the fourth ventricle posteriorly (Fig. 5–25). Since these are smaller lesions, they may not be detected if their diameter is less than one centimeter, as they may dissect longitudinally throughout the brain stem. Large cerebellar infarctions may be diagnosed on the basis of characteristic CT findings, which show a large relatively homogeneous, low-density area in the posterior fossa, which may compress the fourth ventricle and does not usually enhance (Fig. 5–26).

CT is not as reliable in massive cerebellar infarction, as several cases that came to necropsy examination showed no CT abnormality. In addition, enhancement may be seen in posterior fossa infarction; the pattern is round and dense or ringlike and is visualized even if the plain scan is normal (Figs. 5–27 and 5–28). In these cases, differentiation from neo-

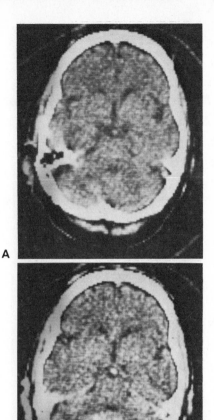

A

B

Figure 5–27. This elderly man had sudden onset of vertigo and inability to walk. Findings included unsteady gait falling to left with horizontal nystagmus. All studies were normal. Pre-infusion study was normal (A) but following infusion a wedge-shaped enhancing lesion was detected in the left cerebellar region (B). The patient's symptoms cleared, and repeat scan was negative.

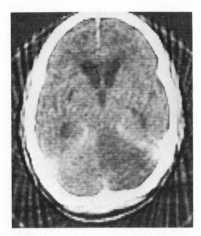

Figure 5–26. This 62-year-old man was evaluated because of increasing clumsiness in using his right hand and somnolence of abrupt onset 48 hours prior to admission. Neurological findings included right-sided Horner's syndrome and cerebellar disturbance, conjugate gaze paresis, left peripheral facial paresis and bilateral Babinski sign. EEG and isotope scan were negative. CT findings: ventricular dilatation with a large low-density region in the right side of the posterior fossa, causing nonvisualization of the fourth ventricle and no enhancement, consistent with cerebellar infarction.

plasm is most reliably determined by serial scans and the clinical course, which is characterized by recovery. CT is less reliable than angiography in diagnosing posterior fossa infarction, and in patients suspected of having this latter condition this is the most sensitive and accurate diagnostic study.[36]

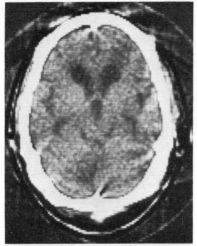

A

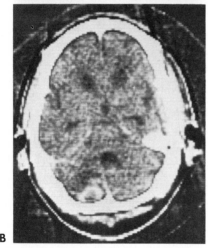

B

Figure 5–28. A hypertensive man presented with headache and inability to stand or walk without assistance. Neurological findings included truncal ataxia, right facial paresis, and gaze paresis to the right. CSF was xanthochromic under high pressure. CT findings: plain scan showed ventricular dilatation with fourth ventricle displaced to right side; a vague low-density lesion is located in the left paramedian region (A) which showed a ring of enhancement (B). The patient rapidly improved without medication and metastatic work-up was negative. Repeat scan four months later showed no abnormal density in the posterior fossa, and this was consistent with an enhancing cerebellar infarction.

INTRAVENTRICULAR HEMORRHAGE

Intraventricular hemorrhage may result from the dissection of blood from intracerebral hematoma through ependymal lining or may occur when there is rupture of blood vessels that are lining the ventricular surface or choroid plexus. The vascular supply of the ventricular structures is derived from the terminal branches of the anterior and posterior choroidal arteries. Primary intraventricular hemorrhage is associated with hemangioma of the choroid plexus or saccular aneurysm of the deep vessels. Clinically these patients present with sudden onset of headache without premonitory symptoms, rapid alteration in consciousness, generalized seizures, truncal rigidity, increased tone and absence of focal neurological signs. Rapid clinical deterioration does not invariably occur, as is usually true of ventricular hemorrhage secondary to intracerebral hematoma. CSF examination reveals bloody fluid, and angiography demonstrates ventricular enlargement, as well as the underlying angioma or aneurysm.

With CT the incidence of intraventricular extension in intracerebral hematoma is higher than previously suspected on a clinical basis, and the outcome is fatal in only 40 percent, a significantly lower rate than determined by necropsy studies. In patients who present clinically with headache and sudden alteration of consciousness and are found to have bloody CSF, the clinical impression of primary intraventricular hemorrhage may be confirmed by CT and subsequent angiography performed to detect aneurysm or angioma. Rarely, this may be caused by choroid plexus papilloma, which may be defined by CT. In two cases of clotted hematoma that were located intraventricularly, CT showed the high-density blood cast but not the specific outline of the clot, and no evidence of angioma, aneurysm or neoplasm was detected by contrast study. Blood resolves from the ventricles usually by three weeks as compared with one week from the subarachnoid spaces and one to two months for an intracerebral hematoma. In all cases of intraventricular hemorrhage due to hypertension, an intraparenchymal hematoma is defined by CT. (See Chapter 9, Figure 9–3.)

CLINICAL PROBLEMS

1. Pure Motor Hemiplegia (PMH) of sudden onset is usually believed to be caused by a small deep infarction located in either the internal capsule or the basis pontis. If the lesion responsible for this syndrome were located more superficially, it would be expected to be large enough to evoke sensory symptoms consistent with the involvement of the postcentral gyrus, although more limited motor deficit, including pure motor monoplegia, facio-brachial paralysis or brachio-crural involvement, may occur without associated sensory symptoms. Fisher and Curry found evidence of healed infarctions in 10 percent of routine necropsy studies, and these were 1 to 4 mm in diameter. In nine cases of pure motor hemiplegia that came to necropsy, six had lacunar cavities in the internal capsule and three in the basis pontis and they reported that this syndrome would be unlikely to be caused by a small hemorrhagic lesion.[38]

Recent evidence has suggested that there may be a more varied etiology: Chokroverty demonstrated abnormal

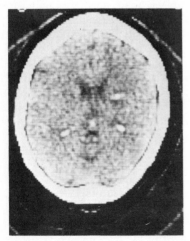

Figure 5–29. A hypertensive patient developed left-sided hemiparesis syndrome without any impairment of consciousness, stiff neck or headache. CSF examination, EEG, isotope scan and angiography were negative. CT findings: a small high-density lesion in the right ganglionic region with surrounding slight amount of edema without mass effect; this was consistent with a small hematoma rather than infarction.

somato-sensory potentials in certain patients and they had more varied pathological lesions, including fronto-parietal metastases, carotid occlusion and medullary pyramid infarction.[39] In one third of patients in another series isotope scan was positive.[40] Since the prognosis rate and completeness of recovery are quite good for lacunar infarctions but less so for larger lesions that present with PMH, visualization of the lacunar infarction by CT would provide the only positive diagnostic technique with which to establish this diagnosis.

The results of CT have confirmed the wide range of pathological conditions associated with PMH. In many instances this was associated with hemorrhagic disorders of markedly varying sizes (Fig. 5–29). In patients with PMH most commonly a single enhancing gyral pattern was detected by CT in the region of the motor cortex, consistent with cortical or subcortical involvement (Fig. 5–30). Ten percent of cases were associated with nonvascular lesions, including subdural hematoma and high parietal tumor. The majority showed no CT abnormality, as is consistent with small size of the lesion, but they may be visualized more clearly by utilizing 8 mm sections. In several cases no abnormality was detected in the acute stage but several months later a small low-density lesion in the region of the internal capsule was detected. If the CT scan was negative, residual impairment was minimal as compared to those with a lesion visible on the scan, and in no case was the isotope scan positive when the CT scan was negative.

2. Reversible Ischemic Neurological Deficit (RIND). These are episodes of focal neurological dysfunction that have an abrupt onset; the symptoms and signs resolve rapidly, usually in less than several days, but last too long to be classified as TIA. The pathophysiological mechanism is reversible but prolonged focal cerebral ischemia, and it is possible that effective collateral circulation becomes operative to pre-

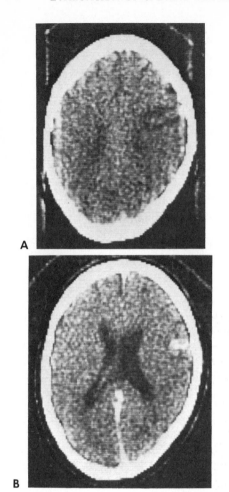

A

B

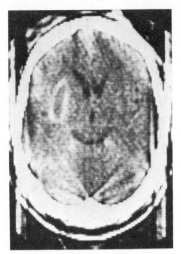

Figure 5–31. A 44-year-old normotensive man suddenly developed right hemiparesis-sensory syndrome without homonymous hemi-anopia or aphasia or a preceding transient ischemic attack. The deficit resolved completely within 72 hours with no pronator drift, reflex asymmetry or sensory disturbance. EEG, performed 48 hours after ictus, was normal, as was isotope scan performed eight days later. CT findings: preinfusion study showed no abnormality but contrast study showed a definite enhancement pattern outlining the putamen, without associated mass effect, consistent with cerebral infarction.

Figure 5–30. A patient with hypertensive and chronic atrial fibrillation awakened with left pure motor hemiparesis. Isotope scan and EEG were negative. CT findings in second week after ictus: a linear area of low density adjacent to the motor cortex (B) that showed a single gyral enhancement pattern consistent with cortical infarction (A).

vent cerebral infarction in both conditions. It is believed that the mechanisms of TIA and RIND are similar, but that the latter represents more prolonged ischemia, although it may be due to embolic phenomena from the internal carotid artery; angiography is necessary to differentiate. If cerebral infarction has occurred in the distribution of the internal carotid artery, EEG and isotope scan should be abnormal, but they are usually negative with ischemia only. With conventional diagnostic studies, it

is not possible to assess cerebral damage in these disorders. Of 10 patients whose neurological deficit cleared completely in two to five days and who had normal EEG and isotope scan, CT was abnormal in five cases. All were studied less than 96 hours after the episode, and three showed a wedge-shaped, low-density pattern, but two showed an unusual enhancement pattern in the ganglionic region (Fig. 5–31).

3. Old Versus New Vascular Insult. In patients who have had a stroke with partial recovery and then several months later present with seizure or recurrence of their neurological deficit, two questions are raised concerning (1) the accuracy of the initial diagnosis, and (2) the presence of a new vascular episode or postictal deficit resulting from a seizure that was not observed. In patients who develop a secondary generalized sei-

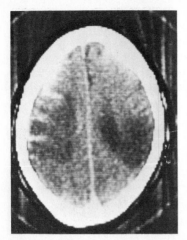

Figure 5–32. This patient had had a left hemiparesis due to cerebral infarction one year previously, and now developed generalized confusion. EEG was diffusely slow and isotope scan was negative. CT findings: a speckled low-density irregularly enhancing lesion causing slight ventricular compression in the left hemisphere, consistent with recent infarction, and a homogeneous well-marginated low-density lesion associated with ipsilateral ventricular dilatation in the right hemisphere, consistent with an old infarction.

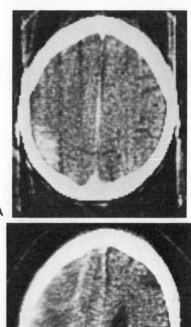

A

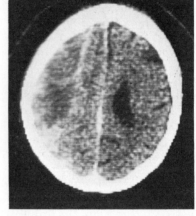

B

Figure 5–33. This patient suddenly developed a profound aphasic disturbance with mild right hemiparesis. CT findings: a wedge-shaped enhancement pattern in the left parieto-temporal region (A). The patient initially improved for four months but then the hemiparesis worsened; repeat study showed an isodense lesion with medially enhancing membrane (B).

zure several months following stroke, CT has enabled us to determine if a new insult has occurred, as it is possible to differentiate a recent from an old infarction or hemorrhage (Fig. 5–32). In addition, if the neurological deficit does not improve or worsens several months later, CT may define subdural hematoma that occurred in association with the infarction (Fig. 5–33).

4. Hypertensive Encephalopathy. This may be defined as an acute clinical condition in which the symptoms result from a sudden and pronounced increase in arterial blood pressure. Symptoms include headache, visual blurring, nausea, vomiting, altered mentation, seizures and occasionally focal neurological deficit. This disorder results from an impairment of the cerebral autoregulatory mechanism with resultant generalized cerebral edema, petechial hemorrhage and microscopic cerebral infarction. This is a reversible disorder and the most important diagnostic criteria to confirm this diagnosis are clinical — a rapid reduction of blood pressure and resolution of clinical symptoms in response to hypotensive drug therapy.[41] If this does not occur, certain other less reversible complications of hypertension or nonvascular etiologies must be considered. In hypertensive encephalopathy, funduscopic examination invariably reveals evidence of spasm of the retinal arterioles, with associated hemorrhage, exudate and blurring of disc margins. This disorder usually occurs in patients with established hypertension but may rarely be an initial manifestation.

If this condition occurs in a patient without pre-existing hypertension, the possibility of a posterior fossa neoplasm should be raised; in two cases CT demonstrated the tumor and thus altered the clinical management. In hypertensive encephalopathy there is severe arteriolar spasm, which may be demonstrated by angiography. This results in cerebral edema and ischemia owing to the decreased cerebral blood flow. With prompt rapid lowering of the blood pressure, the clinical symptoms resolve, and it is presumed that the arteriolar changes clear, but there is little direct evidence for this. With CT we have had the opportunity to follow serially and noninvasively the course of several patients, and the findings have confirmed these pathological inferences, as the generalized edema is visualized with marked compression of the ventricles by a vague low-density lesion (Fig. 5–34).

In patients clinically suspected of having this disorder, CT should be performed before treatment is initiated, because if an intracerebral hematoma or infarction is present, the rapid lowering of blood pressure may significantly decrease generalized or focal cerebral blood flow, since the lower limit of autoregulation is higher in hypertensive than in normotensive patients. In these conditions, the too vigorous treatment of elevated blood pressure may result in extension of the hemorrhage or infarction. If the patient with hypertensive encephalopathy presents initially with focal neurological deficit, differentiation from infarction or ICH may not be possible clinically, and CT may be the only technique with which this is possible.

5. Swallowing Difficulty. The presence of this abnormality in stroke patients is believed to be highest with posterior fossa cerebrovascular disorders. Of patients who had severe

difficulty, at least 50 percent had CT evidence of bilateral hemispheric infarction or hematoma, and no abnormality was detected in the posterior fossa. In the other patients, the scan showed no focal abnormality, and

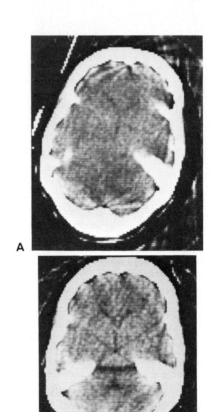

A

B

Figure 5–34. A 35-year-old patient with established hypertension presented with blood pressure of 200/145 mm Hg and was confused, could not walk and had severe headache. Funduscopic examination showed several arteriolar narrowings and blurred disc margins and the patient had horizontal nystagmus and ataxic gait. CSF contained red blood cells and elevated pressure. Angiography showed severe spasm of the basilar artery with only minimal filling and mild generalized spasm of both carotid arteries, but no aneurysm was detected. CT findings: a low-density irregular area in the midline posterior fossa with obliteration of the fourth ventricle and no enhancement (A). The patient's condition rapidly improved with reduction in blood pressure; repeat study three weeks later showed normal size and position of the fourth ventricle, with disappearance of the low density area (B).

these problems were presumed to be caused by a brain stem infarction of a size below the resolving capability of the scan. Of those patients with normal scan, the prognosis for the recovery of function was better than in patients with bilateral cerebral disease. No patient with unilateral infarction had swallowing difficulty that persisted for longer than seven days.

6. Transient Global Amnesia. This disorder is believed to be due to ischemia in the PCA circulation but, rarely, supratentorial and pituitary tumors have been associated with this abnormality, and in one case this was documented by CT[42]. In no case did CT show either low density or enhancement pattern in the temporal or occipital region, but several patients had unequivocal diffuse cerebral atrophy.

7. Aphasia. Previous isotope scan studies have correlated nonfluent aphasic disturbances with lesions located anterior to the Rolandic fissure and fluent aphasia with lesions posterior to this region. Hayward has demonstrated the CT findings in patients with varied aphasic disorders: (1) Nonfluent (Broca's aphasia) patients have a linear-shaped, low-density lesion adjacent to the inferior portion of the frontal horn of the lateral ventricle that may extend from the cortex to the edge of the ventricle. (2) Fluent (Wernicke's aphasia) aphasics with impaired comprehension have lesions in the posterior portion of the superior temporal gyrus; they are visualized by CT as low-density areas lateral to the atrium of the lateral ventricle. (3) Global (mixed) aphasia patients have more extensive lesions involving both the frontoparietal and the temporal region. (4) Anomic aphasics frequently have lesions in the left angular gyrus, but the localization of this language disorder is more variable. (5) Conduction aphasia is due to involvement of the arcuate fasciculus, which traverses the posterior temporal-parietal region and continues anteriorly and inferiorly through the

suprasylvian operculum to Broca's area, but the lesions spare direct involvement of the speech area.[43] The correlation of the low-density patterns with the type of language disturbance is generally reliable, but the location of the enhancement pattern has been less reliable; for example, patients with pure nonfluent Broca's aphasia demonstrated dense linear enhancement in only the posterior temporal-parietal region. Since these speech patterns frequently resolve over time in a characteristic pattern, serial scans may permit more precise in vivo pathological correlation with these changes.

8. Childhood Hemiplegia. This includes acute hemiplegia in which the cause may be infection, trauma, hematological or cardiac disease, cerebral angioma or idiopathic occlusive cerebrovascular disease. Clinically, a previously well child suddenly develops hemiparesis, frequently accompanied by seizures, altered consciousness and fever. Angiography has usually been done to exclude angioma, hematoma or mass lesions or to demonstrate stenosis or occlusion of one or both internal carotid arteries at the basal proximal origin or involvement of the more distal branches. In addition, abundant collaterals are frequently visualized as a prominent telangiectatic network and this then disappears over several months.[17] In other cases, the hemiplegia that was recognized may be of congenital origin or related to perinatal factors and may have been present at birth but gone unrecognized for several months. In these cases, angiography may not show these vascular abnormalities but may show a residual cyst. EEG is usually abnormal but may show a severe bilateral generalized slow pattern or spikes to obscure the focal origin, whereas isotope scan, echoencephalogram and CSF examination are normal unless an angioma is present.

After several months to years, a

skull radiogram may show thickening of the skull with dilatation and over-development of the nasal sinus on the involved side; air study demonstrates ipsilateral ventricular dilatation and cortical atrophy, with a shift of midline structures to the involved side. In these cases CT may demonstrate the low-density infarction pattern and obviate the need for angiography, whereas if hematoma is present angiography is still necessary.

Handa studied CT findings in children less than 15 years old with episodes of acute hemiplegia who showed angiographic findings of severe stenosis of one or both internal carotid arteries with dense vascular telangiectasis (Moyamoya syndrome) and found contrast enhancement in only 8 percent, but the CT scan was performed at least three months after the last episode;[44] enhancement may be more frequent if patients are studied earlier (see Fig. 5–4). The most prominent CT features were cortical atrophy, most marked in the frontal region, and symmetrical dilatation accompanied by single or multiple irregular, low-density lesions in the cortex and periventricular and ganglionic regions (Fig. 5–35).

Other findings in patients with childhood hemiplegia include hemispheric hypoplasia with ventricular dilatation and ipsilateral shift of midline structures or a low-density, wedge-shaped lesion.[45] (Fig. 5–35) In children

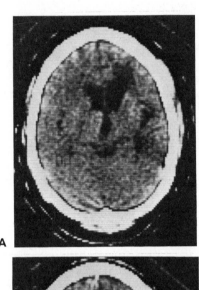

A

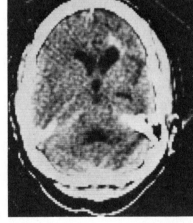

B

Figure 5–36. A 50-year-old woman developed left-sided weakness and was found to have left hemiparesis, which resolved rapidly. EEG and isotope scan demonstrated a lesion in the right frontal parietal region. Six months later she developed a generalized seizure but no worsening of neurological signs. CT findings: mild focal right lateral ventricular enlargement with a periventricular low-density lesion (A) and definite periventricular enhancement (B). Because of CT evidence of recent and active pathologic process, CSF examination was performed; this showed pleocytosis, and elevated protein content; a positive serologic test was consistent with a diagnosis of neurosyphilis.

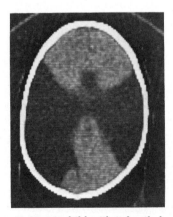

Figure 5–35. A child with infantile hemiplegia and generalized seizure disorder. CT findings: bilateral, homogeneous wedge-shaped low-density areas in the distribution of the middle cerebral artery, consistent with extensive bilateral cerebral infarction.

with acute hemiplegia who had a normal scan one week following the ictus, the recovery was complete; but there was no correlation between prognosis and other CT abnormalities, although those with periventricular or ganglionic infarctions demonstrated by CT improved more rapidly than those children with larger cortical infarctions. In addition, CT may detect expanding porencephalic cysts, which may require surgical intervention.

9. Abnormalities of CSF Examination. The major indication for lumbar puncture in patients with clinical diagnosis of a stroke syndrome is to define a hemorrhagic lesion and exclude an inflammatory condition or meningovascular syphilis. In the majority of nonhemorrhagic infarction, there are no abnormalities in CSF content, although xanthochromia and elevated protein content have infrequently been detected. Of 50 nonhemorrhagic infarctions diagnosed by CT, the protein content was elevated in 40 percent, and this is consistent with previous studies. In 20 percent, the protein content was greater than 100 mg per 100 ml, a rate that is highly suspicious for tumor, but CT findings obviated the need for angiography.

Pleocytosis, including the presence of polymorphonuclear leukocytes, may occur with infarcts that extend to the ventricular or meningeal surface, but this is more characteristic of vasculitis, meningovascular syphilis or an inflammatory process. In patients with a clinical diagnosis of nonhemorrhagic infarction who are found to have pleocytosis, CT may help to establish the explanation for this response (Fig. 5–36).

REFERENCES

1. McKissock W, Richardson A: Primary intracerebral hemorrhage. Lancet 2:221, 1959.
2. Dalsgaard-Nielsen T: Some clinical experience in the treatment of cerebral apoplexy. Acta Psychiat Scanda (suppl) 108:101, 1956.
3. McKissock W, Richardson A, Bloom WH: Subdural hematoma — a review of 369 cases. Lancet 1:1365, 1960.
4. Melamed E, Lavy S, Reches A, Sahar A: Chronic subdural hematoma simulating transient cerebral ischemic attacks. J Neurosurg 42:101, 1975.
5. Daly DD, Svien HJ, Yoss SD: Intermittent symptoms with meningiomas. Arch Neurol 5:287, 1961.
6. Carter AB: Intragravescent cerebral infarction. Quart J Med 29:611, 1960.
7. Groch SN, Hurwitz LJ, Wright IS: Intracranial lesions simulating cerebral thrombosis. JAMA 172:1469, 1960.
8. Bull JD, Marshall J, Shaw DA: Cerebral angiography in the diagnosis of the acute stroke. Lancet 1:562, 1960.
9. Kjellin KG, Soderstrom CE, Cronquist S: CSF spectrophotometry and CT in cerebrovascular disease. Eur Neurol 13:315, 1975.
10. Groch S, McDevitt E, Wright IS: Long term study of cerebrovascular disease. Ann Int Med 55:358, 1961.
11. Glynn AA: Vascular diseases of the nervous system. Br Med J 2:216, 1956.
12. Kinkel WR, Jacobs L: CT in cerebrovascular disease. Neurology 26:924, 1976.
13. Paxton R, Ambrose J: EMI Scanner: brief review of first 650 patients. Br J Radiol 47:530, 1974.
14. Davis KR, Taveras JM, New PFJ, Schnur JA, Roberson GH: Cerebral infarction diagnosis by computerized tomography. Am J Roentgenol 124:643, 1975.
15. Yock DA, Marshall WH: Recent ischemic brain infarctions at computed tomography. Radiology 117:599, 1976.
16. Wing SD, Norman D, Pollock JA, et al: Contrast enhancement of cerebral infarcts in CT. Radiology 21:89, 1976.
17. Solomon GE, Hilal SK, Gold AP: Natural history of acute hemiplegia of childhood. Brain 93:107, 1970.
18. Scott WR, New PFJ: CAT of intracerebral and intraventricular hemorrhage. Radiology 112:73, 1974.

19. Zimmerman RD, Leeds NE, Naidich TP: Ring blush associated with intracerebral hematoma. Radiology 122:707, 1977.
20. Messina AV, Chernik NL: CT: The "resolving" intracerebral hemorrhage. Radiology 118:609, 1975.
21. Welch DM, Coleman RE: Brain scanning in cerebral vascular disease: A reappraisal. Stroke 6:136, 1975.
22. DeLand FH: Scanning in cerebral vascular disease. Semin Nucl Med 1:31, 1971.
23. Gado MH, Coleman E, Merlis AL, et al: Comparison of CT and radionuclide imaging in stroke. Stroke 7:109, 1976.
24. Chiu LC: CT and brain scintigraphy in ischemic stroke. Am J Roentgenol 127:481, 1976.
25. McDowell FH: Cerebral embolism. In: Handbook of Clinical Neurology. (PJ Vinken, GW Bruyn (eds) American Elsevier Company, New York, 1972. p 410.
26. Huckman MS, Weinberg PE, Kim KS, et al: Angiographic and clinico-pathologic correlates in basal ganglionic hemorrhage. Radiology 95:79, 1970.
27. Shea S, Schwartzman RJ: Syndrome of medial versus lateral basal ganglionic hemorrhage. Neurology 25:371, 1975.
28. Hier DB, Davis KR, Richardson EP, Mohr JP: Hypertensive putaminal hemorrhage. Ann Neurol 1:152, 1977.
29. Walshe TM, Davis KR, Fisher CM: Thalamic hemorrhage: computer tomographic-clinical correlation. Neurology 27:217, 1977.
30. McCormick WF, Rosenfield DB: Massive brain hemorrhage. Stroke 4:946, 1973.
31. Scott M: Spontaneous intracerebral hematoma caused by cerebral neoplasms. J Neurosurg 42:338, 1973.
32. Fisher CM, Picard EH: Acute hypertensive cerebellar hemorrhage: diagnosis and surgical treatment. J Nerv Ment Dis 110:38, 1965.
33. Rosenberg GA, Kaufman DM: Cerebellar hemorrhage. Stroke 7:332, 1976.
34. Pressman BD, Kirkwood JR, David DD: Posterior fossa hemorrhage. JAMA 232:932, 1975.
35. Muller HR, Wuthrich R, Wiggli U, et al: The contribution of CT to the diagnosis of cerebellar and pontine hematoma. Stroke 6:467, 1975.
36. Ludwig B, Swerdlow ML: Lethal cerebellar infarction with normal EMI scan. Neurology 27:402, 1977.
37. Doe FD, Shuangshoti S, Netsky MG: Cryptic hemangioma of the choroid plexus: a cause of intraventricular hemorrhage. Neurology 22:1232, 1972.
38. Fisher CM, Curry HB: Pure motor hemiplegia of vascular origin. Arch Neurol 13:30, 1965.
39. Chokroverty S, Rubino FA: Pure motor hemiplegia. J Neurol Neurosurg Psychiatry 38:896, 1975.
40. Richter RW, Brust JCM, Bruun B: Frequency and course of pure motor hemiparesis. Stroke 8:58, 1977.
41. Gifford RW, Westbrook E: Hypertensive encephalopathy. Progr Cardiovasc Dis 17:115, 1974.
42. Lisak RP, Zimmerman RA: Transient global amnesia due to a dominant hemisphere tumor. Arch Neurol 34:317, 1977.
43. Hayward RW, Naeser MA, Zatz LM: CT in aphasia: Correlation of anatomical lesions with functional deficits. Radiology 123:653, 1977.
44. Handa J, Nakano Y, Okuno T, et al: CT in Moyamoya syndrome. Surg Neurol 7:315, 1977.
45. Rothner AD, Cruse R, Weinstein M: CT findings in patients with childhood hemiplegia. Abstract at Child Neurology Society, Carmel, Calif., 1976.
46. Toole JF, Janeway R: Diagnostic tests in cerebro-vascular disease. In: Handbook of Clinical Neurology, Vol 11. PJ Vinken, GW Bruyn (eds). North Holland Publishing Co., Amsterdam, 1972, pp 235–240.

Aneurysms

With CT the diagnostic evaluation of patients with suspected subarachnoid hemorrhage (SAH) has been modified, and the staging of the severity of neurological deficit may be correlated with more direct pathological observation rather than inferred indirectly from angiographic, CSF, isotope scan and EEG findings. Davis compared the results of angiographic and CT findings in 11 cases of suspected intracranial aneurysm, and CT provided additional information that had not been revealed by angiography in nine cases.[1] Since CT is not as sensitive in identifying the presence of small aneurysms and does not define vascular spasm directly, this procedure remains complementary to angiography in evaluation of patients with SAH. In patients who present with headache and stiff neck alone, lumbar puncture and angiography are usually performed to define the presence of subarachnoid blood and to outline the vascular lesion. In these patients an aneurysm is the most likely diagnosis, as patients with SAH due to angioma, neoplasm or ICH are more likely to have accompanying localizing findings. In these neurologically intact patients following aneurysmal rupture, CT is believed to be usually negative; but others have shown evidence of high-density blood in the cisternal spaces, and the site of the bleeding is usually contiguous with the cistern that appears most filled with blood.[2] In addition, since hydrocephalus is a frequent cause of morbidity in aneurysm patients, early CT scan may be used to evaluate baseline ventricular size.

In patients with suspected intracranial hemorrhage who present with headache and stiff neck associated with altered mentation or focal neurological deficit, CT scan may be the initial procedure used to define the location of the hemorrhage as either subarachnoid, subdural, intracerebral or intraventricular; and in many cases CT suggests the most likely underlying etiology by indicating the location and appearance of the hemorrhage. This is extremely important information for the clinician, since the clinical deficit may be nonlocalizing or may inaccurately reflect the location of the hemorrhage.[3] The mortality in the initial 24 hours after rupture of the aneurysm is related to the effect of a localized hematoma; early angiography has been advocated to define the location of the aneurysm as well as the presence of those complicating factors which may require early surgery but are most readily visualized by CT. The location of the hematoma as defined by CT may suggest the vessel which should be initially studied. If angiography is initially performed and demonstrates multiple aneurysms or the presence of both aneurysm and angioma, the pattern and location of the hemorrhage detected by CT may suggest the most probable etiology and location of the vascular lesion. In one fifth of cases of SAH, four-vessel angiography does not demonstrate the source of the bleed, and these cases are presumed to be caused by cryptic microangiomas or saccular aneurysms that have thrombosed completely. CT may visualize these calcified or thrombosed portions with greater sensitivity than angiography and define the pathophysiological vascular lesion in light of a negative angiogram (Fig. 5–37).

Aneurysms that have a diameter of greater than 5 to 8 mm may be identified by CT contrast infusion study, and if lumen is thrombosed or calcified it may be visualized with a plain scan. With CT it may be possible to obtain a more accurate esti-

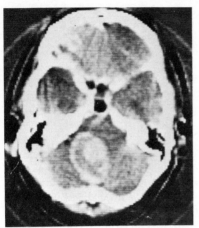

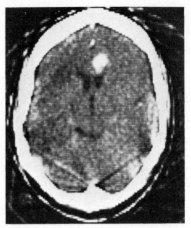

Figure 5–37. A 55-year-old hypertensive man had a marked increase in blood pressure with accompanying symptoms of headache, nausea, dizziness and unsteadiness of gait. Neurological examination showed only minimal unsteadiness of gait with poor tandem gait. With reduction of pressure, all other symptoms resolved but the gait disturbance became more severe; no other abnormalities were detected. CT findings: dilatation of the lateral and third ventricles with anterior displacement of the fourth ventricle, which was normal in size. There was an egg-shaped high-density rim (70 units) with a second round rim of high density located inside this rim. With infusion there was enhancement of the smaller central area to homogeneous high density. Angiography showed ventricular dilatation by an extra-axial posterior fossa mass, but no aneurysm was detected. At operation a large calcified and thrombosed basilar artery aneurysm was encountered.

Figure 5–38. A middle-aged patient with previously known hypertension developed severe headache in the bifrontal region and became confused and agitated. When examined he was normotensive, was inattentive to verbal commands and had mild hemiparesis. CSF was bloody and xanthochromic, with elevated protein content. EEG showed a right frontal-temporal delta pattern; isotope scan was negative. CT findings: contrast infusion study showed a circular homogeneous dense area located immediately anterior to the anterior horn of the lateral ventricle in the midline, this pattern was suggestive of anterior cerebral aneurysm, which was visualized by angiography.

mate of the size of the aneurysmal sac than is possible with angiography, since CT may define the wall with a plain scan and the lumen with contrast infusion; whereas angiography usually defines the lumen only and may underestimate the size of the aneurysm.[4] The mechanism of CT enhancement in aneurysms is not clearly established but may be related to flow of stagnant blood in the aneurysm sac. Aneurysms usually appear as round masses, which may show peripheral or diffuse, round, homogeneous, intravascular, high-density enhancement (Fig. 5–38).

They usually cause little mass effect, although occasionally may be large enough to simulate neoplasm.

Another source of potential diagnostic confusion may be an ectatic vessel, frequently an elongated basilar artery, which may appear in cross-section as a rounded mass rather than an elongated curvilinear density, and angiography may then be necessary to define the course of a tortuous arteriosclerotic vessel (see Fig. 10–4). Because CT is not sensitive enough to detect small aneurysms, angiography remains the definitive procedure to detect their presence and is still required to define the structural anatomy, bleeding points, mass effect

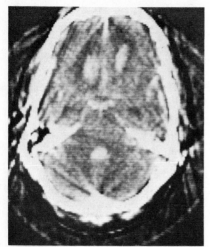

A

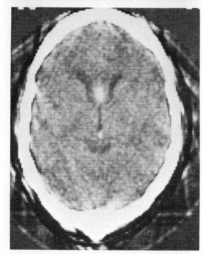

B

Figure 5–39. A 37-year-old normotensive patient suddenly developed headache and stiff neck and became increasingly lethargic. Initial neurological findings included marked stupor and bilateral positive Babinski response with no lateralizing neurological findings. CSF showed a large quantity of blood and EEG had a monorhythmic high-voltage frontal delta pattern. Because of the clinical findings and poor condition of the patient, an intraventricular hemorrhage was suspected. Initial CT findings: A, A bifrontal intracerebral hematoma surrounded by edema; no aneurysm was visualized even with contrast infusion. The patient's clinical condition improved and repeat scan (B) showed no intraventricular blood but persistence in the caval and bifrontal regions. This was most characteristic of anterior cerebral communicating artery aneurysm, which was then demonstrated by angiography.

and relationship of aneurysm to parent vessel and contiguous structures.

The most frequent site for an aneurysm is in the anterior cerebral–anterior communicating artery region, and rupture causes blood to dissect into the caval-collosal region and less frequently into the frontal lobes. With CT, high-density blood may be seen in the septum pellucidum region (Fig. 5–39). More severe neurological deficit may result from hematoma in the frontal lobe. If the hematoma is located in either frontal lobe, the patient may present with monoplegia; if it dissects into both hemispheres, the patient may present with seizures and impaired consciousness (see Fig. 6–1). The presence of blood in the septal region is pathognomonic of an aneurysm, but blood in the frontal lobe may also involve many other etiological entities, and angiography is necessary for diagnosis.[3]

Aneurysms of the internal carotid artery complex occur most commonly at the junction of the posterior communicating artery. The aneurysm enlarges to compress the third nerve, causing complete third nerve paresis with almost invariably the finding of a large nonreactive pupil. Following rupture, CT may visualize blood in the floor of the middle fossa or, less frequently, in the temporal lobe and peribasal region. It is quite unusual for blood to dissect into the region of the head of the caudate with these aneurysms, but in these cases differentiation from hypertensive etiology is usually not possible. Intra- and supraclinoid carotid aneurysms may cause radiographic sella enlargement, optic chiasmal compression and extraocular muscle paresis. These aneurysms may undergo thrombosis and calcification so that they do not fill on angiography and may be detected by plain skull radiogram or

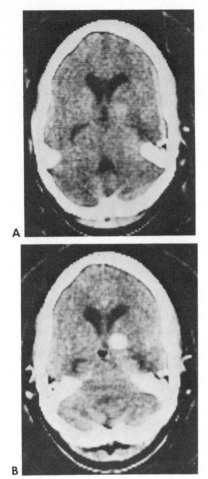

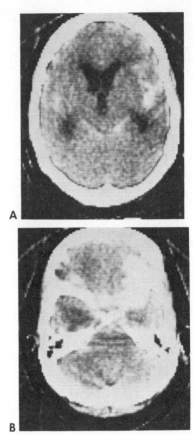

Figure 5–40. A 44-year-old woman developed headache, vomiting and weakness. Neurological finding was left hemiparesis alone. CSF showed bloody fluid, and a skull radiogram showed erosion of the right posterior clinoid, but EEG and isotope scan were negative. CT findings: a nonhomogeneous round dense region in the right paraganglionic region (A), which enhanced as a dense round mass (B) with perfectly round shape, suggestive of aneurysm; angiography visualized aneurysm of distal segment of the internal carotid artery.

Figure 5–41. A 50-year-old woman with severe hypertensive disease suddenly developed headache and gait difficulty. When examined, her blood pressure was 200/140 mm Hg and she had left hemiparesis-hemisensory syndrome with normal level of consciousness. The diagnostic impression was a hypertensive hemorrhage but CT findings suggested another possibility, as there was a comma-shaped high-density region in the right sylvian cistern and in the sulci over the right convexity and quadrigeminal cistern (A). There was also a localized hematoma in the right inferior frontal anterior temporal region (B). This was suggestive of middle cerebral artery aneurysm, which was demonstrated by angiography. In addition, mild communicating hydrocephalus was present.

CT; in which case the high-density wall with lamellated calcified thrombosis is visualized or nonthrombosed aneurysms may be seen most clearly following contrast infusion (Fig. 5–40). In rare instances these aneurysms may rupture and suggest pituitary apoplexy from chromophobe adenoma, and differentiation of an-

eurysm from tumor still requires angiography.

Aneurysms of the middle cerebral artery may cause an intracerebral hematoma in the sylvian fissure. When the aneurysm ruptures, the patient has a focal neurological deficit, usually with preserved consciousness. The cause of this focal dysfunction is an intracerebral hematoma in the temporal or parasylvian region; it may be comma-shaped, following the curve of the sylvian fissure (Fig. 5–41). Less frequently, rupture of this aneurysm may cause no focal deficit and the patient presents with only headache and stiff neck; in several cases the only diagnostic clue was provided by CT finding of blood in the sylvian region. If the aneurysm thromboses and calcifies, it may simulate middle fossa neoplasm, and angiography may detect only an avascular extra-axial mass, without any indication of its vascular nature. With CT the presence of a peripheral high-density rim is suggestive of aneurysm (Fig. 5–42).

Aneurysms of the posterior fossa are less frequent and may involve vertebral, basilar and cerebellar arteries. If they rupture they may mimic a hypertensive cerebellar or pontine hemorrhage, or more frequently they may simulate a posterior fossa neoplasm, causing compression of the fourth ventricle with resultant obstructive hydrocephalus or growing laterally to cause a CPA syndrome. On plain scan they are visualized as a high-density calcified wall and may homogeneously enhance with contrast infusion (Fig. 5–37).

In patients with suspected SAH, the CT finding of blood in the caval and septal regions is characteristic of anterior communicating artery aneurysms, and unilateral blood collection in the sylvian fissure is pathognomonic of middle cerebral aneurysms, but the demonstration of blood in the basilar cisterns, along the cortical sulci or in the interhemispheric fissure is less helpful in localizing the source of the bleed (Fig. 5–43). The frequency of finding extravasated blood in these subarachnoid spaces is dependent upon the amount of blood present and also upon the orientation of these structures to the transverse tomographic plane; most frequently visualization occurs if the structure is perpendicular (interhemispheric fissure and sylvian cistern) and less frequent if parallel (suprasellar and pericallosal cistern).[2, 5] If the patient is neurologically intact with the exception of signs related to direct compressive effect of the aneurysm, diagnostic evaluation may require only CSF examination and angiography. Recent

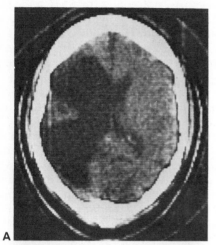

A

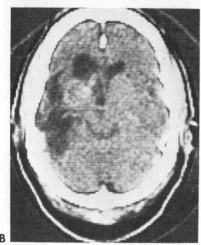

B

Figure 5–42. A middle-aged man had suffered an episode of right hemiparesis accompanied by headache eight years previously. At that time the CSF was xanthochromic and arteriography showed a large left middle cerebral artery aneurysm in the middle fossa. The patient refused surgery and has had only minimal neurological residual deficit. CT findings: marked left lateral ventricular and sylvian cisternal enlargement due to old infarction or hemorrhage (A) in this region; following contrast infusion there is a rim of enhancement consistent with aneurysm of the wall of the giant middle cerebral artery (B).

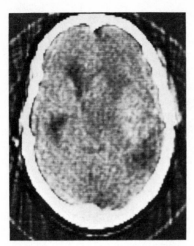

Figure 5–43. A 39-year-old hypertensive man presented with sudden onset of headache, stiff neck, left-sided weakness and double vision. Neurological findings included nuchal rigidity, left hemiparesis and right oculomotor nerve paresis but no papilledema. CSF was bloody and xanthochromic, with elevated opening pressure; EEG showed a slow-wave pattern, and isotope scan was positive in the right temporal region. CT findings: a high-density, irregularly curved area in the right temporal region, surrounded by low-density edema fluid. This was causing marked distortion, compression and displacement of the right lateral and third ventricular structures, with contralateral ventricular dilatation and no visualization of the suprasellar cistern. This hematoma location was consistent with either middle cerebral or internal carotid aneurysm; angiography demonstrated a middle cerebral artery aneurysm.

studies have indicated the efficacy of CT in detecting with almost 100 percent accuracy extravasated blood in cisternal spaces and the importance of establishing baseline ventricular size. If angiography demonstrates spasm, CT should then be definitely indicated to determine if this has resulted in any parenchymal disturbance. When vascular spasm is prominent, angiography may fail to demonstrate filling of the lumen of the aneurysm, but CT may directly visualize the aneurysm or, by the precise location of low-density infarction, suggest the localization of the aneurysm. If neurological deficit is severe, the presence of other complicating factors may be detected with CT, including localized hematoma, edema or ventricular obstruction.

With CT, intraventricular blood has been frequently identified, and although these patients often present with altered mentation and bilateral corticospinal tract signs, they may be asymptomatic. The mortality of this disorder is not as high as previous studies have indicated. A previously unsuspected finding was that 33 to 60 percent of patients with SAH had developed ventricular enlargement within 48 hours of the hemorrhage.[1]

CT is of value in patients who are initially neurologically intact and then clinically worsen, either suddenly or gradually. If early angiography has defined the presence of the aneurysm, it is not necessary to perform serial studies, as CT may define the pathophysiological disturbance. If the patient develops an abducens nerve paresis, hydrocephalus is suspected and CT can reliably define ventricular size. If such dilatation is present, serial scans may be an alternative to immediate shunt procedure, as the ventricles may spontaneously return to normal size. The presence of early hydrocephalus is associated with higher mortality, but not all patients with ruptured aneurysms are routinely studied. The incidence of this finding may be much higher than previously indicated by clinical-pathological studies. Further studies are necessary to investigate the incidence of ventricular enlargement in all clinical groups of aneurysm patients, and to correlate CT finding of cisternal and intraventricular blood with incidence of hydrocephalus.

Following aneurysm rupture, there may be either focal or generalized vascular spasm, which may occur immediately but become maximal five to seven days later. The presence of significant spasm is usually a contraindication to surgery; its resolution determines the optimal time for surgical intervention, and this is determined by serial angiography. Vascular spasm may be localized to the territory of the ruptured aneurysm and may cause focal cerebral ischemia and infarction. In these cases, flow through the region of spasm is reduced, and aneurysm may not be demonstrated angiographically.

The presence of spasm and infarction is associated with significant surgical mortality, and although angiography may suggest resolution of spasm, significant mass effect may still be present and this is more reliably defined by CT. If the spasm develops early, causing edema and infarction, this may mimic an intracerebral hematoma; differentiation is possible with CT and is therapeutically important because hematoma requires surgical intervention, whereas spasm is treated more conservatively. Occasionally generalized vascular spasm occurs and it may produce bilateral cerebral edema with ventricular compression. This may be less reliably visualized by CT because edema fluid is isodense with brain, but the finding of ventricular

nonvisualization is highly suggestive evidence in this clinical setting. In those patients whose clinical condition does not permit surgery initially, recurrence of hemorrhage may occur

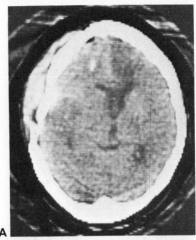

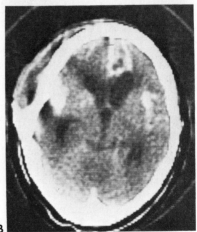

B

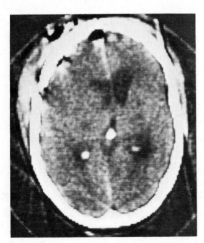

Figure 5–44. A 60-year-old man presented with headache and stiff neck; he was slightly lethargic. Angiography showed aneurysm of the anterior communicating artery with slight spasm. Artery was ligated surgically twelve days after bleed. Six days postoperatively the patient became lethargic with developing right hemiparesis. CSF showed no fresh blood and elevated pressure. CT findings: compression of the left lateral ventricle and third ventricle without any abnormal density, a pattern consistent with edema in the left hemisphere. In addition, there is a subgaleal hematoma. In this case, CT was able to reliably differentiate edema from infarction or hemorrhage.

Figure 5–45. A patient with aneurysm of the anterior communicating artery; after surgical ligation the patient developed right-sided weakness. CT findings (A): the left lateral and third ventricle are shifted from the left to the right side; this appears to be related to a wedge-shaped area of nonhomogeneous low density with punctate areas of high density in the distribution of a branch of the left middle cerebral artery. A second high-density area is surrounded by low density in the left frontal region. In addition, there is a low-density area in the distribution of the right anterior communicating artery (ACA), consistent with infarction. Three weeks later the patient had recurrence of headache and vomiting. CT findings (B): striking enhancement of the ACA infarction and high-density material in both sylvian cisterns and the left ganglionic region, a pattern consistent with recurrent hemorrhage. In addition, the ventricles are moderately dilated.

in 50 percent of cases, and if the patient suddenly worsens, CT may define this occurrence without the need for repeat lumbar puncture. Following surgical ligation, CT is the most accurate study to determine the cause of any postoperative clinical deterioration (Figs. 5–44 and 5–45). Postoperative angiography is occasionally difficult to evaluate because of the presence of surgical changes, metallic clips and shunt tubes, and CT has almost completely replaced angiography in these cases.

REFERENCES

1. Davis KR, New PFJ, Ojemann RG, et al: CT evaluation of hemorrhage secondary to intracranial aneurysm. Am J Roentgenol 127:143, 1976.
2. Lim ST, Sage DJ: Detection of subarachnoid blood clot and other thin, flat structures by CT. Radiology 123:79, 1977.
3. Hayward RD, O'Reilly GUA: Intracranial hemorrhage — accuracy of CT in predicting underlying etiology. Lancet 1:1, 1976.
4. Pressman BD, Gilbert GE, Davis DO: CT of vascular lesions of the brain. Part II. Aneurysms. Am J Roentgenol 124:215, 1975.
5. Scott G, Ethier R, Mclancon D: CT in the evaluation of intracranial aneurysms and subarachnoid hemorrhage. Radiology 123:85, 1977.

Intracranial Vascular Malformations

Vascular malformations are the result of incomplete and abnormal development of embryonic vascular channels. Their classification is dependent upon which level of the vascular tree is dilated and whether there is normal parenchyma separating abnormal vessels and includes the following types: (1) arteriovenous malformation (AVM), consisting of abnormal tortuous dilated arteries that directly connect to "arterialized veins" without an intervening capillary network, with the abnormal vessels separated by atrophic cortex and fibrous tissue; (2) venous angioma, consisting of enlarged single or multiple tortuous veins without abnormal arterial supply; (3) cavernous angioma, consisting of multiple dilated vascular spaces clustered together and separated by neuroglial elements; (4) telangiectasis, consisting of capillary vessels separated by normal parenchyma.[1]

1. Arteriovenous Malformation. AVM are not neoplasms but may increase in size as contiguous vessels are incorporated or recruited into the flow pattern of the angioma and act as a space-occupying lesion even in the absence of intraparenchymal hemorrhage. The majority are located superficially on the cortex but may extend into subcortical structures and into the ventricular walls. The angioma consists of dilated tortuous abnormal vessels, which displace underlying parenchyma and cause infarction and hemorrhage with subsequent atrophy, gliosis, calcification, cyst formation and brownish discoloration from old hemorrhage in the parenchyma and leptomeninges. Ninety percent are located supratentorially with the majority in the fronto-centro-parietal region of the vascular distribution of the MCA, but they may also be perfused and drained by other vascular sources; 10 percent are infratentorial in location or involve the dural vessels.

The clinical pattern of symptoms is highly dependent upon the source from which the case material is derived. In several of the neurosurgical series of AVM, 40 to 78 percent of patients presented with symptoms related to subarachnoid or intracerebral hemorrhage, whereas necropsy studies of all angiomas have indicated that only 10 to 40 percent of these lesions show pathological evidence of hemorrhage.[1, 2] In symptomatic angiomas that do not bleed, focal or generalized seizures are the most common early symptom (42 percent), whereas vascular headache, progressive neurological deficit or the finding of an intracranial bruit occurs less frequently. The progressive focal neurological deficit may be due to increase in size and mass effect of the angioma due to recruitment into the abnormal perfusion and drainage pattern or the ischemia as the angioma shunts or steals blood from the underlying parenchyma. In other instances, patients may present with transient episodes of neurological deficit which resolve completely and then develop apoplectic onset of fixed deficit but without evidence of hemorrhage, and this is presumed to be due to nonhemorrhagic infarction. In rare instances, the angioma may be associated with progressive dementia, which may be related to generalized cortical blood flow steal phenomena or hydrocephalus; or may present predominantly with symptoms of intracranial hypertension.

Subarachnoid and intracerebral hemorrhages are the most life-threatening complications of the angioma and account for 10 to 15 percent of all subarachnoid hemorrhages. Frequently the episode of hemorrhage is the initial clinical symptom of the angioma. Since the bleeding occurs from venous pressure, the neurological deficit may be less severe than from aneurysm with lower mortality; thus a history of repeated bleeding episodes is highly characteristic of angioma. Not all angiomas that cause hemorrhage are of large size and some may not be detected by angiography. These smaller but clinically symptomatic lesions are called "cryptic angiomas."[3, 4] The natural history of AVM is not clearly established; some may be a source of repeated bleeding episodes, whereas others may cause progressive or intermittent neurological deficit, but infrequently some may undergo spontaneous thrombosis with evidence of regression in size on subsequent angiograms.[5, 6]

In patients clinically suspected of harboring an AVM, plain skull radiogram may show faint or irregularly speckled ringlike calcification in 15 to 20 percent of cases. Less frequently there may be enlargement of the meningeal arterial grooves caused by dural arterial supply to the malformation, but the diagnosis is most reliably established by the findings of isotope scan and angiography.[7] EEG findings may identify the involved hemisphere but are not reliable to define the extent of the lesion, since the abnormal EEG pattern may reflect the more widespread cerebral ischemia resulting from arteriovenous shunting.

In 90 to 95 percent of supratentorial symptomatic AVM, the isotope scan is positive. In those cases not associated with hematoma the positive scan is correlated with the increased blood volume in the AVM and with leakage of isotope through the immature blood-brain barrier of the angioma. Dynamic scanning performed immediately after injection shows increased and accelerated flow through the angioma, and the early uptake is due mostly to the increased flow. Therefore, if only a static scan is performed several hours after injection, the angioma may not be detected. Handa *et al.* reported 100 percent accuracy with early scanning, and a fall-off of detection rate with delayed scanning time.[8] If hemorrhage has occurred, the blood flow through the angioma may be decreased perhaps as a result of thrombosis and compression of dilated vessels, and a positive scan may be due to an impaired blood-brain barrier.

Angiography is the most reliable procedure to define the presence, location, extent and vascular supply and drainage of the angioma. If hemorrhage has occurred, it is possible that only an intracerebral hematoma is detected without visualizing the accompanying vascularity, as the hematoma may compress the feeding vessels, slow the circulation and cause thrombosis in the vessels. If the AVM is totally thrombosed, it may not fill with angiography and there may be evidence of only an avascular mass. CT usually shows a high-density calcified mass without enhancement but the diagnosis may frequently not be established preoperatively.

CT has become an important complementary noninvasive procedure with isotope scan to establish the diagnosis of an AVM, and, based upon the results of these two studies, it may be decided that nonoperative management is indicated and angiography may not be necessary. This would be the case if the angioma is extensive and involves the entire hemisphere, is located deeply with extension into the ventricular system or is located in the brain stem. If CT shows a more lateralized and superficially located lesion that has the density characteristics of an angioma and surgery is therefore indicated, preoperative angiography is necessary to establish the precise vascular anatomy and connections to the normal cerebral vessels.

The pattern of density of an AVM in a CT scan is dependent upon the underlying pathological characteristics of the angioma. The noninfusion study may show low, mixed or high density and in almost one fourth of cases may be normal, with identification dependent upon contrast enhancement. The majority of these angiomas initially appear as mixed-density patterns (Fig. 5–46). The density may be consistent with cal-

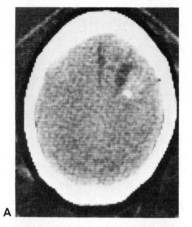

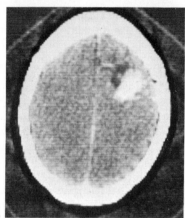

Figure 5–46.   This patient presented with left-sided focal motor seizures. Isotope scan showed uptake in the right fronto-parietal region. CT findings; plain scan showed a dense globular area located medially to a more vaguely defined non-homogeneous high-density area and another surrounding slitlike area in the right fronto-parietal region (A). Following contrast infusion, there was dense consolidated homogeneous enhancement of the speckled high-density regions with no change in the low-density region, a pattern consistent with an atrophic cortex (B).

cification and may correlate with the presence of mural thrombosis within the vessel wall with a lamellated round pattern or may represent calcification within the underlying gliotic parenchyma. There may be an area of dense consolidated high density, round or irregular in shape, which may represent intraparenchymatous hematoma.

Normally, blood vessels are not sufficiently different from surrounding tissue to be detected by plain scan, but in certain angiomas the dilated vessels are large enough to have a density sufficiently higher than normal brain to be detected on the plain scan. The shape of this high-density lesion will be dependent upon the orientation relative to the scan axis.[9] If the abnormal vessels are parallel to the transverse section, they appear tubular or serpentine in shape, but if they are perpendicular to the section, they have a round or oval shape (Fig. 5–47). These vessels almost always show striking contrast enhancement.

The explanation for the low-density

areas is more conjectural, and several hypotheses have suggested that they represent edema or cystic and necrot-

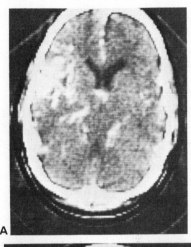

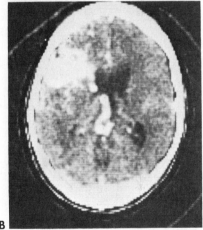

Figure 5–48.   A 40-year-old man presented with left-sided headaches and progressive right-sided hemiparesis-sensory syndrome. Isotope scan showed increased flow with positive static uptake in left fronto-parietal region, and EEG showed a prominent slow-wave pattern over the entire left hemisphere. CT findings; plain scan showed a mixed low- and high-density pattern in the left fronto-parietal region with high density, having M-value of 40 to 45, consistent with calcification. Following contrast infusion, there was definite enhancement in the substance of the angioma as well as prominent tortuous dilated vessels located medially and deeply, consistent with veins, and also a gyral pattern consistent with representation of superficial supplying arteries (A and B). Since the vessels in the angioma are closely packed and there is atrophy of the parenchyma, there is no marked mass effect, although slight left ventricular compression and contralateral ventricular dilatation are present.

Figure 5–47.   Multiple shapes of dilated angiomas, including tubular, serpentine, and ovoid (A). Following infusion, there is dense consolidated enhancement as well as an outline of the deep venous drainage (B).

ic regions resulting from ischemia and infarction or atrophic areas.[10, 11] Since these are sometimes associated with ipsilateral ventricular enlargement, the latter is the likeliest explanation. In those cases in which plain scan is normal, the vessels are not sufficiently enlarged to be visualized, no hematoma formation or atrophy has occurred, and no mass effect of the angioma is present.

Following contrast infusion there is dense intravascular enhancement and this may have a characteristic appearance that is relatively specific for AVM. The vessels show dense and smooth enhancement in either tubular, vermian, or rounded shape, depending on their orientation to the plane of the scan. These vessels are frequently quite serpentine in shape and enlarged, and may show a connection to the normal arterial tree (Fig. 5–48). The arterial supply to the involved hemisphere may be so extensive that infusion study may show a marked asymmetry of the size of the circle of Willis, with the vessels on the involved side denser and thicker than on the opposite side. In addition, the malformation itself may enhance without visualization of specific feeding or draining vessels. The enhancement is usually wedge-shaped, and it has been reported that, if the venous drainage is via the transependymal veins, the apex of the wedge extends toward the lateral ventricle (Fig. 5–49). The venous drainage is frequently seen with the CT scan.[9]

The larger angiomas demonstrate significant mass effect and this is most frequent in those that have developed intracerebral hemorrhage, but this mass effect is seen in less than one fourth of cases — a significant differentiating feature from neoplasms.[12, 13] With contrast infusion, two thirds showed dilated tortuous vessels or a prominent enhancing gyral pattern, whereas one third showed dense homogeneous enhancement. In one fourth of angiomas, the plain scan showed no abnor-

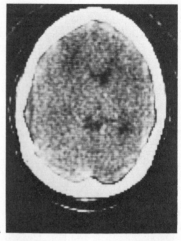

A

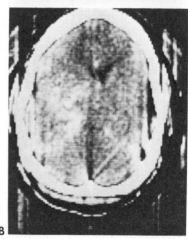

B

Figure 5–49.   A 15-year-old girl suddenly became unable to use her right hand on two occasions but this cleared completely in 30 minutes. Six days later she developed profound right-sided hemiparesis with mixed expressive and receptive aphasia, and had a bruit over the left temporal region. Isotope scan showed hyperperfusion of the left hemisphere with positive uptake in the temporal-parietal region. CT findings; plain scan showed compression of the left lateral ventricle but no abnormal density (A); following infusion there was a nonhomogeneous wedge-shaped high-density area in the left hemisphere with dilated tortuous vessels crossing through the angioma and visualization of deep venous drainage (B). Angiography showed an extensive arteriovenous malformation, with marked narrowing of the proximal left middle cerebral artery, consistent with a shunting effect, away from this vessel.

mal density and enhancement was seen with contrast infusion (Fig. 5–50), In only one case were both plain and contrast studies negative in an-

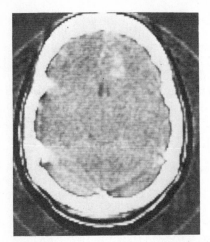

Figure 5–50. This patient presented with generalized seizures but had no headaches, bruit or neurological deficit. EEG and isotope scan suggested a lesion in the right frontal region. CT findings: following contrast there was nonhomogeneous enhancement in the right frontal region, consistent with arteriovenous malformation, which was demonstrated by angiography.

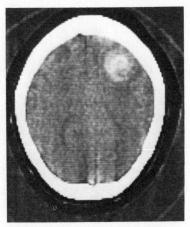

Figure 5–51. This patient developed sudden onset of severe headache and left hemiparesis. EEG showed a delta pattern in the right frontal-parietal region, but isotope scan and CSF examination were normal. CT findings: a high-density lesion in the right frontal-parietal region with several concentric overlapping tubular regions and surrounding edema but no enhancement. Angiography showed an avascular mass but no abnormal vessels, and operative findings showed a recent hematoma with surrounding dilated and tortuous vessels, a pattern consistent with arteriovenous malformation.

giographically documented AVM, but several angiomas were not detected because contrast infusion was not performed. In one case, there was no enhancement but a plain scan had shown a lamellated, round, high-density lesion, and angiography had also shown no opacification of the avascular mass, which pathologically was confirmed to be an angioma (Fig. 5–51). The diagnosis of a thrombosed angioma may be more reliably established by CT than by angiography or isotope scan.[14]

In patients who present clinically with sudden onset of neurological deficit, routine scan may define the presence and location of either an intracerebral hematoma or infarction, and contrast infusion may detect the characteristic enhancement pattern. Alternatively, the scan may show only a high-density lesion in a superficial lobar location or adjacent to the lateral ventricular wall, with extension into the ventricle and evidence of enlarged subependymal veins but no enhancement pattern; angiography

is then necessary to establish the diagnosis.[9]

Hayward reported enhancement in four of five cases in which plain scan showed a hematoma, and therefore all documented cases of ICH should have repeat study with contrast infusion.[11] In several young patients without other precipitating causes of hemorrhage, CT showed evidence of ICH surrounded by low-density edema; all other studies, including isotope scan, CSF examination and four-vessel angiography, were normal. It is possible that this represents hemorrhage from small cryptic angioma.[4, 14]

In other patients, initial scan shows only a slight mass effect and enhancement shows a wedge-shaped area of nonhomogeneous increased density with characteristic vessel abnormalities, and this is consistent with infarction within the angioma. In patients who have a documented angioma and in whom nonsurgical management or embolization is performed, if there is evidence of clinical worsening CT is the procedure of choice to visualize infarction, intraparenchymal or intraventricular hematoma or progressive ventricular dilatation. Hydrocephalus may result from ventricular distortion or previous episodes of hemorrhage as a result of impaired reabsorption through the arachnoid villi or rarely because of ventricular obstruction by the enlarged draining veins located in the ventricular walls.

Pathological processes that may have CT scan characteristics similar to angioma include enhancing infarction, ring enhancement in an intracerebral hematoma, abscess or glioma. If the enhancement within an AVM is dense and consolidated, angiography is required, but several features favor AVM rather than glioma, including prominent regular noncomplex enhancement pattern, presence of intervening low density, serpentine enhancement, wedgeshaped with relatively regular margins. If the plain scan shows only low density and no enhancement, angiography

is necessary to differentiate from a glioma. One fourth of cases of AVM show normal density on plain scan, and there is gyral enhancement which may be confused with cerebral infarction. Dynamic isotope scan may show increased flow in both conditions; serial CT or angiography may be required to differentiate these disorders (Fig. 5–52).

2. Venous Angioma. This angioma consists of tortuous, dilated and irregularly shaped veins, without accompanying abnormal arteries, which course through normal brain parenchyma; these may be located in both the cerebral cortex and cerebellum. The walls of the veins may undergo hyperplasia with fibrinoid change and subsequent calcification but more commonly they do not show any pathological change. There may be atrophy with gliosis and calcification of the underlying cortex. These angiomas are less likely to cause hemorrhage then are AVM and may present clinically with progressive focal neurological deficit or seizures, or the patient may be entirely asymptomatic and routine skull radiogram may show calcification. Isotope scan is more frequently negative than with AVM, and diagnosis is established by angiography, which shows that the abnormal veins have an umbrella radial pattern that is directed toward the central draining vein with usually a normal arterial pattern. Michaels has described the CT findings that reflect the benign appearance of these lesions, in which preinfusion density is normal or high; this was believed to represent an increased blood pool in the central draining vein. Infusion study showed a round or linear enhancement pattern.[15] Other venous angiomas may show densely calcified walls due to degenerative changes and a dense enhancement pattern (Fig. 5–53).

3. Capillary-Venous Malformation. In the characteristic Sturge-Weber syndrome the primary lesion is an angioma involving the meninges without involvement of the vessels of

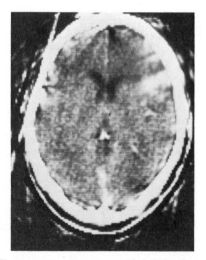

Figure 5–52. A patient with left focal motor seizures but no neurological findings. Isotope scan showed normal flow but positive uptake in the right frontal-parietal region. CT findings: preinfusion study is normal, but infusion study shows dense consolidated enhancement without any associated ventricular abnormality, a pattern consistent with angioma or infarction; angiography demonstrated an angioma.

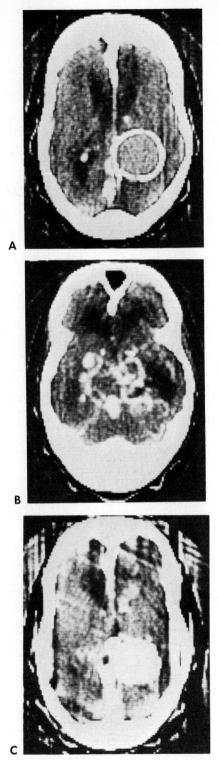

Figure 5–53. This patient was initially evaluated because of a calcification detected in the right parietal area on plain skull radiogram. Pertinent neurological findings included mild organic brain syndrome and mild left hemiparesis. CT findings: a huge round calcified mass in the high parietal region, which appeared as rimlike calcification at lower section (A). Following contrast infusion, serpentine dilated vessels located in the midline were seen, consistent with venous drainage (B and C). Angiography demonstrated venous angioma.

the underlying cortex located in the posterior temporal-parietal and occipital region. This may be associated with cortical atrophy in the involved hemisphere. There is a gyriform, tramlike calcification pattern that is demonstrated by plain skull radiogram and is pathognomonic for this syndrome. This pattern may be absent before the age of two but becomes more frequent after this time.

Angiography demonstrates an abnormal venous pattern with diversion of flow from the superficial cortical veins and superior sagittal sinus into the deep venous system. The cortical arterial flow to the involved hemisphere is decreased, probably as a result of cortical atrophy. Other reported angiographic features include the presence of venous angiomas and telangiectasia, arterial thrombosis, anomalous veins and venous sinuses. In addition, the isotope scan may be positive but flow is not increased, and this is taken as evidence that there is a nonspecific defect in the blood-brain barrier rather than increased circulating blood volume as in AVM. The clinical symptoms include: (1) facial angioma in the ophthalmic division of the trigeminal nerve; (2) seizures, frequently of focal nature; (3) radiographic evidence of calcification.

The CT findings reflect the underlying angiomatous lesion and the pathological cerebral abnormalities more accurately and with greater sensitivity than do skull radiogram or angiography.[16] There is definite evidence of cortical gyriform calcification over the involved hemisphere, which may also be associated with ipsilateral ventricular enlargement and cortical atrophy. In addition, there may be parallel tramlike calcifications similar to those visualized on plain skull radiogram. With contrast enhancement there may be either a diffuse homogeneous haze over the involved hemisphere or tortuous dilated vessels, which may represent the dilated deep venous sys-

tem and not angioma itself (Fig. 5–54). Less frequently the longstanding cortical atrophy is associated with reduced size of the hemicranium (Davidoff-Dyke-Masson syndrome), and others have reported enlargement of the hemicranium due to an associated syndrome. CT has shown characteristic findings even in cases in which facial angioma or radiographic calcification was absent. In the Klippel-Trenannay-Weber syndrome there are venous and arteriovenous abnormalities that lead to hemihypertrophy of the cranium but are not usually associated with intracranial

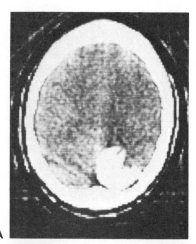

A

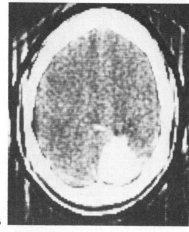

B

Figure 5–54.   This 12-year-old boy with both generalized and focal motor seizures had no facial angioma but definite tram-like calcification on skull radiogram. CT findings: gyriform calcification in the right occipital region (A) with slight enhancement following contrast infusion (B).

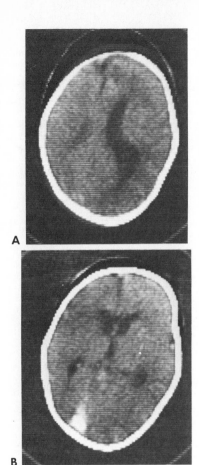

Figure 5–55. A five-month-old child with multiple hemiangiomata over his entire body but not in the trigeminal facial distribution. In addition he had right-sided hemihypertrophy. CT findings; right side of cranium is larger than left; with right-sided ventricular dilatation (*A*). In left occipital region there is dense calcification, and area adjacent to it enhances with contrast infusion (*B*).

angioma. CT may show dense calcification in the occipital region with a diffuse enhancement pattern (Fig. 5–55).

4. Vein of Galen Malformation. In certain angiomas there may be aneurysmal dilatation of this large deeply located midline vein, and this may cause symptoms by compressing the adjacent structures including the brain stem (Perinaud syndrome) or the posterior third ventricle–proximal aqueductal region (hydrocephalus). These may present in three patterns: (1) congestive heart failure due to arteriovenous shunts in the neonatal period; (2) hydrocephalus due to ventricular compression in infants; (3) compression of the midbrain tectal region with ocular and cerebellar symptoms in young children or adults. Diagnosis may be established by air study, which shows midline posterior third ventricular mass, but its vascular nature can be defined only by angiography. The malformation is supplied by the posterior cerebral, superior cerebellar and meningeal vessels with arterialization of the deep venous system. CT may demonstrate a large round regularly shaped central varix located in the midline that shows marked intravascular enhancement. The diagnosis may usually be suspected from CT and isotope findings, but the vascular nature of the lesion is dependent upon angiography (see Fig. 19–9).

References

1. McCormick WF, Schochet SS: Atlas of Cerebrovascular Disease. WB Saunders, Philadelphia, 1976. pp 72–87.
2. Paterson JH, McKissock W: Clinical survey of intracranial angioma with special reference to mode of progression and surgical treatment. Brain 79:233, 1956.
3. Crawford JV, Russell DS: Cryptic arteriovenous and venous hamartomas of the brain. J Neurol Neurosurg Psychiatry 19:1, 1956.
4. McCormick WF, Nofzinger JD: "Cryptic" vascular malformations of CNS. J Neurosurg 24:865, 1966.
5. Kamrin RB, Buchsbaum HW: Large vascular malformations of the brain not visualized by serial angiography. Arch Neurol 13:413, 1965.
6. Eisenman J, Alekoumbides A, Pribram H: Spontaneous thrombosis of vascular malformation of the brain. Acta Radiol (Diagn) 13:77, 1972.
7. Rumbaugh CL, Potts DG: Skull changes associated with intracranial AVM. Am J Roentgenol 98:525, 1966.

8. Handa J, Handa H, Torizuka K, et al: Radioisotopic study of arteriovenous anomalies. Am J Roentgenol 115:751, 1971.

9. Kendall BE, Clavaria LE: The use of CAT for diagnosis and management of intracranial angioma. Neuroradiol 12:141, 1976.

10. Pressman BD, Kirkwood JR, Davis DO: CT of vascular lesions of the brain. Part I Arteriovenous malformations. Am J Roentgenol 124:208, 1975.

11. Hayward RD: Intracranial arteriovenous malformation; experience with CT. J Neurol Neurosurg Psychiatry. 39:1027, 1976.

12. Goree JA, Dukes HT: Angiographic differential diagnosis between the vascularized malignant glioma and intracranial AVM. Am J Roentgenol 90:512, 1963.

13. Terbrugge K, Scotti G, Ethier R, et al: CT in intracranial AVM. Radiology 122:703, 1977.

14. Kramer RA, Wing SD: CT of angiographically occult cerebral vascular malformations. Radiology 123:649, 1977.

15. Michels LG, Bentson JR, Winter J: CT of cerebral venous angiomas. J Comput Assist Tomog 1:149, 1977.

16. Enzman DR, Hayward RW, Norman D: CT scan appearance of Sturge-Weber disease. Radiology 122:721, 1977.

6 Progressive Neurological Deficit

Localization

FRONTAL LESIONS

Frontal lesions produce distinctive symptoms according to their location: lateral convexity lesions present with focal motor or sensory seizures; para-sagittal lesions may cause generalized seizures and contralateral monoparesis, usually involving the leg; basal and inferior lesions result in papilledema, psychiatric disturbance, dementia, olfactory impairment; bifrontal and callosal lesions lead to hydrocephalus, generalized seizures, disordered consciousness and gait disorder.[1] The development of an organic brain syndrome without accompanying neurological signs other than the presence of certain reflex abnormalities, including grasp, palmo-mental, suck and snout, is most likely the result of a frontal lesion. Apathy, confusion and incontinence are prominent with middle or superior frontal involvement, whereas excitement, psychosis and hallucinosis are associated with basal frontal lesions.[2] Disturbances of gait and balance may falsely suggest a cerebellar lesion.[3] Extracerebral lesions may grow to large size but produce minimal symptoms whereas intracerebral lesions (glioma, metastasis, abscess) usually spread through deep white matter to cause more rapid development of neurological symptoms.

The more superficially located frontal lesions cause a prominent unilat-eral, continuous, high-voltage, slow wave pattern, whereas the deeply infiltrating tumors may cause a bilateral polymorphic or monorhythmic delta pattern.[4] The presence of nonfocal or negative EEG does not exclude a frontal lesion, and this has been reported in subdural hematoma or cystic lesions. Angiographic diagnosis of a frontal lesion usually depends upon the characteristic vascular displacement, stain pattern in mass lesions, or abnormalities of the arterial or venous pattern in vascular disorders. From this pattern it is usually possible to distinguish intra- from extracerebral and vascular from avascular lesions. With CT it is possible to identify frontal lesions based upon density pattern, shape, location, extension and ventricular distortion and displacement. In certain cases CT may obviate the need for angiography.

The following guidelines apply:

1. Anterior cerebral artery occlusion with frontal lobe infarction shows a rectangular or triangular-shaped, low-density lesion extending to the midline. It may also be bilateral. It has minimal mass effect, and a linear enhancement pattern. (See page 93, Fig. 5–45).

2. Intracerebral hemorrhage appears as a homogeneous, consolidated, high-density lesion that extends deeply into the white matter and ventricle, with significant ventricular displacement and distortion, and usually no enhancement. With certain large

105

anterior cerebral aneurysms, there may be dissection of blood into both frontal lobes and into the interhemispheric fissure (Fig. 6–1).

3. Extracerebral hematoma or empyema usually has a concave or convex shape, is contiguous with bone, and may compress the lateral ventricle and bow the falx posteriorly. It is associated with edema in the frontal region and demonstrates a medial rim of enhancement.

4. Cysts may be intra- or extracerebral in location and, although well visualized by CT, their precise location usually requires angiography and air study. The presence of dense enhancement is most consistent with a cyst associated with neoplasm, whereas non-neoplastic cysts rarely may show a faint rim of peripheral enhancement.

5. Malignant neoplasms usually have irregular frondlike projections extending deeply into white matter, corpus callosum and basal ganglia,

and may cause marked distortion and displacement of the lateral and third ventricles. They show irregular contrast enhancement (Fig. 6–2), and CT is the most reliable means to detect a multiplicity of lesions.

6. Meningiomas are located peripherally with contiguity to bone or dura, and have less surrounding edema, ventricular distortion or displacement than gliomas. Meningio-

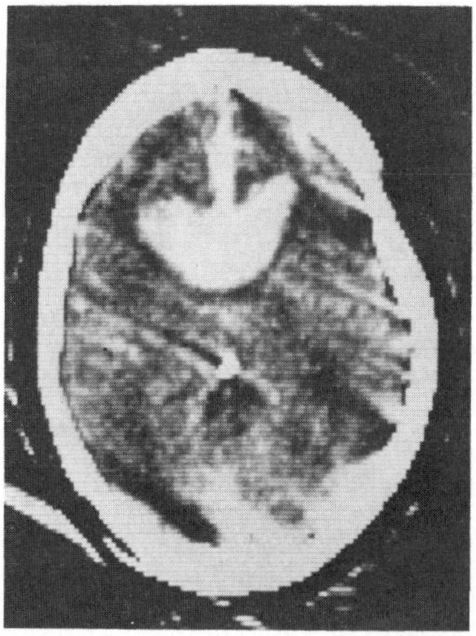

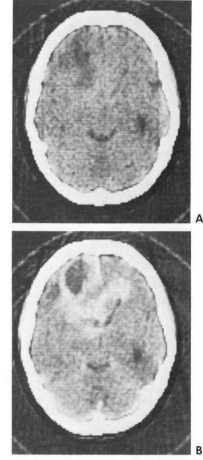

A

B

Figure 6–1. A 50-year-old normotensive man developed severe headache and suddenly became unresponsive. He was found to have bilateral Babinski sign; CSF was bloody and xanthochromic. CT findings: high-density hematoma in both frontal regions, with blood penetrating into the interhemispheric fissure, but no aneurysm was identified with contrast infusion. Angiography showed severe spasm of anterior cerebral arteries, but no aneurysm was visualized.

Figure 6–2. Patient was a chronic alcoholic who had two generalized seizures following alcoholic binges; EEG was diffusely slow and isotope scan was negative. CT findings: preinfusion scan shows irregularly shaped low-density lesion in left frontal region (A). Following infusion there is dense enhancement in left frontal region, which spreads across the corpus callosum to the right frontal, ganglionic and thalamic region (B). Operative diagnosis: malignant glioma of the corpus callosum.

mas frequently have a surrounding lucent collar, are round and regular in shape, are calcified in 50 percent of cases, and have a dense enhancement pattern. The thickening of the falx adjacent to tumor is highly characteristic of a meningioma (Fig. 6–3). In rare instances, CT may not be able to differentiate intra- from extracerebral lesions. Diagnosis depends upon the angiographic pattern with characteristic vascular displacement and stain.

7. Cerebritis and abscess formation may simulate a malignant neoplasm and differentiation may be most de-

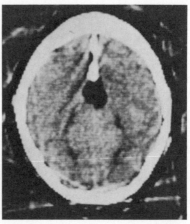

Figure 6–4. High-density round calcification in the region of the corpus callosum with very low-density (− 10) round area consistent with pattern of fat and no enhancement; this is characteristic of a lipoma of the corpus callosum.

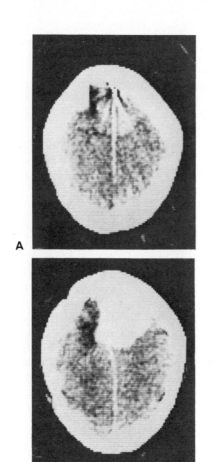

A

B

Figure 6–3. A and B, Patient previously had falx meningioma removed surgically. CT scan shows dense homogeneous enhancement pattern contiguous with anteriorly thickened falx, which is suggestive of meningioma originating from this structure.

pendent upon clinical symptomatology. Ring hematoma may also be seen.

8. Aneurysm and angioma without hematoma formation may show characteristic changes of calcification and enhancement, but usually require angiography for diagnosis.

9. Lipoma of the corpus callosum may be detected by visualization of a mixture of high-density calcification and low-density fat, but the extent of the lesion requires coronal and sagittal reconstructions (Fig. 6–4).

TEMPORAL LESIONS

Lesions located in the temporal region may be either intracerebral (hematoma, abscess, metastasis, glioma) or extracerebral (middle fossa or sphenoid wing meningioma, subtemporal subdural hematoma, epidermoid cyst, lateral extension of pituitary adenoma, incisural tumor). Extracerebral lesions cause characteristic angiographic findings, including elevation and medial displacement of the MCA, medial displacement of the anterior choroidal artery and midline shift of the ACA and internal cerebral vein; but the mass effect of edema and actual tumor mass may not be distinguished.

Intracerebral lesions cause elevation and stretching and draping of superficial vessels around a deeply located intratemporal mass, but angiography is not as sensitive in detecting mass effect as is air study, which may define the outline and position of the body and tip of the temporal horn.[5]

With computed tomography, the shape, density characteristics and pattern of ventricular displacement may define the presence and location of the mass in the temporal region. Intracerebral lesions are usually rounded in shape, more medially located

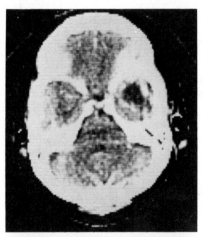

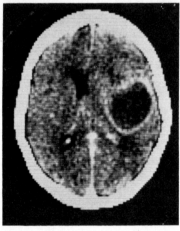

B

Figure 6–5. A and B, Patient with left-sided weakness; isotope scan was positive in the right temporal region, and EEG showed bitemporal slow wave pattern. CT findings: circular rim of enhancement surrounding lower-density core, causing marked shift of the septum pellucidum and third ventricle, with compression of the right lateral ventricle, a pattern consistent with malignant neoplasm.

and not contiguous with bone; they cause significant distortion and displacement of the septum pellucidum and third ventricle and compress the ipsilateral portion of the suprasellar cistern (Fig. 6–5). If the lesion is located in the inferior temporal region, the major vector of expansion may be in an upward direction and there may be minimal lateral shift. Extracerebral lesions may be contiguous with bone and conform to the shape of the extracerebral space, demonstrate less mass effect and surrounding edema, are less likely to distort the suprasellar cistern and are usually located below the sylvian fissure, but angiography or air study may be required. Isotope scan is less reliable than CT in the temporal region because of the obscuring effect of the overlying temporalis muscle and the problem of spatial resolution with the isotope scan. An EEG pattern of unilateral or bilateral temporal abnormalities may not always be indicative of a structural lesion in the temporal region,[4] as this may reflect a more distant lesion.

PARIETAL LESIONS

These may extend into adjacent regions; and the symptoms depend upon this extension and also upon the spread into deep white matter and central nuclear structures. Superficially placed lesions may cause motor or sensory seizures, frequently with numbness, electrical sensation or a pins-and-needles feeling; whereas more deeply penetrating lesions that extend into the thalamic region cause a sensation of pain and hyperpathia. Dominant parietal involvement results in aphasic disturbance, especially if the lesion is contiguous to the temporal region; nondominant lesions cause disorders of body schema perception, denial of illness (anosognosia) and constructional apraxia. An inferior homonymous quadrantanopia is characteristic of a parietal lobe lesion, and hemiparesis is invariably present unless the lesion is located in the posterior parietal region. Twenty-five percent of parietal tumors have no characteristic neurological findings.[6] The major diagnostic problem with lesions in this region involves differentiation of branch occlusion of MCA with infarction from a mass lesion. With CT, it may be possible to make this diagnosis accurately though it is not always possible with EEG and isotope scan. Infarction is visualized as a wedge-shaped low-density lesion with minimal mass effect, sometimes with extensive enhancement confined to its vascular distribution by sharp boundaries, and angiography is rarely now necessary. In both the temporal and parietal regions, edema appears as three fingerlike low-density projections extending from the deeper white matter to the superficial cortical area.

OCCIPITAL LESIONS

Homonymous hemianopia is the most characteristic presenting sign of occipital lobe involvement. In one fourth of cases this finding is not demonstrated because of other disturbances of mentation that make visual field testing difficult; in 10 percent of cases visual field study is entirely normal if the lesion involves the lateral convex occipital surface.[7] In one third of cases focal seizures with flashing colored lights moving from the peripheral to the central visual field are present, and there is an associated headache; in these cases the diagnosis of migraine may be raised. Other findings with occipital involvement may falsely localize to a distant region and these include the following: (1) paralysis of conjugate gaze or dementia is characteristic of deep frontal lesions; (2) incoordination and cerebellar signs may indicate an infratentorial location; (3) hemiparesis due to compression of the cerebral peduncle by the edge of the tentorium. Furthermore, homonymous hemianopic defect may result from compression of the posterior cerebral artery against the tentorium,

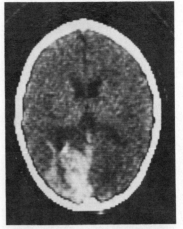

A

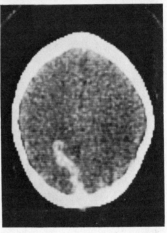

B

Figure 6–6. A two-year-old developed sudden onset of bilateral blindness, one week after head truma to occipital region. EEG showed bilateral delta pattern, which was most pronounced over left hemisphere, with complete absence of alpha rhythm. CT finding: dense gyral (A) and serpentine (B) enhancement pattern in left occipital region without mass effect, and minimal nonenhancing low-density area in the right occipital region, consistent with bilateral occipital infarction.

with resultant occipital lobe infarction as a consequence of transtentorial herniation by neoplasms not involving the occipital region.

The most frequent lesions involving the occipital cortex are gliomas and metastases; angioma, meningioma and porencephalic cyst occur less frequently. Based upon the results of EEG and isotope scan, it may not be possible to differentiate these lesions from infarction or hematoma.

EEG is a sensitive indicator of the

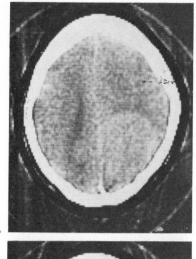

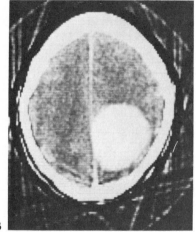

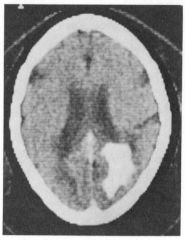

Figure 6–8. Patient developed left homonymous hemianopia. Both isotope scan and EEG were negative, but skull radiogram showed calcification in the occipital region. CT findings: round, irregularly shaped high-density (45 to 50) lesion in the right occipital region, which is displacing and distorting the occipital horn; no change following infusion. Repeat study nine months later showed no interval change — this was consistent with oligodendroglioma.

Figure 6–7. This elderly patient developed progressive loss of vision and intermittent scotoma in right eye. Examination showed papilledema and incomplete incongruous left homonymous hemianopia. Isotope scan was positive in right occipital region. CT findings: preinfusion study shows almost isodense lesion displacing the right occipital horn and choroid plexus, with obliteration of posterior portion of lateral ventricle (A). Following infusion there was a dense round consolidated enhancement, with sharply marginated borders, which extends to the falx medially (B). Operative finding: medial falx meningioma.

presence of a lesion by showing abolition of alpha background rhythm or a polymorphic delta pattern, but it may be negative in one fourth of cases. The findings with isotope scan are dependent upon the specific pathological condition. With CT, it is frequently possible to detect the lesion and define its specific pathologi-

cal characteristic without angiography. In occipital infarction there is initially a wedge-shaped low-density pattern with its base oriented to midline; later there may be a gyral or serpentine enhancement pattern, which may extend to the inferior temporal and thalamic region, remaining within the vascular distribution of the PCA and causing minimal mass effect (Fig. 6–6). The presence of a ring pattern of enhancement may suggest malignant neoplasm, but lack of mass effect and the absence of surrounding edema are more consistent with infarction, whereas extension into the parietal and temporal region with surrounding edema is more consistent with malignant neoplasm. Differentiation of intra- and extra-axial occipital lesions may be difficult, but meningiomas are usually attached to or contiguous with bone or falx and have sharp edges and a round shape (Fig. 6–7), whereas oligodendrogliomas have a more irregular shape, are not attached to bone and cause more ventricular displacement and surrounding edema (Fig. 6–8).

THALAMIC LESIONS

Primary thalamic tumors may cause symptoms which simulate supratentorial, intraventricular or posterior fossa lesions. If there is lateral extension, early involvement of the internal capsule causes hemiparesis-sensory syndrome; medial expansion causes early obstruction of the third ventricle with intracranial hypertension, altered mentation and dementia; posterior expansion causes impaired ocular movement, pupillary disturbance, visual field involvement related to the upper brain stem, or geniculate body involvement.[10]

Prior to CT, the diagnosis of thalamic tumor was dependent upon air study or angiography. In patients who present without intracranial hypertension, EEG may frequently be normal, but if this finding is present the majority have focal EEG abnormality; in some cases this is located contralateral to the tumor.[11]

Isotope scan is positive in more rapidly growing tumors but overall accuracy is 30 percent. Four-vessel angiography is sometimes required to demonstrate thalamic tumors because vessels that are displaced and show tumor stain are derived from both carotid and vertebral circulation. The characteristic changes include elevation of the MCA with lateral displacement to widen the arc between the MCA and pericallosal area, stretching elongation and enlargement of the anterior choroidal artery, enlargement of the curvature of the lateral posterior choroidal arteries and elevation and shift of the internal cerebral and thalamostriate veins.

From the angiographic findings it may be difficult to determine primary thalamic tumor from one that has secondarily infiltrated deeply from the parietal or temporal region. With thalamic tumors air study demonstrates elevation of the floor of the lateral ventricle on the involved side, usually with medial shift, bowing of the third ventricle to the opposite side, and downward and slight lateral dis-

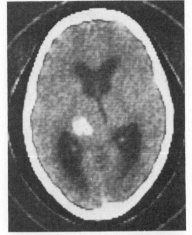

A

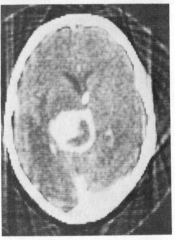

B

Figure 6–9. This ten-year-old presented with signs of increased intracranial pressure and had impairment of upward gaze. EEG was diffusely slow and isotope scan was negative. CT findings: high-density, irregularly shaped nonenhancing lesion in left thalamic region, causing posterior displacement of choroid plexus, with elevation and displacement of third ventricle to the right side (A). Following insertion of shunt, the ventricular size decreased, but the tumor mass has increased in size and shows enhancement, with extension posteriorly into the splenium and inferiorly into the brain stem (B).

location of the temporal horn. These studies define the presence of the thalamic mass but do not determine its pathological nature. The majority of lesions are astrocytomas or glioblastomas; these are best managed with shunt and radiotherapy. Poor results have been obtained in patients who underwent craniotomy with evacuation of cyst, biopsy or an attempt at partial removal of the lesion.[12] In rare instances, the thalamic mass may be a granuloma, abscess, hemorrhage or vascular malformation; with CT, preoperative diagnosis may be possible, as well as defining the primary location and direction of extension.[13]

As mentioned previously, thalamic tumors cause narrowing, bowing, elevation and contralateral deviation of the third ventricle to the opposite side (Fig. 6–9). As the tumor expands further, it may obliterate the third ventricular cavity, encroach upon the retrothalamic cistern, displace posteriorly and laterally the choroid plexus of the lateral ventricle, com-

press the atrium and occipital region of the ipsilateral ventricle and cause contralateral lateral ventricular dilatation. In addition, the tumor may expand into the splenium of the corpus callosum, septum pellucidum, quadrigeminal cistern, floor of the lateral ventricle, basal ganglia, and laterally into the superficial cortical region (Fig. 6–10).

CT clearly defines the presence of a large cystic component and there is usually a peripheral edge of enhancement; this cystic component was present in 30 percent of cases and was responsible for a mass effect which resolved following drainage in 10 percent (Fig. 6–11). Medially located tumors compress the mid and

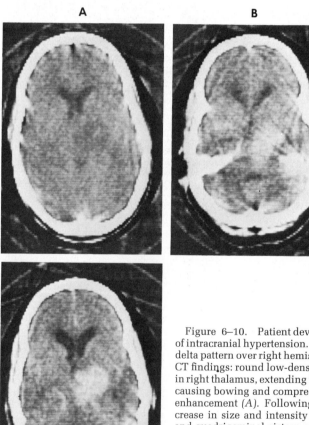

A   B

C

Figure 6–10.   Patient developed left hemiparesis without signs of intracranial hypertension. EEG showed high voltage rhythmical delta pattern over right hemisphere, but isotope scan was negative. CT findings: round low-density area with one high-density region in right thalamus, extending to putamen and medial temporal area, causing bowing and compression of third ventricle with minimal enhancement (A). Following radiotherapy, CT scan showed increase in size and intensity of enhancement, involving ambient and quadrigeminal cistern as well as temporal region (B and C).

A   B

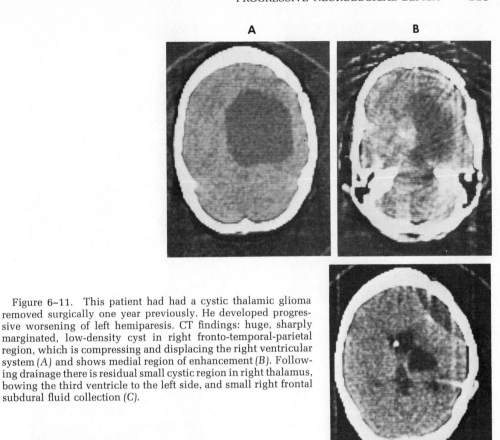

C

Figure 6–11. This patient had had a cystic thalamic glioma removed surgically one year previously. He developed progressive worsening of left hemiparesis. CT findings: huge, sharply marginated, low-density cyst in right fronto-temporal-parietal region, which is compressing and displacing the right ventricular system (A) and shows medial region of enhancement (B). Following drainage there is residual small cystic region in right thalamus, bowing the third ventricle to the left side, and small right frontal subdural fluid collection (C).

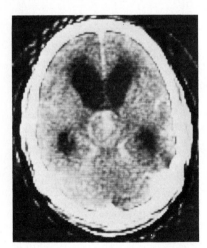

Figure 6–12. A 26-year-old man developed right-sided weakness and apathy one month following an automobile accident and was found to have papilledema and right hemiparesis. Bilateral carotid angiography showed evidence of ventricular dilatation only. CT findings: symmetrical lateral ventricular dilatation with anterior bowing of midportion of third ventricle by round enhancing lesion, consistent with medial thalamic tumor; these findings were confirmed by ventriculography.

posterior portion of the third ventricle forward and the pineal body posteriorly with resultant hydrocephalus (Fig. 6–12). Based upon the density characteristics, it is possible to classify thalamic glioblastomas, which are initially of mixed density with dense complex enhancement (Fig. 6–13). Thalamic hemorrhages may have similar spatial and density characteristics but usually do not enhance, and this, combined with the clinical presentation, makes differentiation possible; but angiography may still be indicated in some instances to exclude an underlying angioma (Fig. 6–14). The finding of a smooth, regular and completely round enhancing area suggests the possibility of an abscess, and needle aspiration should be performed prior to initiation of radiotherapy (Fig. 6–15).

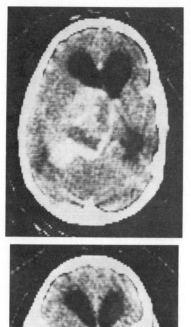

A

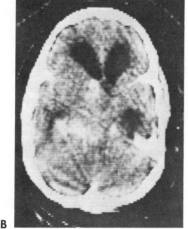

B

Figure 6–13. Patient with rapidly progressive right-sided weakness. EEG showed delta focus over the entire left hemisphere, and isotope scan was positive in left temporal region. CT findings: large mixed-density lesion in left thalamus, extension into temporal and parietal region with complex and extensive enhancement pattern *(A)*. There is lateral ventricular enlargement with distortion and displacement of third ventricle to the right and lateral displacement of left temporal horn *(B)*

TUMORS OF THE POSTERIOR THIRD VENTRICULAR REGION

The majority of these tumors are pathologically classified as pinealomas, but they may occasionally be teratomas, medulloblastomas, metastases or gliomas. The pinealoma causes early obstructive hydrocephalus and these patients present with

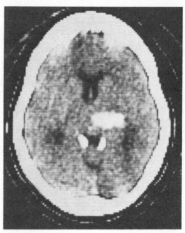

Figure 6–14. Patient with history of poorly controlled hypertension who suddenly became obtunded. Findings included left hemiparesis sensory deficit, downward and right-sided eye deviation. CT Findings: rectangularly shaped consolidated homogeneous lesion, which did not enhance, consistent with thalamic hemorrhage.

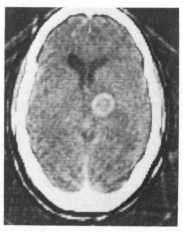

Figure 6–15. Patient had previously undergone posterior fossa and parietal craniotomy for brain abscess, and had recently developed left hemiparesis and dysarthria. EEG showed extensive right-sided delta pattern but isotope scan was negative. CT findings: density enhancing homogeneous lesion with higher-density peripheral rim in the right thalamic region. Angiography demonstrated an avascular thalamic mass, which was surgically demonstrated to be an abscess.

increased intracranial pressure without localizing signs. As the quadrigeminal plate region is compressed, limitation of upward gaze, dilated pupils with poor reactivity to light and diplopia develop. More severe compression of the midbrain may cause ataxia, nystagmus and pyramidal tract signs, and these later findings may suggest primary posterior fossa neoplasm.[14, 15]

The diagnosis of pinealoma is suggested by the radiographic finding of calcification in the pineal region in patients less than 10 years of age, and is established by ventriculography, which demonstrates symmetrical hydrocephalus with a smoothly rounded defect directed convex and anterior in the pineal region. If this diagnosis is suspected but not confirmed by air study, positive contrast material may be necessary to outline the posterior region of the third ventricle to detect more sensitively any filling defects.[15, 16] Because of their location, direct operative removal has been associated with high operative mortality, and treatment usually involves shunt and radiotherapy without tissue biopsy. With this diagnostic and therapeutic approach, it is not always possible to define those tumors which have secondarily involved the pineal region, or to verify the specific macroscopic and histological features of the lesion, including the presence of its cystic component, or to assess response to treatment without involving further invasive procedures.

With CT, the diagnosis of posterior third ventricular tumor may be established and the direction of expansion visualized. The correlation of clinical and CT scan features may help to suggest certain histological features without the necessity for surgical biopsy.[13] These tumors distort, indent and compress the posterior third ventricle from the caudal aspect and usually expand into the quadrigeminal cistern and then into the superior cerebellar cistern (Fig. 6–16). There is symmetrical enlargement of the lateral ventricles, and the posterior third ventricle may be elevated, laterally displaced, or enlarged by the tumor. If the third ventricle is dilated an im-

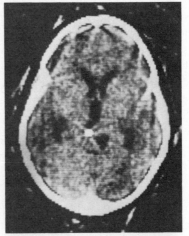

A

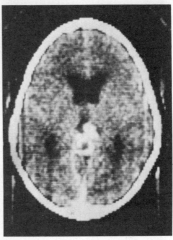

B

Figure 6–16. This ten-year-old presented with paralysis of upward gaze, dilated and nonreactive pupils and papilledema. Skull radiogram showed pineal calcification. CT findings: plain scan shows dense, large eccentrically placed pineal calcification and triangularly shaped low-density region elevating and distorting the posterior third ventricle and extending into the quadrigeminal cistern, with lateral and third ventricular dilatation (A). Following infusion there is dense enhancement within the pineal and quadrigeminal cistern region, consistent with pinealoma (B).

portant sign of a mass is anterior concavity of the posterior third ventricle, and this differentiates from nontumorous aqueductal stenosis in cases in which the tumor is isodense and does not enhance. The tumors have a round and multilobulated shape and are usually dense; occasionally a cystic component is present. Pinealomas

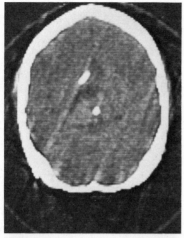

A

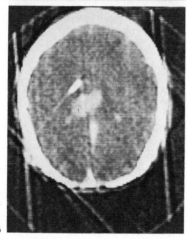

B

Figure 6–17. This 16-year-old had been shunted and irradiated following diagnosis of pineal tumor, established by ventriculogram and biopsy one year previously. Patient has now developed ataxia, bilateral pyramidal tract signs and lethargy, but no papilledema was demonstrated. CT findings: shunt tube is seen, and ventricles are small in size and poorly visualized (A). There is shift of pineal to the right side by a dense, but not consolidated, enhancing mass in the pineal region, extending laterally and posteriorly (B).

and teratomas calcify but glial tumors and metastases do not, and this may be determined from the plain scan density characteristics. Following contrast infusion the majority of pinealomas and teratomas enhance, although this may be difficult to identify if the tumor is densely calcified, and the glial tumors may also show little enhancement. If the patient

clinically has papilledema only and CT scan shows a calcified and enhancing mass of the posterior third ventricle, the diagnosis of pinealoma-teratoma is most likely. If there are signs of infiltration of the midbrain tegmentum before evidence of intracranial hypertension and CT shows a noncalcified and nonenhancing lesion, a glioma is more likely. Paraventricular extension and spread into the subarachnoid spaces may be detected with CT infusion studies.

Following shunt and irradiation, the ventricular size and reduction in tumor size and enhancement may be evaluated, and the need for further surgical treatment established without need for ventriculography or angiography (Fig. 6–17). Less frequently, tumors with histological features of pinealoma-teratoma are most prominent in the anterior third ventricular–hypothalamic region and may cause diabetes insipidus, hypopituitarism of precocious puberty and bitemporal hemianopic defect. CT may readily define the major location of the tumor.

TUMORS OF THE LATERAL VENTRICLE

These tumors are quite rare and usually consist of choroid plexus papillomas, ependymomas, gliomas, meningiomas, dermoids or epidermoids.[18] Symptomatology is related to CSF pathway obstruction with intracranial hypertension. Focal neurological signs may result from localized dilatation of an obstructed or loculated portion of the ventricular system distal to the tumor, infiltration of the tumor through the ventricular wall into the underlying parenchyma, or from the distant effect (false localizing sign) of increased intracranial pressure. Meningiomas and choroid plexus papillomas bulge into the ventricular cavity and are therefore primarily intraventricular, whereas other tumors may also infiltrate into underlying paren-

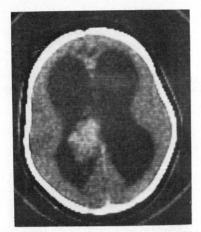

Figure 6–18. This eight-month-old child had increasing head size. CT findings: symmetrical ventricular dilatation with a coarsely lobulated round and nonhomogeneous high-density lesion in the posterior region of the left lateral ventricle. Operative diagnosis: choroid plexus papilloma.

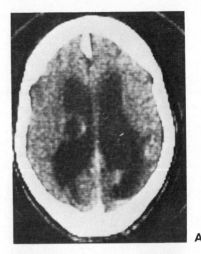

A

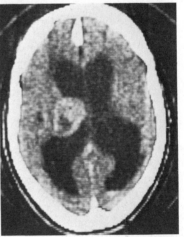

B

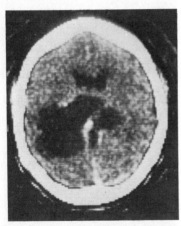

Figure 6–19. CT findings: ventricular enlargement associated with focal dilatation of the left lateral ventricle, extending into the left temporal parietal region. Operative diagnosis: cholesteatoma of the left lateral ventricle.

Figure 6–20. A and B, Fifty-year-old normotensive man developed generalized seizures, and on examination had only right pronator drift. EEG was diffusely slow and isotope scan was negative. CT findings: symmetrical ventricular enlargement with a high-density mass in posterior portion of the body of the left lateral ventricle, projecting inferiorly into the floor of the ventricle and the thalamic region. At operation this was proved to be a thalamic hemorrhage which did not project into the lateral ventricle.

chyma to cause seizures, dementia and focal deficit. If the tumor infiltrates into one hemisphere, EEG and isotope scan may suggest a primary hemispheric or deep thalamic tumor.

Angiography has been the initial contrast study, and the intraventricular location of the tumor may be indicated by characteristic changes of choroidal arteries and veins. Combined pneumography-ventriculography will outline the air–tumor interface, and the specific pattern of lobulation may differentiate meningioma from epidermoid tumor. Problems in diagnosis may be encountered if air does not fill the ventricle because of tumor obstruction. The ventriculogram needle may puncture the tumor, or cystic dilatation of the occipital horn may result from tumor obstruction, and the diagnosis of cystic occipital tumor may be erroneously made.[19, 20]

The CT diagnosis of an intraventricular tumor may be suggested by the finding of hydrocephalus, which is usually symmetrical with a high-density mass protruding into the lumen, or there may be localized distention of the ventricular shape with extension into the underlying parenchyma. Choroid plexus papilloma and meningioma cannot be differentiated by CT characteristics, as both are round, speckled, nonhomogeneous, high-density, intraventricular lesions, which show marked contrast enhancement (Fig. 6–18). The epidermoid or dermoid tumors may have a smooth or lobulated appearance, with high-density calcified material in the wall and a low-density core. Since they usually infiltrate into surrounding tissue, there is localized distention of the ventricle (Fig. 6–19). It is not always possible to differentiate a thalamic pathological process from primary intraventricular tumor with a two-dimensional scan, and sometimes requires air study or coronal and sagittal CT reconstructions (Fig. 6–20). In addition, intraventricular hemorrhage may have the appearance of a tumor, but these usually conform more to the shape of the ventricular cast.

CEREBELLAR TUMORS

These may be classified as arising in either the vermal or hemispheric region. Patients with medulloblastoma present with characteristic "vermal syndrome," consisting of truncal and gait instability with evidence of early obstruction of the fourth ventricle. These neoplasms originate from cells of the external granular layer of

the inferior medullary velum and grow anteriorly to fill the lumen of the fourth ventricle, posteriorly into the vermis or laterally into the cerebellar hemispheres. Pathologically, medulloblastomas are well marginated, highly vascularized tumors, with a propensity to seed into the cisternal spaces, but hemorrhage, cyst formation and calcification are uncommon. Diagnosis has depended upon a ventriculogram, which usually

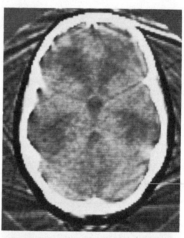

A

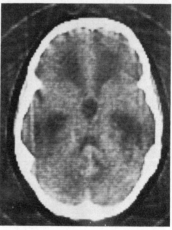

B

Figure 6–21. Patient presented with headache, nausea, vomiting and papilledema. Skull radiogram, EEG and isotope scan were negative. CT findings: forward displacement and splaying of the fourth ventricle by a round, low-density midline mass, with nonhomogeneous enhancement (A). Following infusion, the large extent of the low-density surrounding edema is more clearly visualized, as several areas with the tumor enhance (B). Operative diagnosis: medulloblastoma.

demonstrates dilated lateral and third ventricles, with distortion and upward displacement of the aqueduct and fourth ventricle and other less characteristic findings. These include upward extension into the third ventricle, intraventricular expansion and lateral expansion into the cerebellar hemisphere, which is seen less frequently. Vertebral angiography may show vascular displacement and delicate stain without early draining veins,

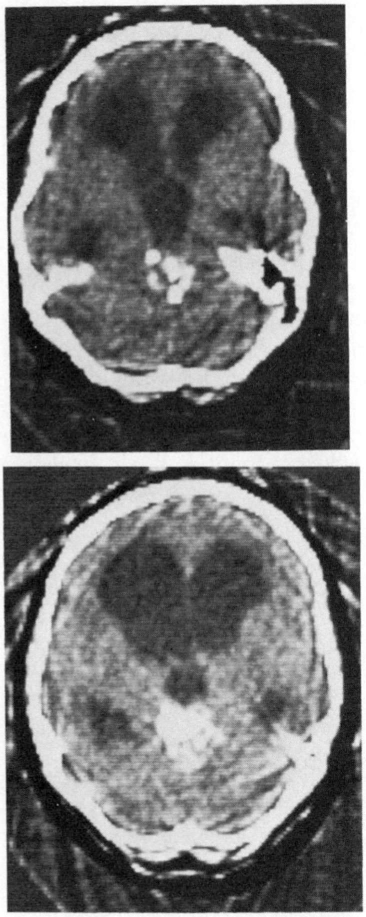

A

B

Figure 6–22. Preinfusion scan shows round, lobulated, high-density (25 to 35) lesion in the anterior and superior cerebellar region with non-visualization of the fourth ventricle and reversal of usual shape of posterior third ventricle (A) and definite enhancement (B). The third and lateral ventricles are markedly enlarged. Necropsy finding: cystic microglioma of the anterior superior cerebellum, not invading the fourth ventricle.

but preoperative pathological diagnosis is not always possible.

With CT the medulloblastoma may cause characteristic changes in the ventricular and cisternal spaces, and frequently the density characteristics permit definitive pathological diagnosis preoperatively.[21-24] These tumors always cause significant change in the fourth ventricle that may consist of two patterns: (1) splaying apart with increase in width but no change in height, as the vector of growth is to expand the lumen; (2) obliteration of the lumen of the fourth ventricle, with the neoplasm surrounded by a low-density rim (Fig. 6–21). This latter pattern may be also present if there is an anterior midline cerebellar tumor, which results in a CT pattern of nonvisualization of the fourth ventricle, although it is not obliterated by tumor (Fig. 6–22). In 90 to 95 percent of medulloblastomas, there is ventricular dilatation. The density characteristics may be low, isodense or high density, and the lesion is surrounded by a peripheral zone of edema. There is usually no evidence of calcification or hemorrhage, but 40 percent have a central lucency suggestive of cyst formation, although this is not pathologically confirmed in 50 percent. In these latter cases it is believed that the central portion of the lesion does not enhance as well as the periphery (Fig. 6–23). The majority of medulloblastomas show dense nonhomogeneous enhancement, whereas others enhance only in the peripheral portion and 10 to 20 percent show no enhancement.

Ependymomas arise from the floor of the fourth ventricle and enlarge to fill this cavity. They may extend exophytically into the basal cisterns and compress the brain stem; this accounts for the failure to visualize the fourth ventricle. These tumors are multilobulated and highly vascularized and frequently contain small cystic components, which are visualized by CT; but differentiation of these cysts from a distorted fourth ventricle is not

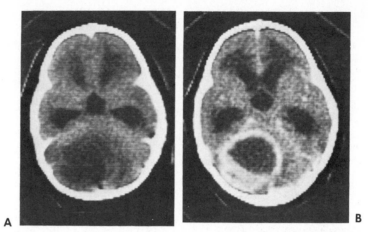

Figure 6–23. Plain scan demonstrates homogeneous, irregularly shaped low-density area in left cerebellar hemisphere that extends across the midline and obliterates the fourth ventricle *(A)* and shows irregular dense peripheral ring enhancement *(B)*. Operative finding: medulloblastoma.

always possible preoperatively (Fig. 6–24). These tumors show microscopic calcification, and the CT evidence of calcification or hemorrhage is more indicative of ependymoma than of medulloblastoma. Other than more frequent evidence of degenerative change, the density and enhancement patterns are similar to those of medulloblastoma (Fig. 6–25).

Cerebellar hemangioblastoma may be solid or cystic, with a mural nodule.[25] The solid tumors may be pathologically indistinguishable from posterior fossa meningioma, and the CT pattern may reflect this similarity, since they initially may be isodense or high-density, with calcification, and demonstrate dense homogeneous enhancement with sharp margination.

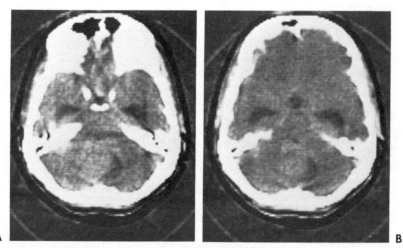

Figure 6–24. *A* and *B*, Plain scan shows nonvisualization of the fourth ventricle by a mottled high-density round nonenhancing lesion with semicircular lucent collar to the right of the lesion, a pattern consistent with a small cyst and accompanying ventricular dilatation. Operative diagnosis: ependymoma.

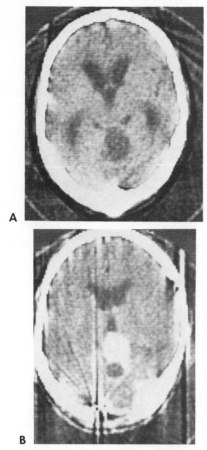

A

B

Figure 6–25.   CT scan shows lateral and third ventricular enlargement, with poor visualization of the fourth ventricle by a low-density mass in the middle of the posterior fossa (A). Following infusion, there is dense enhancement with a second region of low-density core and enhancing rim (B). This was surgically proved to be an ependymoma.

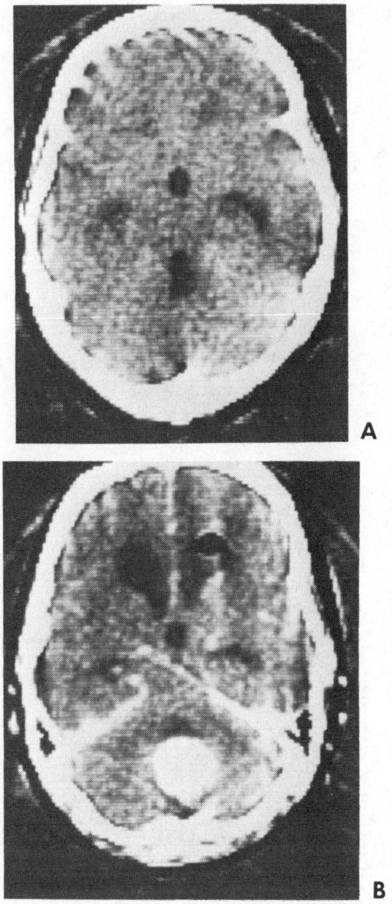

A

B

Figure 6–26.   Plain scan shows tilting and anterior displacement of the fourth ventricle only (A); infusion study shows homogeneously dense, well-marginated mass, which is not in continuity with bone (B). This was proved operatively to be a solid hemangioblastoma.

Contiguity to bone by the lesion is most consistent with meningioma (Fig. 6–26). If a cyst is present, contrast infusion is necessary to attempt to demonstrate the mural nodule, which may also be seen in cystic astrocytoma. If there is no enhancement, angiography is indicated, but occasionally the nodule may be present at surgery even though it was not defined by CT or angiography. This cyst without a mural nodule may not be differentiated from porencephalic cyst (Fig. 6–27).

Midline cerebellar tumors cause forward displacement and tilting of the fourth ventricle, whereas unilateral hemispheric tumors cause flattening and contralateral displacement of the ventricle (Fig. 6–28). Solid or microcystic anterior midline cerebellar tumors cause nonvisualization of the fourth ventricle. Because of their location they obliterate or distort the quadrigeminal cistern and extend further forward, causing truncation of the posterior third ventricle, with loss of its characteristic convexity. Tumor

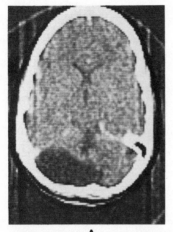

A

Figure 6–27. Oval-shaped, sharply marginated low-density lesion extending from the left side of the posterior fossa across the midline, with contralateral and slight forward displacement of the fourth ventricle, a pattern consistent with porencephalic cyst or nonenhancing cystic astrocytoma (A). This may be contrasted to a similarly shaped lesion that showed peripheral nodule of enhancement, consistent with cystic astrocytoma (B and C).

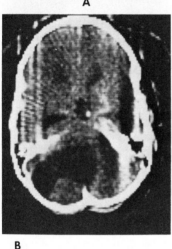

B

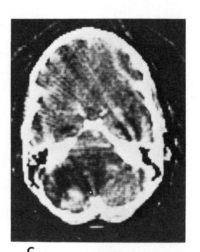

C

in the midline cerebellum and fourth ventricle may seed into the cisternal spaces and outline the brain stem cisterns.

In children, the astrocytoma and medulloblastoma are the most frequent cerebellar hemispheric tumors, whereas in adults metastases and hemangioblastoma predominate. In almost one half of cases the astrocytoma contains a large cystic component with a small tumor nodule, usually located in the periphery of the tumor; the others are either solid or microcystic. The prognosis is best for the cystic lesions. The CT appearance of the astrocytoma depends upon the pathological characteristics and includes the following

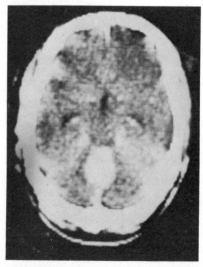

Figure 6–28. Dense, enhancing round lesion with nonvisualization of the fourth ventricle. It was surgically proved to be a solid cerebellar astrocytoma.

patterns: (1) a large low-density, laterally placed cyst, which may be irregular in shape and cause contralateral displacement of the fourth ventricle; there may be evidence of a small nodule of enhancement; (2) a large cyst with a nodule too small to be detected by CT. Gado has reported that 60 percent of low-grade astrocytomas show no contrast enhancement and may not be preoperatively differentiated from benign cysts, except that astrocytomas usually have a mottled or speckled appearance with less well-defined margins and are more irregular; exophytic growth may occur into the CPA. Laterally located medulloblastoma may show denser and more irregular ring enhancement, similar to astrocytoma. Metastases may be solitary and located laterally or in midline; other than multiplicity, there is no characteristic appearance that distinguishes them from primary tumor.

FOURTH VENTRICULAR TUMORS

In addition to the medulloblastoma and ependymoma, other tumors may involve this region, including choroid plexus papilloma, meningioma dermoid and epidermoid. The initial symptoms of these latter tumors may be positional, with intermittent obstruction of the ventricle. The detection of these lesions may be accomplished with CT, but the outline of the position of the neoplasm within the cavity of the fourth ventricle is best accomplished by air study. These tumors may expand and fill the fourth ventricular lumen, but this may be difficult to differentiate from a high-density lesion that is surrounded by lucent periphery. Intraventricular tumors usually have well-defined sharply marginated and smooth edges. Meningiomas and papillomas usually demonstrate enhancement, but cholesteatomas and dermoids usually do not.

BRAIN STEM TUMORS

Primary intramedullary brain stem tumors occur most frequently in childhood whereas metastatic deposits and gliomas occur with equal frequency in adults.[26, 27] Initial symptoms include facial and abducens nerve paresis and cerebellar disturbance. One half of patients present with symptoms consistent with intracranial hypertension, but nausea and vomiting may be due to direct vagal medullary nuclei compression, and frontal headache may be caused by traction on the ophthalmic branch of the trigeminal nerve.

Cranial nerve involvement is present in 93 percent, pyramidal tract and cerebellar signs in 75 percent, and papilledema in 33 percent. In the absence of intracranial hypertension, skull radiogram and EEG are negative, and these lesions are rarely detected by isotope scan.[28] The diagnosis is established by air study, as there is symmetrical enlargement of the brain stem with obliteration of the mesencephalic, pontine and medullary cisterns. There may be eccentric growth, which is usually anterior but may be lateral or posterior; less commonly the tumor may grow exophytically and appear as a mass in the cerebellopontine angle cistern or medially in the fourth ventricle, and in these cases air study findings may simulate an extra-axial mass. In one series air study confirmed the diagnosis of intrinsic brain stem mass in 32 of 35 cases, but in three patients findings were most consistent with an extra-axial lesion, and the diagnosis of exophytic brain stem lesion was confirmed by surgery. Vertebral angiography is necessary to exclude posterior fossa angioma, aneurysm or ectatic vertebral-basilar artery, and if tumor is present the demonstration of stain pattern or vessel encasement is indicative of malignant tumor. A contrast study may define the presence of brain stem lesion but, although it usually defines the size of the mass, it does not exclude other possible causes of brain stem enlargement, including focal encephalitis, angioma, granuloma, demyelinating disorder, and intrapontine cysts, or can it differentiate primary from metastatic tumors.

The diagnosis of brain stem tumor can usually be established by CT and this will obviate the need for air study or angiography. These tumors appear as paramedian abnormal densities in the posterior fossa and cause characteristic displacement of the fourth ventricle and the basilar cisterns. Brain stem tumors are intraaxial in location and expand the brain stem concentrically, but occasionally may be eccentric in location, simulating an extra-axial mass. They usually show maximal enlargement of the brain stem in the midpontine level but may grow in a serpentine manner into the medulla or upward into the midbrain and thalamus. The most characteristic change is posterior displacement of the fourth ventricle with anterior flattening and blunting of its apex, and if there is eccentric growth there may also be lateral displacement (Fig. 6–29). In rare instances there is nonvisualization of the fourth ventricle; this may be a genuine phenomenon due to obstructive hydrocephalus or it may be artifactual, as a result of partial volume effect. Rarely, the fourth ventricle may appear normal in the case of a small tumor, and the only CT sign is the abnormal density pattern. The earliest sign is deformity and obliteration of the pontine cistern and posterior portion of the suprasellar cistern. At this stage diagnosis may be more definitively established by air study, although the utilization of coronal and sagittal scans should obviate the need for this procedure. As the tumor expands into the medulla or into the white matter of the cerebellum, the fourth ventricle is displaced posteriorly, and as the tumor grows into the midbrain and posterior

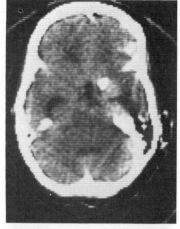

A

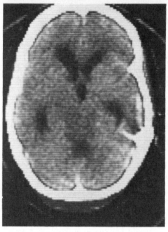

B

Figure 6–29. Patient with history of slurred speech, vertigo and gait unsteadiness. Findings included bilateral abducens paresis, right hemiparesis and consistent falling to the left. EEG showed left posterior temporal delta focus, and isotope scan was negative. CT findings: midline low-density nonenhancing lesion with anterior displacement of third ventricle (A). Posterior to this mass is triangular-shaped structure that was believed to be the fourth ventricle (B). Subsequent ventriculogram showed posterior displacement and obstruction of the aqueduct, consistent with brain stem tumor; it was proved by surgical biopsy to be a glioma.

thalamic region, there is deformity of the quadrigeminal cistern with alteration in convexity of the posterior third ventricle (Fig. 6–30). Hydrocephalus was present in only one third of brain stem tumors as compared with 90 percent for cerebellar and fourth ventricular tumors.

The   density   and   configuration

A   B

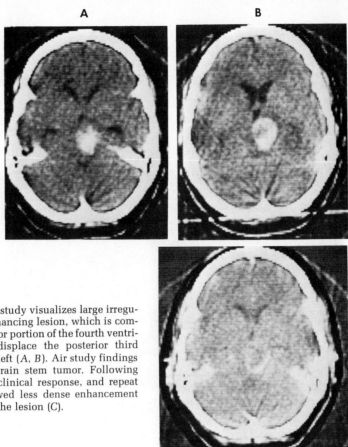

C

Figure 6–30. Preinfusion study visualizes large irregularly shaped high-density enhancing lesion, which is compressing and distorting anterior portion of the fourth ventricle and has expanded to displace the posterior third ventricle upward and to the left (A, B). Air study findings were also consistent with brain stem tumor. Following irradiation, there was good clinical response, and repeat scan four months later showed less dense enhancement and slightly reduced size of the lesion (C).

characteristics of brain stem tumors are quite variable and it is not possible to distinguish glioma from metastases. Gado has reported isodense or high-density lesions in 80 percent of tumors, with surrounding low density in the cerebellum or midbrain; this is believed due to exophytic extension and surrounding edema. Of ten brain stem gliomas, eight were initially low-density areas with irregular margins that caused mass effect and six enhanced following contrast infusion. In three cases there were ring enhancement patterns, and these were due to either glioma or metastases, but could not be differentiated without surgical or necropsy confirmation. The best prognosis and response to radiotherapy occurred in tumors which showed the most intense enhancement, and most poorly responsive neoplasms showed no enhancement. Pontine hemorrhage appears as a round high-density mass located posterior to the dorsum sella but does not enhance; most brain stem infarctions are wedge-shaped low-density lesions, but occasionally an enhancing infarction may have an appearance identical to that of brain stem glioma. Angiography is usually necessary to differentiate between angioma, aneurysm and ectatic basilar artery, although CT appearance is sufficiently characteristic in most cases. CT provides an excellent technique to monitor response to radiotherapy and to avoid the necessity for surgical biopsy, which has been performed by several centers. In all cases, good clinical response correlated with decrease in size of the lesion and enhancement pattern (Fig. 6–31).

A   B

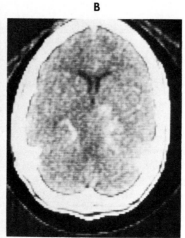

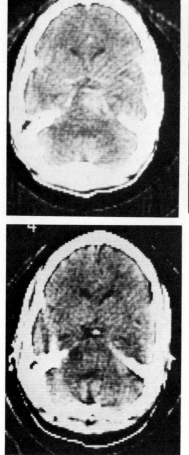

C

Figure 6–31. This 20-year-old initially presented with bilateral abducens nerve and right facial paresis. EEG, skull radiogram and isotope scan were negative. CT findings: an enhancing, irregularly marginated and nonhomogeneous lesion in right pontine, midbrain and thalamic region (A). There is posterior displacement and flattening of the apex of the fourth ventricle, distortion of the posterior portion of the suprasellar cistern, obliteration of the quadrigeminal cistern and truncation of the posterior portion of the third ventricle, a pattern consistent with brain stem glioma (B). Following radiotherapy, there was an excellent clinical response, and CT showed less compression of the fourth ventricle and minimal enhancement (C).

In one case, clinical worsening was related to development of hydrocephalus rather than tumor recurrence.

TENTORIAL LESIONS

Tentorial meningiomas may arise from either a supra- or infratentorial location, and these patients frequently present with signs of trigeminal nerve involvement, difficulty in walking or intracranial hypertension. Because of the sometimes vague, poorly defined nature of the findings, the average duration of symptoms may be two to five years, and occasionally longer, before the diagnosis is made.

With CT, the average duration of symptoms has been six to eight months, and this earlier diagnosis should result in improved surgical results. The tumor may originate from the lateral tentorium and is visualized as a complex but regularly shaped mass with a round medial border and flattened lateral border, which is in continuity with the tentorium; these lesions have sharply defined borders with a surrounding lucent collar. They may expand to the incisural region and appear comma-shaped, with flattening in the posterolateral region, and round configuration more anteriorly (Fig. 6–32). Other CT signs of transincisural extension include: (1) obliteration, distortion or elevation of the quadrigeminal cistern; (2) compression of the posterolateral portion of the suprasellar cistern; (3) eleva-

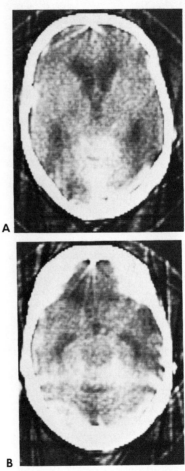

A

B

Figure 6–33. Plain scan showed only nonvisualization of the fourth ventricle with dilatation of other portions of the ventricular system. Following infusion there is dense enhancement in brain stem cisterns with widening of tentorial arc and dense enhancement, consistent with tumor in superior cerebellar cistern and midbrain region (A and B).

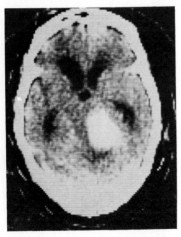

Figure 6–32. This patient rapidly developed right-sided hearing impairment, numbness and inability to walk. Skull radiogram showed enlarged internal auditory canal on the right side. CT findings: dense homogeneous and consolidated enhancing mass in right CPA with base directed toward petrous bone. The anterior round portion of the mass extends transincisurally with elevation and lateral displacement of the third ventricle and anterolateral displacement of the dilated temporal horn, consistent with tentorial meningioma.

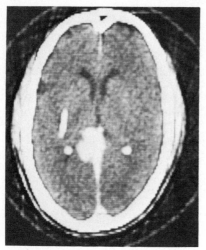

Figure 6–34. Postinfusion study visualizes densely enhancing lesion attached to the tentorium; this was proved surgically to be tentorium meningioma.

tion and lateral displacement of the posterior third ventricle; (4) anterolateral displacement of the dilated ipsilateral temporal horn, as there is usually hydrocephalus.[29] Tentorial lesions are always located medial to the tentorial margins, whereas occipital and posterior temporal supratentorial lesions are located lateral to these structures (Fig. 6–33 and 6–34). The midbrain and superior vermis are located medial to the tentorial folds, and tumors involving these structures cause bulging and expansion in this region; an important point of differentiation is that midbrain tumors displace the quadrigeminal cistern posteriorly, and superior vermal tumors displace it anteriorly.

REFERENCES

1. Botez MI: Frontal lobe tumors. In: Handbook of Clinical Neurology, Vol 17, PJ Vinken, GW Bruyn (eds). North Holland Publishing Co., Amsterdam, 1974. pp 234–280.
2. Hunter R, Blackwood W, Bull J: Three cases of frontal meningiomas presenting psychiatrically. Br Med J 3:9, 1968.
3. Meyer JS, Barron DW: Apraxia of gait. Brain 83:261, 1960.
4. Joynt RJ, Cape CA, Knott JR: The significance of focal delta activity in adults. Arch Neurol 12:631, 1965.
5. Taveras JM, Wood EH: Diagnostic Neuroradiology. Williams and Wilkins, Baltimore, 1975. pp. 1613–1615.
6. Suchenwirth RMA: Parietal lobe tumors. In; Handbook of Clinical Neurology, Vol 17, PJ Vinken, GW Bruyn (eds), North Holland Publishing Co., Amsterdam, 1974. pp. 290–307.
7. Gassel, MM: Occipital lobe tumors. In: Handbook of Clinical Neurology, Vol 17, PJ Vinken, GW Bruyn (eds). North Holland Publishing Co., Amsterdam, 1974. pp 310–349.
8. Parkinson D, McCraig W, Kernohan JW: Tumors of the occipital lobe. J Neurosurg 7:555, 1950.
9. Bilodeau L, Hanafee W: Roentgen findings in occipital pole tumors. Calif Med 106:112, 1967.
10. McKissock W, Paine KWE: Primary tumors of the thalamus. Brain 81:41, 1958.
11. Cheek WR, Taveras JM: Thalamic tumors. J Neurosurg 24:505, 1966.
12. Lawrie BW: Radiology of thalamic tumors. Clin Radiol 21:10, 1970.
13. Messina AV, Potts G, Sigel RM, et al: Computed tomography: evaluation of the posterior third ventricle. Radiology 119:581, 1976.
14. Poppen JL, Marino R: Pinealomas and tumors of the posterior portion of the third ventricle. J Neurosurg 28:357, 1968.
15. Cole H: Tumors in the region of the pineal. Clin Radiol 22:110, 1971.
16. Tod PA, Porter AJ, Jamieson KG: Pineal tumors. Am J Roentgenol 120:19, 1974.
17. Cummins FM, Taveras JM, Schlesinger EB: Treatment of gliomas of the third ventricle and pinealomas. Neurology 10: 1031, 1970.
18. Bartlett JR: Tumors of the lateral ventricles. In: Clinical Neurology, Vol 17, PJ Vinken GW Bruyn (eds). North Holland Publishing Co., Amsterdam, pp 596–609.
19. Bohm E, Strang R: Choroid plexus papilloma. J Neurosurg 18:493, 1961.
20. Boudreau RP: Primary intraventricular tumors. Radiology 75:867, 1960.
21. Gado M, Huete I, Mikhael M: CT of infratentorial tumors. Semin Roentgenol 12:109, 1977.

22. Naidich TP, Lin JP, Leeds NE, et al: CT in the diagnosis of extra-axial posterior fossa masses. Radiology 120:333, 1976.
23. Baker HL, Houser DW: CT in the diagnosis of posterior fossa lesions. Radiol Clin North Am 14:129–47, 1976.
24. Boltshauser E, Hamalatha H, Grant DN: Impact of CT on the management of posterior fossa tumors in childhood. J Neurol Neurosurg Psychiatry 40:209, 1977.
25. Jeffreys R: Clinical and surgical aspects of posterior fossa haemangioblastoma. J Neurol Neurosurg Psychiatry 38:105, 1975.
26. White H: Brain stem tumors occurring in adults. Neurology 13:292, 1963.
27. Panitch HS, Berg BD: Brain stem tumors of childhood and adolescence. Am J Dis Child 119:465, 1970.
28. Burrows EH: Clinical reliability of posterior fossa scintography. Clin Radiol 27:473, 1976.
29. Naidich TP, Leeds NE, Kricheff I, et al: The tentorium in axial Section. II. Lesion localization. Radiology 123:639, 1977

Meningioma

The diagnosis of intracranial meningioma may be suggested by plain skull radiographic and isotope scan findings and established by characteristic angiographic patterns, which visualize a superficial extracerebral mass with a dense persistent stain and an abnormal vascular supply derived from the dural vessels. Air study localizes 95 percent of clinically symptomatic meningiomas but is presently utilized only in detection of certain parasellar, intraventricular and posterior fossa tumors.[1] Plain skull radiograms will detect bony lesions or calcification in 30 to 60 percent of meningiomas, and this may be more sensitive if tomography is also performed. These bony changes include sclerosis or hyperostosis of the overlying bone, thinning of bone due to pressure erosion, presence of prominent vascular grooves which increase in diameter as they extend toward the region of the tumor, and calcification within the tumor.[3]

Isotope scan usually detects 70 to 90 per cent of meningiomas; this is most sensitive for supratentorial tumors (90 to 95 percent), but false negative studies occur most frequently with parasellar, tentorial, intraventricular and posterior fossa tumors (50 to 60 percent). Meningiomas appear as well-circumscribed areas of isotope uptake, which show maximal uptake on the static scan immediately after injection, and on the dynamic study there is accumulation during the late arterial and capillary phases, with persistence during the venous washout phase.[1, 3] There is a direct correlation with results of dynamic scan and the presence of characteristic angiographic stain. The static scan is sensitive enough to detect meningiomas as small as one centimeter in size, but does not detect microscopic foci of meningioma, which are frequent incidental necropsy findings. Angiographic studies, usually performed as common carotid injections, demonstrate a mass in 95 percent of cases and show specific angiographic features of meningioma in 73 percent.[4]

Angiography usually defines the presence of an abnormal circulatory pattern, the most common exceptions being the intracerebral and parasellar meningiomas, which may be avascular. The stain is usually a homogeneous opacification within the tumor that begins to appear in the early arterial phase, and persists into and may even increase in the mid and late venous circulation. The tumor vessels show regular alignment with little discrepancy between size of vessels, and the stain is well marginated. This vascular pattern is consistent with the noninfiltration and histologically benign nature of these tumors, but the angioblastic meningiomas show nonhomogeneous opacification, irregularly aligned vessels, and early draining veins, a pattern more suggestive of malignant lesion.[5, 6]

In rare instances pathognomonic angiographic signs of meningioma may be caused by other tumors. Superficial cortical glioma may reach and infiltrate the dura and derive part of the vascular supply from dural vessels; the presence of a homogeneous stain pattern may be seen in certain malignant tumors, but the feeding vessels are irregularly arranged, tortuous and of varying size. Angiographic determination of tumor size may not always be entirely accurate, as estimation based on vascular displacement may suggest a larger dimension because this reflects tumor and edema, whereas size determined by diameter of the stain may underestimate size because the tumor may be partly avascular or cystic.[4] In all patients suspected of having intracranial meningioma, angiography is necessary because the surgeon needs to know the source of the abnormal vascular supply and the relationship of tumor to the contiguous arteries, veins and venous sinuses as well as

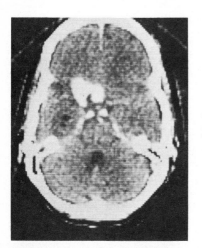

A

Figure 6–35. Homogeneous, consolidated, irregularly shaped lesion with sharp borders is contiguous with the medial sphenoid ridge and appears to distort the anterolateral border of the suprasellar cistern (A). Compare to more extensive, densely enhancing right sphenoid wing meningioma (B and C).

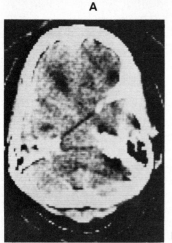

B

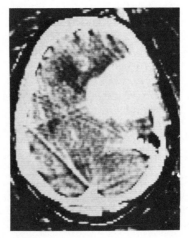

C

defining the presence of arterial encasement. Examples of the importance of the relationship include the following: certain meningiomas may invade the superior sagittal or lateral sinus; sphenoid wing meningiomas may invade the middle or anterior cerebral artery; and encasement of the internal carotid artery by parasellar meningiomas may occur.

Initial studies with CT in evaluating patients with clinical symptoms suggestive of meningioma in whom surgical findings later confirmed this diagnosis have demonstrated 100 percent accuracy and 90 percent specificity in anticipating the finding of a meningioma.[7, 8] In addition, CT has detected meningiomas that were later surgically proven in patients who had no abnormal neurological findings, a normal skull radiogram and a negative isotope scan. Careful necropsy studies have shown that CT was able to detect all meningiomas with a diameter of more than 1.5 centimeters if contrast infusion was performed.

Meningiomas usually show several characteristic density patterns and spatial characteristics in non-infusion studies and with contrast infusion, but those located in the parasellar region, cerebellopontine angle, and orbital and intraventricular regions cannot be differentiated from other tumors without angiography. In 60 percent of meningiomas plain scan shows a homogeneous, densely consolidated, sharply marginated high-density lesion, which is located in the superficial region close to bone, falx or tentorium. In addition, because of the superficial location there are less prominent mass effect and white matter edema than visualized with more deeply infiltrating neoplasms (Fig. 6–35). If the tumor is noncalcified the density is usually 20 to 35 units and if calcified may be greater than 45 units. The attenuation coefficient of the calcification may be as high as 300 but may be only 25 to 40 owing to the partial volume effect. There

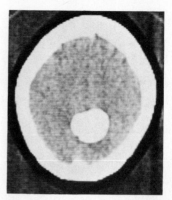

Figure 6–36.   Dense (70 to 100) round, sharply marginated lesion located slightly to the right of the midline over the parietal convexity, with no enhancement. Isotope scan was negative but plain skull radiogram showed prominent hyperostosis and calcification. A densely calcified meningioma with psammomatous calcifications was removed at operation.

may be a mottled or speckled appearance to the high-density region, which may be quite faint. Pathologically, these tumors are highly cellular with minimal psammomatous body formation. Whereas other tumors had densities consistent with calcification these were less cellular and had more dense calcification demonstrated pathologically (Fig. 6–36). The tumor appears to be separated from the un-

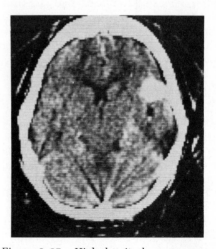

Figure 6–37.   High-density, homogeneous enhancing lesion is contiguous with bone and extends across the sylvian fissure. It does not cause significant ventricular compression and was found to be lateral sphenoid wing meningioma.

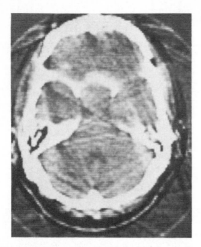

Figure 6–38. Patient had planum sphenoidale meningioma resected one year previously. Plain scan shows large area of midline hyperostosis and low density in the right frontal region. With infusion there is a faint parasellar enhancement but no definite evidence of significant tumor recurrence.

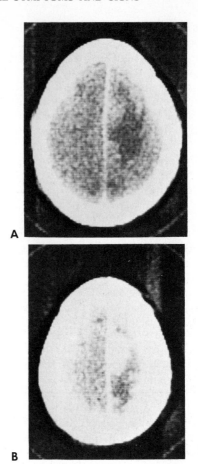

Figure 6–39. CT findings: routine sequence showed a low-density lesion in the right parasagittal area with suggestion of high-density lesion confluent with the falx (A), which was then clearly visualized on additional higher sections (B). The diagnosis of meningioma was confirmed by angiographic and operative findings.

derlying brain and may be contiguous with bone (Fig. 6–37) and, rarely, there may be scan evidence of bone destruction and hyperostosis (Fig. 6–38). Occasionally the meningioma may be located in the high parietal convexity or parasagittal region, in which case the standard scan sections may be normal or show minimal abnormality, consisting of a low-density region. Unless additional sections extending to the vertex are performed, the enhancing lesion may not be detected (Fig. 6–39).

In 30 percent of cases the meningioma appears as a low-density area relative to surrounding parenchyma, and this is most frequent with parasellar, parietal convexity and cerebellopontine angle lesions. Following infusion there may be a dense consolidated or speckled enhancement. In 10 percent of cases the tumor is initially isodense and the only clue to its presence may be dense calcification in the falx and dense enhancement of the meningioma adjacent to the falx (Fig. 6–40). Two angioblastic meningiomas were of low density on plain scan and showed ring-like enhancement, simulating a malignant glioma, but the diagnosis was established by angiography. Cyst formation is rare and evidence of hemorrhage was not seen in unoperated tumors. Surrounding the meningioma is a low-density, crescent-shaped collar or more irregular frondlike extensions that project more deeply and represent cerebral edema. In the majority of cases the edema surrounding meningioma is minimal, and treatment with corticosteroids does not usually alter the clinical symptoms. Pneumographic analysis has suggest-

increment may be 100 percent. The enhanced area sharply delineates the meningioma from the surrounding parenchyma (Fig. 6–41). In rare instances the enhancement pattern is more faint, but the sharp margination and superficial location are most indicative of meningioma. In the

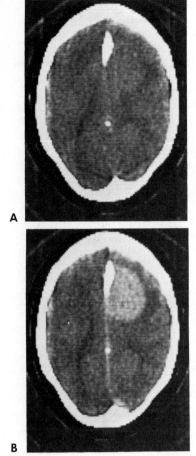

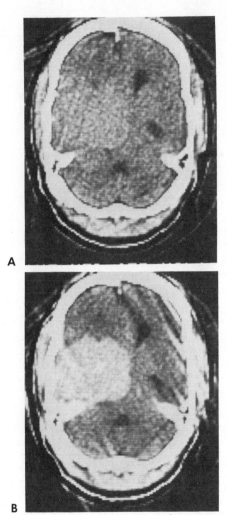

Figure 6–40. Plain scan *(A)* shows dense calcification in the anterior falx but no other region of abnormal density is visualized; following infusion, well-circumscribed nonhomogeneous high-density (25 to 35) area was visualized, mainly in right parasagittal region with slight extension to the left side. Located laterally to this dense lesion is a crescent-shaped lucent collar *(B)*. Angiography showed dense persistent stain with supply from middle meningeal artery.

ed that the lucent collar represents a localized and widened subarachnoid space resulting from the mechanical compression of underlying parenchyma by the tumor.[9]

Following contrast infusion there is dense enhancement, which is immediately maximal and fades rapidly; this is compatible with the density changes due to an enlarged intravascular component. The pattern appears visually homogeneous and the

Figure 6–41. Patient with left-sided rubral tremor. Plain scan *(A)* shows large but only faintly high-density mass occupying the entire left middle fossa, with slight extension to the right of midline. It is compressing and displacing the lateral ventricle to the right side. Following infusion *(B)*, there is dense nonhomogeneous enhancement and no surrounding low-density regions. At operation, an encapsulated meningioma was removed almost entirely, with only slight extension into the left cavernous sinus.

densely calcified lesions there is frequently no evidence of contrast enhancement, and this may be due to less prominent neovascularity in these tumors or to the masking of the

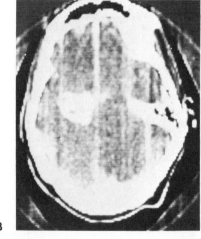

A

B

Figure 6–42. A 37-year-old patient with primary amenorrhea and syncope had experienced possible psychomotor attacks of 12 years' duration and visual disturbance of two years' duration. Findings include evidence of hypopituitarism and bitemporal hemianopia. Skull radiograph showed an enlarged eroded sella; isotope scan was positive in left temporal region. CT findings: a calcified irregularly shaped lesion (A) in inferior temporal region; a dense ring of enhancement (B) was visible. Angiography showed a slight elevation of the middle cerebral artery. At operation no extracerebral lesion was found, but biopsy of calcified area of temporal region showed evidence of an intracerebral meningioma.

enhancement by initial high-attenuation coefficients of the calcification. There is direct correlation between the density of enhancement and the presence of an angiographic stain pattern. Contrast infusion is necessary to differentiate from intracerebral hemorrhage, oligodendroglioma and vascular malformations.

In making the CT diagnosis of meningioma, certain sources of error may arise. In rare instances multiple meningiomas may be present, but the location of the lesion and the pattern of enhancement should permit differentiation from metastatic deposits. Low-density cysts and ringlike enhancement rarely occur in meningioma, especially that of angioblastic type, and in certain instances the presence of a complex ring pattern in a deep-seated intracerebral meningioma may suggest the diagnosis of a glioma (Fig. 6–42). Parasagittal meningiomas and gliomas may present identical CT characteristics and in rare instances may be differentiated only by operative findings. Oligodendrogliomas also appear on the plain scan as high-density calcified masses, but are more irregular in shape than meningiomas, and the nonhomogeneous enhancement, mass effect and deeper location are also points of differentiation from meningioma. Lobar intracerebral hematomas do not enhance or they show only a peripheral rim of enhancement, and their temporal evolution helps to differentiate them from meningioma. Aneurysms usually show ringlike or dense calcification on plain scan with round globular enhancement.

In certain locations, the CT findings are less specific for meningioma, and if angiography does not detect a dural supply or stain, preoperative diagnosis is not possible. Parasellar meningiomas are usually more laterally located in the anterior portion of the suprasellar cistern, show denser homogeneous enhancement and are less likely to show cystic or

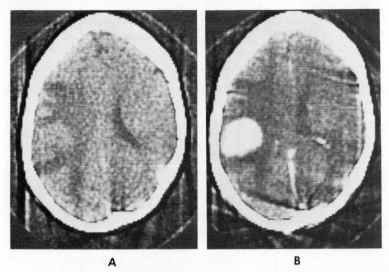

A   B

Figure 6-43. Plain scan (A) shows extensive low-density area with fingerlike projections into the white matter, causing significant left lateral ventricular compression. In addition there is a vague, round, high-density area in the left parietal region, which enhances densely and appears continuous with bone. Although there was dense homogeneous and superficial enhancement, the presence of extensive edema and ventricular compression was less consistent with meningioma (B). Angiography showed dense stain pattern, mostly derived from internal carotid artery, and operative findings demonstrated metastatic adenocarcinoma from the lung. The wide-spread edema would be most unusual for meningioma.

hemorrhagic change than pituitary adenoma. Meningiomas of the cerebellopontine angle may be contiguous with bone, have a lucent collar, and may be visualized only with enhancement study. Intraventricular meningiomas cause ventricular dilatation and appear as high-density, well-circumscribed round lesions but may not be differentiated from other tumors in this location. Hemangioblastomas, which are solid, are highly vascular and may be difficult to differentiate pathologically from angioblastic meningiomas. These tumors occur predominantly in the posterior fossa. On CT they appear as round enhancing dense lesions with margins that are slightly less sharp than those of meningiomas, but angiography is required for differentiation. Despite the relative specificity of the CT findings of meningioma, it must be remembered that metastases and gliomas may occasionally have identical appearances, and although it was hoped that CT would be specific for tumor diagnosis, this is not always the case (Fig. 6-43).

CT is the most reliable diagnostic study to evaluate both the immediate postoperative complications and the adequacy of surgical resection and evidence of tumor recurrence. Differentiation of residual meningioma from intracerebral hematoma or necrotic postoperative brain change may be difficult because all may show evidence of enhancement, but in the latter conditions this is characteristically peripheral ring enhancement (Fig. 6-44). The presence of high-density metallic clips may produce a sunburst artifact, which may obscure evidence of tumor recurrence. Following surgical resection, seizures or progressive deficit may develop and this may be evidence of a postsurgical defect or recurrence. The CT finding of a low-density area without enhancement or mass effect is 100 percent effective in excluding tumor recurrence.

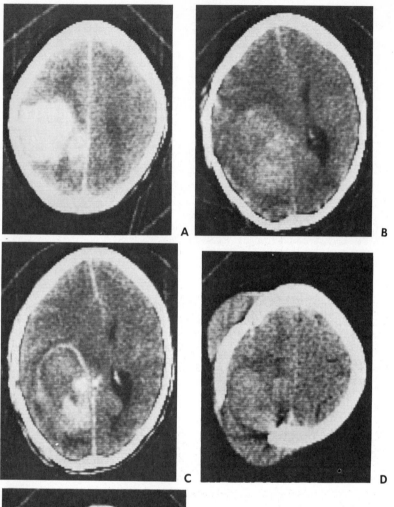

A   **B**

C   **D**

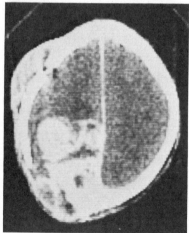

E

Figure 6–44.   A 35-year-old man who initially presented with a history of episodic headache of several months' duration and paresthesias in right arm, on examination, had bilateral papilledema. Isotope scan showed an uptake in left parietal region. Initial CT scan showed large, round, homogeneous high-density enhancing lesion in the left parietal region, with surrounding low density. The lesion produced ventricular displacement and compression (A). Angiography showed homogeneous stain with supply from dural vessels, and a large parietal convexity meningioma was surgically removed. Post-operatively, the patient's level of consciousness did not improve and the craniotomy site was tense and slightly bulging. Ten days after surgery, CT scan showed vague high-density area with surrounding low-density region, causing bulging of falx and left ventricular compression on plain scan (B) and ring enhancement with one large dense area of enhancement (C). This was compatible with residual tumor and ring hematoma. Despite treatment with corticosteroids the patient did not improve, and repeat study showed extracranial bulging enhancing mass and dense intracranial enhancement, causing significant mass effect consistent with possible malignant sarcomatous neoplastic transformation (D and E), and this was confirmed by pathological findings.

REFERENCES

1. Sauer J, Fieback D, Otto H, et al: Comparative studies of cerebral scintography, angiography, and encephalography for diagnosis of meningioma. Neuroradiology 2:102, 1971.
2. Gold LH, Kieffer SA, Peterson HD: Intracranial meningiomas: a retrospective analysis of the diagnostic value of plain skull films. Neurology 19:873, 1969.
3. Sheldon JJ, Smoak W, Gargano FP: Dynamic scintography in intracranial meningiomas. Radiology 109:109, 1973.
4. Banna M, Appleby A: Some observations on the angiography of supratentorial meningiomas. Clin Radiol 20:375, 1969.
5. Stattin S: Significance of some angiographic signs of intracranial meningiomas. Acta Radiol (Diagn) 5:530, 1966.
6. Newton TH, Potts DG: Radiology of the Skull and Brain. CV Mosby, St. Louis, 1971. pp 2265–2275.
7. Claveria LE, Sutton D, Tress BM: The radiological diagnosis of meningiomas; the impact of EMI scanning. Br J Radiol 50:15, 1977.
8. New PFJ, Scott WR, Schnur JA: CT in the diagnosis of primary and metastatic intracranial neoplasms. Radiology 114:75, 1975.
9. Sigel RM, Messina AV: CT: The anatomic basis of the zone of diminished density surrounding meningiomas. Am J Roentgenol 127:139, 1976.

Glioma

The histological classification of cerebral hemispheric gliomas presents many problems because the majority of these tumors do not show uniform pathological characteristics. Biopsy specimens obtained from one area of the tumor may indicate low-grade malignancy, while excluding an adjacent area that has extensive changes indicative of malignant neoplasm. These astrocytomas infiltrate deeply and irregularly with fingerlike projections into the region of the corpus callosum, septum pellucidum, basal ganglion and thalamus. Low-grade gliomas frequently contain dense clumps of calcification and uncommonly undergo necrosis or hemorrhage. If cysts are present, they consist of a single smooth-walled cavity with a mural nodule of tumors; this occurs most commonly with cystic cerebellar gliomas.[1] The malignant astrocytomas also show degenerative cystic spaces that result from breakdown of tumor tissue, forming a confluence of microcysts with xanthochromic proteinaceous fluid.

In low-grade gliomas microscopic cellular density and morphology are only slightly different from those of surrounding tissue, and these tumors are not highly vascularized as are more malignant astrocytomas. The presence of neovascularity is not always evidence of malignant degeneration because pilocytic astrocytomas of the hypothalamus, optic chiasm and third ventricle may be highly vascularized but remain well circumscribed with little tendency to degenerative change or cellular anaplasia.

Gliomas of the brain stem resemble low grade diffusely infiltrating hemispheric astrocytomas but may show extensive vascularity, with interspersed areas of hemorrhage and necrosis. Despite their usually benign cellular architecture, even low-grade hemispheric and pontine gliomas may show some degree of anaplastic change, whereas this is rarely present in cerebellar astrocytomas.

The more malignant gliomas frequently contain multiple confluent areas of microcysts, hemorrhage, necrosis or infarction.[1, 2] If these pathological changes are extensive enough, the tumor is classified as glioblastoma multiforme. This highly malignant tumor arises in the deep white matter and extends deeply into surrounding nuclear masses and to superficial cortical areas. Grossly, the tumor may appear to be well circumscribed, but the margins are poorly defined without any encapsulation and the most characteristic feature is a highly variegated multiform surface showing solid tumor interspersed with degenerative changes.

Diagnosis of the low-grade glioma may not always be achieved with isotope scan and EEG. As the biological activity, vascularity and degree of anaplasia increase, so does the probability of localized scan uptake. Since 25 to 50 percent of gliomas are scan-negative, this limits its use as a sensitive and reliable screening procedure for these neoplasms.[3] Morena reported results of isotope scan in the diagnosis of glioma: Grade I was positive in only 50 percent, Grade II in 75 percent, Grade III in 80 percent and Grade IV in 96 percent. In these cases the presence of tumor stain seen with angiography correlated with positive isotope scan only in Grade IV glioma.[4] Despite the presence of a high degree of anaplasia, biological activity and neovascularity in glioblastoma multiforme, 11 percent of patients initially had a negative isotope scan when the patient was symptomatic, and this became positive over several weeks to months. Not infrequently there may be rapid progression of symptoms, and the scan suddenly becomes positive, which is suggestive of tumor apoplexy, but pathological analysis may fail to detect evidence of hemorrhage.

EEG shows a polymorphic delta slow wave pattern in 93 percent of cases of glioblastoma but occasionally bilateral EEG abnormalities may make localization and lateralization difficult. With low-grade glioma focal spike and spike–slow wave discharges are more common than a polymorphic slow wave pattern, and in some patients who harbor low-grade glioma and present with generalized seizures EEG may be normal or show a diffuse slow wave pattern. Twenty-five percent of low-grade gliomas show radiographic calcification, whereas this is seen in only 2 percent of glioblastomas, and this finding may suggest the location of the neoplasm.[5] There is no relationship between morphology or the extent of the calcification and the degree of malignancy. In addition, histological evidence of dense calcification occurred in 11 percent of gliomas, twice the number that demonstrated radiographic evidence of calcification (5.5 percent).

In hemispheric gliomas, angiography usually shows the major mass effect but does not demonstrate the full extent of the tumor. Since these tumors are more extensively infiltrating, they may require air study to delineate the full extent of tumor growth. Several studies have emphasized that negative air study and angiogram do not exclude the presence of glioma.[6, 7] In 25 percent of patients who have been found to harbor a glioma and who initially presented with seizures without any other neurological findings, initial studies were negative, but when focal neurological findings develop, the angiogram usually becomes positive.

Characteristic angiographic findings in low-grade glioma include evidence of an avascular mass without abnormal tumor vessels and prolongation of circulation time through the tumor. If the tumor is more diffuse and infiltrating there may be minimal local mass effect and diagnosis may require air study. Anaplastic astrocytoma and glioblastoma multiforme show an extensive vascular pattern with abundant irregularly sized feeding vessels and prominent early-draining veins. In one third of tumors, abnormal vessels are located at the periphery and surrounding the avascular masss. In other cases the only manifestation of abnormal circulation is the presence of an early-draining vein, which may occur in metastatic lesions and in non-neoplastic vascular conditions. In rare instances, malignant gliomas have a diffuse homogeneous stain, but the presence of irregularity in the vessels supplying the tumor permits differentiation from meningioma. In 15 percent of glioblastomas angiography shows only an avascular mass without abnormal circulation, and specific pathological diagnosis requires surgical biopsy.[6]

Initial studies utilizing CT in the diagnosis of supratentorial glioma reported a diagnostic error of 35 percent, and this compared with a false-negative incidence of 16 percent with conventional neurodiagnostic studies, especially for the low-grade glioma.[7] Comparison of CT with other neurodiagnostic studies in the diagnosis of malignant glioma showed that CT was capable of earlier diagnosis, as 50 percent of patients had no localizing neurological signs or evidence of intracranial hypertension, whereas isotope scan was negative in 40 percent, and 30 percent had no localizing or lateralizing EEG findings. Of the low-grade gliomas documented by CT, isotope scan was negative in 60 percent and EEG showed no lateralized abnormality in 50 percent. The most frequent presenting clinical sign was generalized seizure without any other neurological findings. In no case was CT negative and the presence of glioma confirmed by EEG and isotope scan findings.

Huckman attempted to correlate the CT pattern of plain and contrast studies with the degree of malignancy of the glioma. Glioblastoma showed the most marked variation in density pattern and enhancement characteristics within the same tumor, and this reflected its pathological multiformity. Grade II and III gliomas showed more homogeneous density charac-

teristics on plain scan, with diffuse and homogeneous or ringlike patterns of enhancement. Frequently there were cystic components. Low-grade gliomas were of low density with irregular margins and showed minimal enhancement and mass effect.[8] Thomson analyzed the results of 100 gliomas diagnosed by CT and classified the plain scan features. In 78 percent there was mixed high and low density, 8 percent had homogeneous high density, 14 percent homogeneous low density, and none were isodense. The mixed-density pattern was most characteristic of the malignant glioma, and low density was visualized in more low-grade gliomas. The finding of a homogeneous high-density pattern may also occur in malignant glioma, but when it occurs it is more consistent with meningioma or metastatic lesion. Contrast infusion utilizing 50 ml of Conray was performed in 77 per cent and enhancement was detected in 96 percent. The malignant glioma showed rimlike or patchy dense enhancement, whereas low-grade glioma showed less intense and occasionally no enhancement.[9]

Experience with CT has indicated that the low-grade and malignant gliomas may be reliably differentiated. The less malignant gliomas are usually of low density, which is usually homogeneous but may be speckled; they infiltrate deeply into the white matter with frondlike projections. Less frequently these lesions may have sharp and well-defined margins and show variable degrees of mass effect and enhancement. Despite their frequent large size and significant mass effect, there may be minimal accompanying edema (Fig. 6–45). These gliomas frequently show pathological evidence of calcification; but skull radiograph infrequently detects this. The high density areas on plain scan consistent with calcification are visualized by CT in 40 percent of low-grade gliomas (Fig. 6–46). Enhancement is detected in 35 percent of low-grade gliomas and may consist of a diffuse faint pattern or

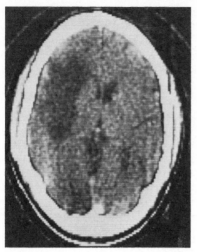

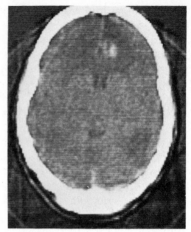

Figure 6–45.   A 32-year-old man initially presented with single right focal motor seizure but had no abnormal neurological findings. EEG showed a large delta pattern involving most of left hemisphere but isotope scan was negative. Angiography showed an avascular mass in the left temporal region, and air study demonstrated compression and displacement of anterior frontal and temporal horn, which was presumed to be due to an infiltrating glioma. Because of its location in the dominant hemisphere, the patient was irradiated without obtaining histological diagnosis, and the patient's seizures increased in frequency. CT findings: large irregularly shaped nonhomogeneous low-density lesion in left frontal-temporal region, causing significant ventricular compression and displacement. This is consistent with low-grade infiltrating glioma.

Figure 6–46.   Patient presented with headache and progressively increasing difficulty with gait. Findings included early bilateral papilledema and spasticity in the legs, with bilateral Babinski sign. Skull radiograph and isotope scan were negative, and EEG showed monorhythmic frontal delta pattern. CT findings: bifrontal mottled low-density pattern with compression of the anterior frontal horn of the lateral ventricle, with single high-density calcified region and no enhancement. Operative finding was extensive infiltrating Grade I glioma.

well-delineated low-density cyst with a dense superficial nodule of enhancement (Fig. 6–48). The malignant astrocytoma and glioblastoma show a more characteristic pattern,

a focal, round, small high-density nodule, whereas this is absent in 65 percent of cases (Fig. 6–47). If the enhancement is superficial and nodular, differentiation from meningioma or metastases is not always possible.

Our findings confirm the results of other centers that since the introduction of CT the incidence of low-grade glioma is 20 to 30 percent of all gliomas compared to 5 to 7 percent demonstrated with conventional studies. Grade II and III gliomas show a more variable appearance but usually show more significant ventricular distortion and displacement with irregular frondlike projections of low density interspersed with high-density regions and more prominent enhancement. A second pattern shows a

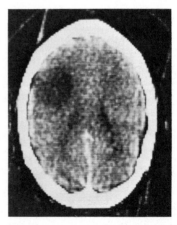

Figure 6–47.   Patient who developed generalized seizures only; EEG and isotope scan were negative. CT findings: speckled nonhomogeneous well-marginated round mass, which was causing no ventricular displacement and does not enhance. Operative finding was Grade II cystic astrocytoma.

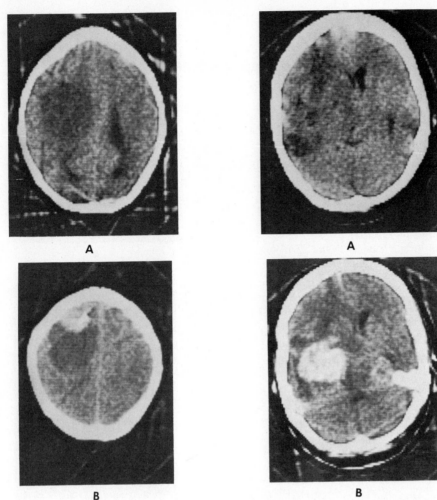

A

B

Figure 6–48. Patient initially presented with several episodes of sudden onset of weakness involving right and left arms, which rapidly cleared. Isotope scan was negative and EEG showed large left frontal-parietal slow wave pattern. CT findings: large round low-density lesion compressing body of lateral ventricle (A). Note striking dense superficial cortical enhancement pattern of lesion, which appears contiguous to bone (B). At operation a cystic glioma was found.

A

B

Figure 6–49. Plain scan shows admixture of low- and high-density regions, which cause significant mass effect (A). Following infusion, there is dense, globular, deeply located enhancement pattern (B), consistent with diagnosis of glioblastoma multiforme.

which includes the following features: (1) mixed high- and low-density regions in both superficial and deep areas on plain scan; (2) irregular margins with significant mass effect and surrounding edema, consisting of cystic regions with mottled low-density admixed with high-density hemorrhagic and necrotic components; (3) enhancement that may be dense, irregular, complex or ring pattern. The heterogeneous low- and high-density pattern is quite characteristic of the glioblastoma (Fig. 6–49). Quite surprisingly 15 percent of glioblastomas showed CT evidence of calcification (Fig. 6–50). Frequently, the CT pattern predicts the multiformity of the pathological specimen and delineates the cystic, necrotic

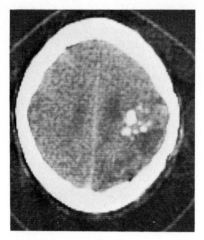

Figure 6–50. Patient with pathologically proven glioblastoma multiforme, which had been surgically treated; the tumor showed evidence of calcification. CT findings six months later: low-density lesion in right parieto-temporal region with one area of enhancement and several contiguous regions of round dense calcification.

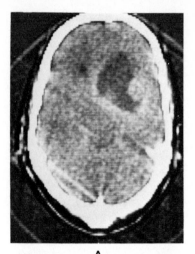

A

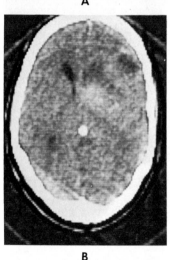

B

Figure 6–51. A and B, Patient presented with headache and change in personality over two-month interval. On examination there were no focal neurological findings. Isotope scan was negative and EEG demonstrated delta focus in right temporal region. CT findings: following infusion, there was diffuse enhancement pattern in superficial region and enhancement along medial border of a cyst. At operation biopsy and cyst drainage of glioblastoma multiforme were performed.

and hemorrhagic regions of the tumor (Fig. 6–51).

The ring or rim pattern of enhancement surrounding central low density is not a specific finding, but several features differentiate the ring of malignant glioma from that seen in infarction, hematoma, abscess or metastases. The malignant glioma shows either multiple irregular or complex rings with variable thickness of the enhancement in different portions of the ring (Fig. 6–52). The central low-density core may be a cyst component, in which case the enhancing rim is thin or contains necrotic material and the rim is more dense. In addition, Davis has indicated that the centrally nonenhancing region may not be necrotic or cystic but may represent failure of contrast to perfuse through to the center of solid tumor.[10]

A retrospective study of 50 cases in which CT scan showed a single enhancing lesion and in which the diagnosis was further established by angiography, surgical biopsy or necropsy study revealed that there were no absolute criteria for diagno-

sis of glioma. In 12 percent of cases glioma was confused with sarcoma, meningioma, metastases or abscess, but in no case was an infarction or intracerebral hematoma confused with glioma by CT analysis. In all cases, glioma showed an abnormality on plain scan with ventricular distortion or displacement, and no glioma

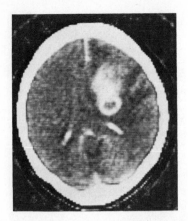

Figure 6–52. Patient presented with progressive left-sided weakness; EEG was consistent with right frontal parietal lesion, and isotope scan was positive. CT findings: preinfusion study shows large irregularly shaped low-density region in right hemisphere with fingerlike projections, compressing and displacing the lateral ventricle to the right side. Following infusion there are several thick complex circular enhancing rings with lucent core. Pattern is consistent with malignant astrocytoma, and this was confirmed by surgical biopsy.

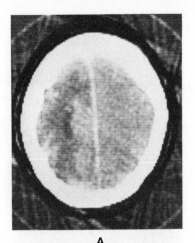

A

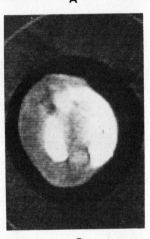

B

Figure 6–53. Patient presented with episodes of stiffening of right leg; EEG and isotope scan demonstrated an abnormality in the left parasagittal region. CT findings: irregular low-density area in left parasagittal region (A) which shows dense enhancement on highest section (B). At operation this was found to be a glioma attached to the dura rather than meningioma.

was isodense, as has been reported by others.[11]

In addition, a nonenhancing cystic glioma cannot be differentiated from a non-neoplastic cyst, and this requires surgical biopsy. Conversely, some epidermoid cysts may show a thin rim of enhancement adjacent to the cyst in the compressed normal parenchyma and not in a nodular or ring pattern, as in glioma. Rarely, gliomas have regular edges with a wedge shape, but this is more consistent with infarction, and the dense enhancement of an infarction is confined to specific vascular territory and has little mass effect. If an angioma spontaneously thromboses, it may be confused with glioma, and this may account for some long-term radiation responses in astrocytoma.[12] If the lesion occurs in a superficial location, it may be identical to meningioma, and differentiation requires angiography (Fig. 6–53). In very extensive gliomas there may be a single nodule of enhancement located superficially, a large amount of edema, and linear gyral enhancement, and differentiation from metastatic tumor is not possible (Fig. 6–54).

Ependymomas have CT features similar to those of malignant glioma, but these are frequently intraventricular in location and may not be differentiated from centrally located glioblastoma. Gangliogliomas are usually well-circumscribed and marginated masses, which may be located supratentorially or in the third

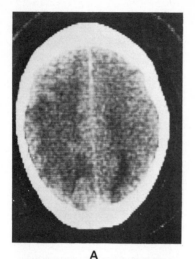

A

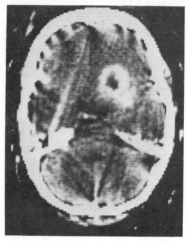

Figure 6–55. Patient had left hemiparesis; EEG showed right frontal delta focus with spike pattern, and angiography showed deep right frontal avascular mass. CT findings: preinfusion study demonstrated round thick walled mass with lucent core distorting the right side of the suprasellar cistern; lesion did not enhance. At operation, a well-circumscribed cystic ganglioglioma without calcification was removed from the interior surface of the right frontal lobe.

Oligodendrogliomas are a distinct type of glial tumor which has certain characteristic pathological features that contribute to its CT scan appearance. The majority of tumors are intracerebral but occasionally they may be adherent to dura. These tumors may be well vascularized and this

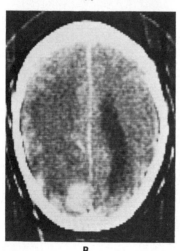

B

Figure 6–54. This patient developed mild right-sided weakness and right-sided headache. Findings included right hemiparesis and homonymous hemianopia. EEG showed large left hemispheric delta pattern, and isotope scan was positive in left occipital region. CT findings: extensive mottled low-density lesion with irregular edges causing marked ventricular displacement (A). With infusion there is dense round enhancement in occipital region and linear enhancement more anteriorly (B). At operation a solid intracerebral tumor located in the left paramedian occipital region and well demarcated from the normal parenchyma was removed. Pathological findings suggested either primary intracranial teratoma or metastatic tumor of testicular origin.

ventricular region. CT appearance is that of a high-density round mass with a lucent core (Fig. 6–55). Primary sarcoma also appears similar to malignant glioma, and in one case angiography was necessary to define its extra-axial location.

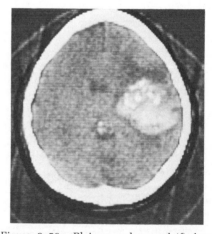

Figure 6–56. Plain scan shows calcified mass in right temporal region (40 to 50), surrounded by irregularly shaped low-density region, with marked shift of lateral ventricular system to the left side. Following contrast infusion there is no enhancement; at operation an oligodendroglioma was found.

may account for the occurrence of hemorrhagic episodes. Cystic degeneration occurs in 20 percent.[13] The frontal region is the most usual location and they may extend bilaterally via the corpus callosum or into the temporal lobe. The most characteristic feature is the dense calcification which occurs in 70 percent of these tumors and is a relative indicator of the tendency for oligodendrogliomas to progress very insidiously.

Despite the histological findings of mitosis, anaplasia and vascular proliferation, these tumors are slow-growing. Patients may initially present with a seizure disorder, which may be well controlled for many years until focal neurological signs develop. Plain skull radiograph shows calcification within the tumor in 50 percent of cases, but the incidence of microscopic calcification is even higher. Because of the slow growth pattern, results of isotope scan have been disappointing. Angiography usually shows an avascular mass but occasionally early-draining veins, which are dilated, may be detected, but no arteriovenous shunting is seen. Preoperative diagnosis is not always possible. CT appearance is relatively characteristic: plain scan shows clumps of high-density areas, which reflect calcification, and these may be interspersed with low-density

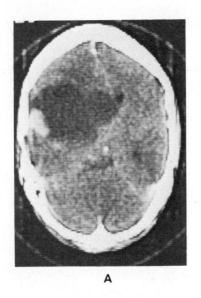

A

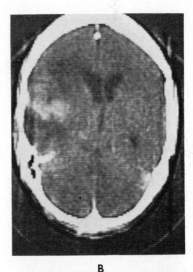

B

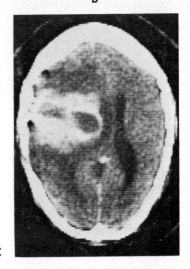

C

Figure 6–57. Patient presented with rapidly progressive right-sided weakness and headache. Neurological findings included right hemiparesis, confusional state, motor aphasia and papilledema. Isotope scan showed uptake in left temporal region, and EEG showed large slow wave pattern involving entire left hemisphere. Initial CT findings: large well-marginated low-density area in left hemisphere; this extended across the midline and was consistent with large cyst. Following contrast infusion there was dense homogeneous enhancement adjacent to lateral border of cyst (A). At operation, cyst drained and glioblastoma multiforme was subtotally removed. The patient also received irradiation and steroids, but there was little change in his clinical condition. Repeat study showed smaller size of the cyst but dense enhancement (B). The patient progressively became more obtunded and scan showed increased size and density of enhancement with increase in the size of the lesion (C).

areas. With contrast there is faint enhancement in the surrounding area (Fig. 6–56). Since hemorrhage may occur in oligodendroglioma, determination of attenuation value of plain scan is important.

Following surgery, radiotherapy or chemotherapy, CT is the most reliable study to detect tumor recurrence or progression; in several instances detection preceded clinical signs of neurological deterioration. An increase in tumor size, ventricular distortion and displacement, central lucency and contrast enhancement correlate most directly with clinical evidence of recurrence and deterioration (Fig. 6–57). In 50 percent of patients with a malignant glioma, neither EEG nor isotope scan showed evidence of progression of the tumor, whereas CT was 95 percent reliable. This compares with only 40 percent detection rate for isotope scan, and this latter study did not permit the clinical-anatomical-pathological correlation which is possible with CT. This compares to the 85 to 90 percent correlation of results of CT scan and clinical pattern of neurological deterioration reported by Norman.[14] In patients who have previously undergone craniotomy and radiotherapy and who develop neurological symptoms, the lack of mass effect or enhancement is strongly against tumor recurrence.

REFERENCES

1. Russell DS, Rubenstein LJ: Pathology of Tumors of the Nervous System. Arnold Ltd, London, 1971. pp 109–160.
2. *Ibid.* pp 134–135.
3. Finkemeyer H, Pfingst E, Zulch KJ: Astrocytomas of the cerebral hemispheres. *In:* Handbook of Clinical Neurology, Vol 18, PJ Vinken, GW Bruyn (eds). North Holland Publishing Co., Amsterdam, 1975. pp 29–33.
4. Moreno JB, DeLand FH: Brain scanning in the diagnosis of astrocytomas of the brain. J Nucl Med 12:107, 1971.
5. Kalan C, Burrows EH: Calcification in intracranial gliomata. Br J Radiol 35:589, 1962.
6. Weinberg P: Neuroradiologic aspects of gliomas. *In:* Recent Results in Cancer Research. J Hekmatpanah (ed). Springer-Verlag, New York, 1975. pp 65–78.
7. Di Giovanni C: Relative value of air studies, angiography and radioisotope scanning in the diagnosis of glial introcranial tumors. Progr Neurol Surg 2:292, 1968.
8. Huckman MS: CT in relation to diagnosis of gliomas. *In* Recent Results in Cancer Research. Gliomas. J Hekmatpanah (ed). Springer-Verlag, New York, 1974. pp 79–87.
9. Thomson JLA: CT and the diagnosis of glioma. Clin Radiol 27:431, 1976.
10. Davis DO: CT in the diagnosis of supratentorial tumors. Semin Roentgenol 12:97, 1977.
11. New PFJ, Scott WR: Computed Tomography of the Brain and Orbit. Williams and Wilkins, Baltimore, 1975. p 441.
12. Kramer RA, Wing SD: CT of angiographically occult cerebral vascular malformations. Radiology 123:649, 1977.
13. Mansuy L, Thierry A, Tommasi M.: Oligodendrogliomas. *In:* Handbook of Clinical Neurology, Vol 18, PJ Vinken, GW Bruyn (eds). North Holland Publishing Co., Amsterdam, 1975. pp 81–103.
14. Norman D, Enzmann DR, Levin V, et al: CT in the evaluation of malignant glioma before and after therapy. Radiology 121:85, 1976.

Chapter 7

Studies in Patients with Suspected Metastatic Disease

The relative incidence of intracranial metastatic disease is dependent upon whether the data is derived from necropsy or neurosurgical studies. Complete necropsy studies in patients who died of cancer revealed that 38 percent had brain metastases, whereas Posner reported that 10 percent of patients with systemic cancer have necropsy manifestations of CNS involvement.[1, 2] These findings are contrasted with the lower incidence of 2 to 4 percent of metastatic lesions obtained from certain neurosurgical reports. They include cases that have been selected for surgery based on clinical evidence and neurodiagnostic studies that indicate the patient is in good general medical condition and is believed to have a solitary intracerebral lesion.[3, 4] With refinement of diagnostic techniques, including isotope scan and angiography, a similar incidence of 11.2 percent of proven metastatic disease was reported, based on necropsy studies obtained from a neurology service and biopsy specimens from a neurosurgical service.[5] This recent increase in operative cases reflects an alteration in the early belief that surgery was of no potential benefit and carried a high operative mortality.

The critical clinical problems that dominate the study of brain metastases are the detection of the presence and location of the intracranial mass, determination of whether it is a solitary or multiple lesion, and analysis of its pathological features to determine if it is a primary intracranial lesion. Paillais and Pellet believe that 20 percent of patients clinically suspected of having an intracranial mass will be found to have a metastatic lesion, and 60 percent of these will be judged to be operable with surgical results benefiting the quality and length of patient survival.[5]

Garde combined the results of 10 large series of metastases and found that of 420 necropsy examinations 260 had multiple lesions and 160 had single lesions.[5] In 17 to 28 percent of cases, the CNS is the only source of secondary involvement, and this is most frequently observed in carcinoma of the lung; in 5 percent of surgically documented metastatic lesions no primary source may be detected even with careful necropsy examination.[3, 5]

Metastatic deposits may involve either the meninges, the parenchyma or both; meningeal involvement is most common with reticular and breast neoplasms, whereas parenchymal metastasis is most frequent in carcinoma of the lung, breast, skin and kidney. It is believed that tumor cells embolize through the arterial system and this explains their propensity for the middle cerebral artery distribution, with 55 percent located posterior to the Rolandic fissure, 26 percent in the anterior temporal lobe and 19 percent in the frontal region. Approximately 20 percent occur in the posterior fossa, but if a cerebellar metastasis is present there are frequently accompanying supratentorial deposits; this has important surgical implications because cerebellar metastases have been removed with good results.

The frequency with which certain visceral carcinomas metastasize to the CNS is quite variable. In 10 to 40 percent of cases the CNS lesion is the first manifestation of the systemic carcinoma. In certain neoplasms, including those of breast and renal origin, CNS involvement may not be detected until many years after detection and treatment of the primary carcinoma. In some cases the interval may be so remote (10 to 20 years) that a primary intracranial tumor may be suspected rather than a metastasis. In addition, 32 percent of patients with visceral carcinoma have asymptomatic lesions demonstrated at necropsy; one half of those with breast tumors and one fifth of those with lung tumors have clinically unsuspected intracranial deposits.

The clinical presentation may cause diagnostic difficulties, as the patient presents with either quite rapid (47 percent) or insidious (53 percent) onset of neurological symptoms.[5] Seizures are presenting symptom in 20 percent of cases but may be of nonfocal onset with no interictal neurological deficit. In those patients who present with a more slowly progressive onset fewer than one half complain of focal weakness or language disturbance; one third are aware of no presenting symptoms and are brought to the hospital by relatives who complain that the patient has had a marked personality and behavioral change. Neurological signs depend upon the location of the metastatic lesion, but frequently mentation is altered owing to extensive cerebral edema or multiple small metastatic deposits. Other patients present with cranial nerve dysfunction or hydrocephalus due to carcinomatous infiltration of the meninges and ventricular obstruction.[1] Recent CT studies of intracranial metastases have demonstrated a much higher incidence of patients who have no neurological findings, and the presence of a clinically silent intracranial lesion alters treatment and prognosis.

The clinical course is frequently characterized by progressive worsening but may be more varied, with a relatively characteristic three-stage illness.[5] Initially there is sudden onset of focal or generalized neurological deficit caused by an arterial neoplastic embolism, which is followed by dramatic remission for several weeks as the acute vascular insult resolves (Fig. 7–1). Tumor growth continues and there is then a gradual worsening which may be exacerbated by the development of cerebral edema. This course may occur in 21 percent of cases, and a similar clinical pattern has been observed with other neoplasms, intracerebral hematoma and subdural hematoma. Less commonly, metastatic lesions may simulate transient ischemic episodes due to exacerbations of edema and dynamic pressure shifts which resolve. In other patients the course may simulate that of stroke syndrome, as a result of hemorrhagic foci in the tumor. Conventional neurodiagnostic studies may detect the presence of metastatic lesions that are symptomatic and rarely may detect clinically silent metastatic lesions, but the abnormalities are frequently not specific enough to differentiate from primary intracranial tumors or non-neoplastic conditions. Plain skull radiograms may show bone lesions in patients who do not also have parenchymal involvement, and only the presence of a pineal shift and erosion of the stella, consistent with increased intracranial pressure, is indicative of an intracerebral lesion. In patients who have metastasis to the sella, radiographic sella changes may be similar to those of

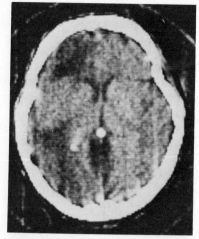

A

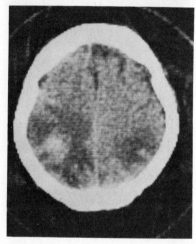

B

Figure 7–1. A 60-year-old man had several transient episodes of numbness in his right hand lasting five minutes. They resolved completely, but then he suddenly developed right hemiparesis several days later that did not resolve. EEG showed focal slow-wave pattern over the left parieto-occipital region, but isotope scan was negative. Initial CT scan showed two separate wedge-shaped low-density regions in the left frontal and parieto-occipital region which did not enhance (A). The patient's deficit cleared, but chest radiograph showed a hilar mass consistent with bronchogenic carcinoma. After initial improvement, the weakness became progressively more severe, and scan showed definite enhancement consistent with metastatic neoplasm, with a third lesion in the right parieto-occipital region (B).

increased intracranial pressure. Since the course of symptomatic metastatic intracranial disease is frequently short, the incidence of abnormal skull radiographic findings is low; Posner reported that only 11 percent had radiographic evidence of metastases and only 6.2 percent had sella erosion or pineal shift.[1]

EEG may detect the presence of a focal lesion, but unless two or more independent focal abnormalities are detected, there are no specific findings to suggest metastasis. In patients with suspected metastatic disease who have altered mentation with lateralizing neurological signs this may be due to a metabolic, toxic, or electrolyte abnormality not directly related to the neoplasm, and EEG findings may demonstrate a focal abnormality. EEG has been used as a noninvasive screening procedure in patients with systemic carcinoma who are neurologically asymptomatic, but results of several studies have shown that focal EEG abnormalities correlate only with the presence of a clinically symptomatic lesion.

Strang reported that in patients with a single supratentorial metastatic deposit, the size of the lesion and the presence of neurological findings were the most important factors in determining the frequency of EEG abnormalities. Among those with a lesion more than 2 cm in diameter, 81 percent had neurological signs and an accompanying focal delta slow wave pattern. Of five metastatic lesions of this size not detected by EEG four were neurologically silent. Of those cases correctly lateralized by EEG examination, all were larger than 2 cm except for one, which consisted of a 1.5 cm nodule associated with a larger area of hemorrhage and edema. In several cases of suspected metastatic lesion, the patients had focal neurological signs but EEG was negative and necropsy examination showed no tumor.[6]

In patients with clinically symptomatic supratentorial lesions, 4.2 percent had normal EEG and 16 percent had bilateral or diffuse abnormalities, whereas 80 percent showed a characteristic focal delta pattern. The delta pattern was most well defined in neoplasms that involved both gray and white matter. In lesions with a superficial cortical location with minimal deeper extension, there was frequent absence of a delta pattern and normal EEG or only a focal spike pattern; this was seen in 17 percent of cases. In infratentorial metastasis, EEG is usually normal although there may be rhythmic temporal or occipital slow wave disturbances, usually due to intracranial hypertension.

Isotope scan may detect and localize the presence of single or multiple lesions more reliably than EEG. The finding of multiple lesions makes the diagnosis of metastases most likely, although differential diagnosis must include abscesses, cerebral emboli, hemorrhages and demyelinating disorders. If isotope scan localizes a single homogeneous uptake, differentiation from other conditions is not always possible, and even the relatively specific "doughnut" pattern suggestive of central necrosis is sometimes seen in other conditions.[7]

Isotope scan may detect 70 to 90 percent of symptomatic lesions; false negatives occur with lesions located in the temporal or midline region, including the posterior fossa and sella region. The sensitivity is dependent upon the size of the lesion — visualization is poor with deposits less than 2 cm. Boller determined that the lower limit of sensitivity was 10 cubic centimeters, equivalent to a sphere 2.67 cm in diameter, with 95 percent accuracy for lesions exceeding this size. Multiple smaller and confluent lesions may be detected even if individually they are smaller than the usual lower limit of detectability.[8] Isotope scan is less sensitive in detecting clinically silent lesions. In patients with carcinoma of the lung McCormick found only one positive study in 43 neurologically intact patients; this is in agreement with other studies which have shown 2 percent positive studies in these patients.[9]

With demonstration of a single lesion, isotope scan is rarely diagnostic, but sequential scans may demonstrate a characteristic temporal profile for metastases, with maximal uptake occurring at 24 hours. Schlesinger demonstrated the value of sequential scanning in metastatic disease, with additional information available at 24 hours that was not obtained in the 3-hour scan in 73 percent of cases. The 24-hour scan was positive in 29 percent of those with a negative 3-hour study; additional lesions were detected in late scan in 20 percent, and the 24-hour study more effectively demonstrated tracer localization in 24 percent when early scan had been only suspicious. The images of the cerebellar and temporal lesions were more definitive, since overlying temporal muscle uptake and vascular uptake in the posterior fossa had washed out when delayed scan was performed. Sequential scans are helpful in evaluating patients who present with sudden onset of neurological deficit and who have a history of carcinoma, since in cerebral infarction the 3-hour uptake is greater.[10] Isotope scan is more sensitive than angiography in detection of metastasis. This may be positive before mass effect or abnormal vascularity are visualized. In one series angiography was positive in 85 percent compared to 88 percent for isotope scan.[1]

If isotope scan demonstrated a single lesion, angiography has previously been required to make an accurate preoperative diagnosis. In one study there was angiographic evidence of multiple lesions in only 10 percent of cases, and this technique only rarely detects clinically silent lesions. Angiography may show an avascular mass, but 50 percent have an abnormal vascular pattern including a nodular stain with homogeneous opacification seen in the arterial capillary phase, the pattern pseudoglioblastomas form with early-draining veins and irregular nonhomogeneous stain, an irregular poorly margined stain seen in the capillary-venous stage, and an avascular nonopacified central portion with peripheral ring stain.[3]

There is no correlation between the extent and pattern of vascularity and the primary tumor, with the exception that metastatic hypernephroma appears as a highly vascular lesion with abundant tortuous vessels and a homogeneous peripheral stain surrounding an avascular core. Based on the angiographic findings of abnormal vascularity and multiplicity of lesions, Zacherson found that diagnosis of metastases was possible in 70 percent, whereas in 7 to 30 percent the angiogram may be negative.[11] With infratentorial lesions ventriculography and vertebral angiography may be necessary.

With CT, the detection of both clinically symptomatic and silent lesions may be more reliably established than with other conventional neurodiagnostic studies. New reported that there were no false negative diagnoses in 24 metastatic lesions; CT was superior to angiography and isotope scan, both of which failed to detect the presence of multiple lesions in several cases.[12] Paxton reported the CT detection of 34 of 35 histologically proven metastases; the only missed lesion was a solitary tumor located high on the parietal convexity. In patients with suspected metastatic disease the role of CT is being evaluated in a number of clinical situations including the following: (1) the ability to detect and accurately establish the pathological diagnosis of metastatic tumor in patients whose neurological findings, EEG and isotope scan findings are suggestive of a single lesion; (2) specificity of CT appearance and density characteristic for different primary systemic carcinomas that produce intracerebral metastases; (3) sensitivity for detection in patients without any neurological findings; (4) correlation of clinical response with corticosteroids, surgery, chemotherapy and radiotherapy.

The CT appearance of the metastatic lesion closely correlates with the pathological features of the tumor. These neoplasms may be located superficially in the gray matter and may vary in size from only microscopic foci to a large multilobulated mass. They are hard and nodular masses, which may be encapsulated and delineated from the surrounding brain, or alternatively the tumor may be soft and necrotic, with infiltration into the normal tissue, simulating an infiltrating glioma. The tumor nodule is usually surrounded by edema fluid, which may be quite widespread despite the small size of the tumor nodule. If the tumor is highly cellular it may have a firm consistency, but it may also undergo degenerative change, with necrotic, cystic or hemorrhagic areas, or have a gelatinous consistency frequently seen in tumors originating in the digestive tract.[5]

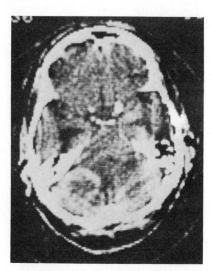

Figure 7–2. An elderly man who had atrial fibrillation and was being treated with anticoagulants suddenly developed headache and confusion and became unable to walk. Chest radiograph showed left hilar mass; isotope scan was positive, and angiography showed an avascular mass in the left cerebellar hemisphere consistent with primary intracerebral hematoma or hemorrhage into neoplasm. CT findings: a large round mass with a thick capsule with a nonhomogeneous low-density core was seen; at higher level it had a mottled high-density appearance consistent with hemorrhage into metastatic adenocarcinoma. This was confirmed at operation.

In all patients with suspected metastatic lesions both plain and contrast infusion studies must be performed. Several studies have demonstrated that melanoma, chorionic carcinoma, colonic carcinoma and osteogenic sarcoma have high-density characteristics, whereas lymphoma and lung, breast and kidney carcinoma are low-density metastases but may show increased density following contrast enhancement. Unfortunately these patterns are not sufficiently different to be of diagnostic value.[13] To obtain maximal pathological information from a CT scan, both plain and contrast infusion studies must be performed, as several false negatives have occurred when only a plain scan was done. If only contrast study is done, it is not possible to differentiate an enhancing lesion from hemorrhage within a tumor (Fig. 7–2). This latter distinction is of therapeutic significance since radiotherapy should be avoided if the lesion is hemorrhagic (Fig. 7–3).

The smallest tumor nodule defined by CT was 6 mm, and visualization of small lesions is dependent upon their location and the presence of surrounding edema. If a small high-density nodule is encompassed by edema, it may be more easily visualized than if surrounded by normal parenchyma because of the partial volume averaging effect. In suspected metastatic lesions, extra sections through the parietal region may visualize small metastatic nodules that are not detected with routine sections. In several cases patients had clinical symptoms suggestive of a

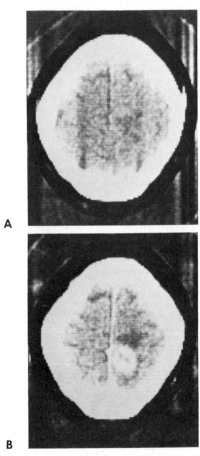

A

B

Figure 7–4. This patient presented with left focal motor seizure involving the left hand only. EEG, isotope scan, CT (A) and angiography were negative, but repeat study two weeks later showed a high-density nodular area in high right parietal convexity region (B), which was a metastatic deposit secondary to adenocarcinoma of the lung.

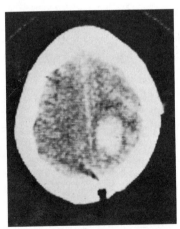

Figure 7–3. A patient with a history of malignant melanoma treated with chemotherapy several years previously suddenly developed left hemiparesis and left homonymous hemianopia. EEG and isotope scan localized an abnormality in the right parieto-occipital region. CT findings: a high-density round lesion in the right occipital region, which did not enhance with contrast or show any additional lesions. Necropsy revealed hemorrhagic melanoma.

parietal convexity lesion, but CT and isotope scan were negative; a repeat study less than two weeks later clearly showed the lesion (Fig. 7–4). In rare instances, CT has detected hydrocephalus with no definite evidence of a lesion, but a small metastatic deposit was subsequently found in the aqueductal region (Fig. 7–5). Of those lesions that were proved to be metastatic by surgical biopsy or necropsy, 35 percent showed evidence of a solitary metastatic lesion by CT scan, and in 55 percent of cases multiple lesions — frequently less than 1.5 cm in diameter — were detected by CT. Eighty percent of metastases demonstrated by CT

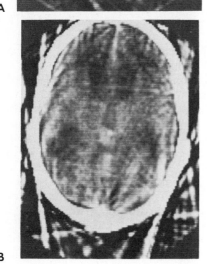

A

B

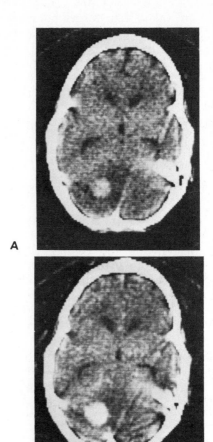

A

B

Figure 7–5. A patient with a history of chronic alcoholism was admitted in a confused state. Neurological findings included unsteadiness of gait and vertical and horizontal nystagmus. Following treatment with thiamine, the confusion and nystagmus cleared, but gait disturbance and organic brain syndrome with recent memory impairment persisted. CT findings: dilatation of lateral and third ventricle with no visualization of the fourth ventricle (A); small round high-density lesion, faintly seen at posterior end of third ventricle (B). Necropsy revealed a small metastatic adenocarcinoma partially obstructing the aqueduct.

Figure 7–6. A 40-year-old woman with anaplastic carcinoma of the lung developed occipital headache and gait unsteadiness. CT findings: plain scan showed round high-density area surrounded by low-density edema in the left cerebellar hemisphere; this obliterated the fourth ventricle and caused ventricular enlargement (A). Following contrast infusion, there was dense enhancement but no increase in the size of the lesion (B).

showed evidence of surrounding edema with accompanying evidence of mass effect in two thirds. In only rare instances did a proven metastatic lesion show no evidence of enhancement. With evidence of multiple discrete high-density tumor nodules in one hemisphere and intervening low-density edema, differentiation of metastatic tumor from multicentric glioblastoma is not always possible.

Adenocarcinoma of the lung may appear as dense nodules (20 to 30 units) of small size surrounded by frondlike low-density edematous areas; there is usually definite enhancement in these nodules (Fig. 7–6). In some instances the small mural nodule is not sufficiently dense to be visualized; plain scan shows only a low-density region until contrast enhancement is performed. Oat cell carcinoma and adenocarcinoma frequently undergo necrosis or hemorrhages in which case the scan shows a thick irregular peripheral high-density rim with a low-density core. Squamous cell carcinoma usually appears as a round central region of homogeneous low density, surrounded by a thin continuous high-density peripheral rim (Fig. 7–7). The scan shows less edema and the tumor nodules are larger than with adenocarcinoma. Retrospective studies of 20 consecutive CT scans from patients with biopsy-proven lung carcinoma permitted differentiation of epidermoid from adenocarcinoma on the basis of these CT scan patterns, but this finding has not been confirmed by other studies.

It should be remembered that the presence of peripheral ring enhancement with central lucency does not always correspond to capsule formation and a necrotic core; it may represent solid tumor with failure of contrast to be taken up in the central portion of the tumor. Malignant melanoma and choriocarcinoma also show this ringlike enhancement pattern. Both of these neoplasms may also appear as high-density lesions

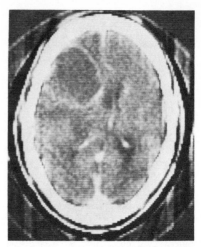

Figure 7–7. A 50-year-old man with proven diagnosis of squamous cell carcinoma of the lung developed right hemiparesis and aphasia. Isotope scan was positive in left frontal region. CT findings: a low-density speckled round core with a peripheral rim of enhancement in left frontal parietal region, with surrounding areas of edema, causing significant mass effect consistent with solitary metastasis.

because of their highly cellular architecture and their tendency to undergo hemorrhage.

Because of their more rapid development, it is unusual for metastatic lesions to show evidence of calcification. Metastatic breast carcinoma usually has a low-density appearance that becomes nodular with contrast infusion. This neoplasm may also have a flat en plaque or concave shape consistent with epidural neoplasm. Based on the characteristic angiographic appearance of metastatic hypernephroma, it was expected that it would appear on CT as a low-density area with peripheral enhancement, but in all cases it has appeared as a low-density irregularly shaped lesion with dense homogeneous enhancement.

In evaluating 50 patients who presented with focal neurological deficit and whose EEG and isotope scan findings were suggestive of a solitary lesion, CT demonstrated multiple lesions in 18, obviating the need in these for angiography or surgical bi-

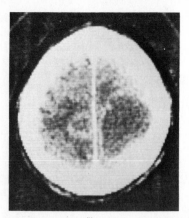

Figure 7–8. A 50-year-old man developed headache and progressive left hemiparesis. EEG and isotope scan were consistent with lesion in right parietal region. CT findings: large low-density round mass with enhancing peripheral rim in right parietal region, compressing the lateral ventricle, and second lesion in region of left high parietal convexity.

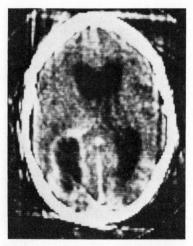

Figure 7–9. This patient presented with increasingly severe headache and 30-pound weight loss. Neurological findings included bilateral Babinski signs with increased tone in lower extremities but no visual field abnormality. Isotope scan was negative, and EEG was diffusely slow. CT findings: marked ventricular dilatation with peripheral enhancement pattern surrounding the left occipital region, suggestive of cystic loculation with subependymal growth of tumor. At operation, loculated cystic fluid collection was found in the left occipital lobe, with sheets of tumor layering the wall of the lateral ventricle.

opsy. In these 18 cases, diagnostic studies had shown no evidence of a primary tumor and the CT findings correctly indicated the metastatic origin of the tumor (Fig. 7–8). In no case did isotope scan demonstrate additional lesions not detected by CT. This may be because many nuclear diagnostic laboratories now utilize technetium with a short half-life which does not permit sequential delayed scan studies.

In 15 other cases in which CT demonstrated a lesion with scan characteristics most consistent with metastatic deposit, there was a known primary systemic cancer, and the presumptive diagnosis was made by CT; 9 cases have been correctly verified by surgical biopsy or necropsy (Fig. 7–9). In 15 cases, reliable differentiation from abscess, glioma or meningioma was not definitely possible, and in 7 of 15 cases preoperative diagnosis was correct based on the following characteristics: (1) a large amount of edema fluid with less significant ventricular distortion and displacement than with malignant glioma; (2) the presence of a small superficially located tumor nodule;

(3) a thin rim or bulls-eye enhancement pattern. In one case initial scan showed several wedge-shaped lesions without enhancement, more consistent with infarction, but serial scan demonstrated enhancement due to metastatic neoplasm. In five patients the clinical symptoms were indicative of a posterior fossa lesion, and both isotope scan and EEG were negative, but the diagnosis of multiple lesions was established by CT (Fig. 7–10). In one additional case, initial study had indicated only hydrocephalus but no abnormal density, and vertebral angiography also indicated hydrocephalus, but a CT scan two months later demonstrated the lesion.

In patients with bronchogenic carcinoma who have no neurological symptoms isotope scan is positive in only 2 to 3 percent of cases, but at necropsy 15 to 32 percent have macroscopic foci of intracranial metastases.[14] The yield with isotope scan is

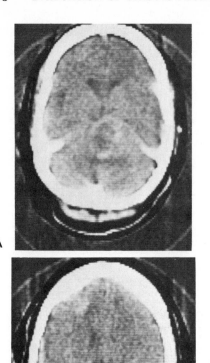

A

B

Figure 7–10. This patient developed right-sided weakness and confusional episodes, which became more severe over a three-week interval. Neurological findings included bilateral facial paresis, right abducens nerve palsy, right gaze paresis, right hemiparesis and left-sided cerebellar deficit. Isotope scan and EEG were normal. CT findings: on plain scan there was a round rim of high density in the region of the brain stem; lesion enhanced slightly (A). In addition, there was a second lesion of low density in the left frontal region (B). Necropsy revealed a mid-pontine metastatic lesion from epidermoid carcinoma of lung and a second lesion 2.5 cm in diameter in the left frontal region. A third lesion measuring 1.7 cm in the right frontal region had not been visualized by scan.

visceral neoplasms is not known. In addition, a false positive isotope scan may result from skull lesions without parenchymal lesions, but skull radiogram and bone scan should allow differentiation. In 10 percent of patients with bronchogenic carcinoma who were neurologically asymptomatic, CT scan showed evidence of parenchymal metastases; three quarters of these were single and one quarter multiple. The incidence of positive CT findings in patients with malignant melanoma was 20 percent, but since patients were neurologically normal and were referred because of headache, they cannot be considered neurologically silent lesions. Of 50 patients with known visceral carcinoma who had neurological symptoms including headache, confusion, weakness, dizziness and visual disturbance, but in whom there were no neurological findings, CT scan demonstrated evidence of metastases in 30 cases; 60 percent had multiple and 40 percent had solitary lesions. Of those with lesions detected by CT,

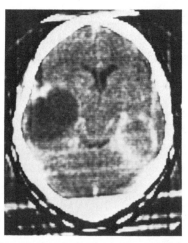

Figure 7–11. A 52-year-old man became confused and agitated. EEG showed bitemporal slow wave pattern, and isotope scan showed bitemporal uptake. CT findings: plain scan showed low-density areas in both temporal regions; following contrast infusion, there is a peripheral rim of enhancement in both lesions. Chest radiogram showed a hilar mass, and bronchoscopy revealed epidermoid carcinoma.

so low with breast carcinoma that this procedure is believed to be unnecessary in the neurologically intact patient when planning therapy. The incidence of clinically silent lesions detected by isotope scans for other

one had a negative isotope scan and 25 percent had normal or nonfocal EEG abnormality (Fig. 7–11).

CT is less sensitive in establishing the diagnosis of carcinomatous meningitis, but in rare instances the findings may be quite striking.[15] The most frequent pattern is to outline the cisternal spaces following contrast enhancement, most likely due to extravasation of contrast through an impaired blood-brain barrier. Less frequently, there may be evidence of deposits of tumor in the cisternal spaces, causing mass effect (Fig. 7–12). In most cases of this neoplastic basilar meningitis, there is an accompanying hydrocephalus.

Necropsy studies have demonstrated that cerebral metastases are associated with considerable amounts of edema, and that the edematous reaction may involve a much greater area than would be expected for a small tumor nodule. In many cases the neurological disturbance is related to cerebral edema, ventricular compression and herniation. Studies of the effectiveness of glucocorticoids have indicated that they are most effective in patients with symptoms of recent onset and least effective in those with more longstanding symptoms, which are believed due to direct compressive effect of the neoplasm.[16] With the use of CT we have had the opportunity to obtain a clinical-pathological correlation of this hypothesis, and in a limited number of patients definite clinical improvement was associated with finding of significant edema formation; minimal clinical response occurred in those patients with nodular deposit and minimal edema formation.

The response to corticosteroids may be detected within 12 to 24 hours and usually lasts for four weeks, although in rare instances it may be sustained for as long as six months. The drug acts to decrease cerebral edema, without any specific anti-tumor effect, as it restores arteriolar tone and capillary membrane impermeability. Several recent studies have evaluated the effect of dexamethasone on the size of the metastatic lesion detected by isotope, and shrinkage in size correlated with clinical improvement.[17, 18] This may have resulted from a decreased localization

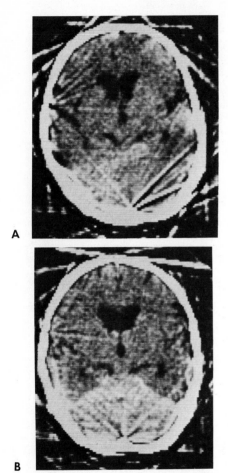

A

B

Figure 7–12. A patient who had been previously well became lethargic and dizzy. Findings included broad-based unsteady gait but no papilledema, truncal rigidity or cranial nerve dysfunction. CT findings: plain scan shows oval-shaped low-density posterior to the quadrigeminal cistern with nonvisualization of the fourth ventricle (not shown) and forward displacement and distortion of the quadrigeminal cistern (A). Following infusion, there is dense enhancement outlining the cerebellar folia, a pattern consistent with carcinomatous meningitis (B). Angiography showed diffuse blush but no mass effect in the posterior fossa. CSF examination revealed many large anaplastic cells, low sugar and elevated protein content.

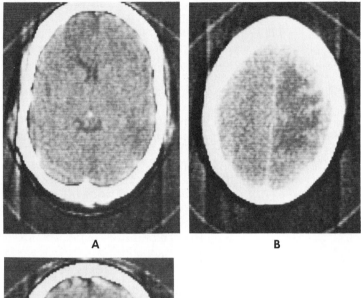

Figure 7–13. This patient had had carcinoma of the colon resected two years previously. He had recently developed clumsiness in using his left hand and lethargy. EEG showed diffuse slow wave pattern, and isotope scan was positive in right parietal region. CT findings: compression of right lateral ventricle by low-density area in right frontal parietal region (A), with gyral enhancement (B). Six weeks following corticosteroid therapy, there is no evidence of ventricular compression (C), but lesion size and enhancement are essentially unchanged.

of isotope within the tumor cells or in the extracellular area of peritumoral edema, as the isotope uptake in neoplasms is believed related to increase in tumor vascularity or in the extracellular space. If the patient is begun on steroids prior to isotope scan, there may be suppression of accumulation in the tumors, and this may lower the sensitivity of the scan in detecting these lesions.[17, 18] Utilizing CT, it is possible to demonstrate definite effects, including (1) a decrease in the low-density edematous region with concomitant diminution of ventricular distortion and displacement, and (2) a decrease in the intensity of the contrast enhancement within the tumor without any change in the size of the lesion (Fig. 7–13). In patients

treated with corticosteroids, clinical improvement always preceded scan evidence of decrease in edema; the change in size of the low-density region and mass effect was not detected until seven to 10 days later.[19]

In patients who are treated surgically, CT is the most effective technique to evaluate the completeness of surgical removal of the lesion. Following complete removal there may be no abnormal density or only a low-density cystic region, but if there is evidence of recurrence, mass effect and contrast enhancement are prominent findings. In one third of recurrent lesions, the isotope scan had not reverted to negative and in one fourth it was not positive in the abnormal area, whereas CT adequately showed definite enhancement indicative of recurrent tumor. In those patients treated with radiotherapy who manifest clinical improvement, there is definite CT evidence of decrease in the size of tumor and diminution of enhancement pattern (Fig. 7–14). Radiotherapy causes necrosis and edema with further breakdown in the blood-brain barrier, and in some instances may be associated with clinical worsening, with the CT scan showing contrast enhancement and mass effect. Preliminary evidence indicates that radiation or occasionally postsurgical-induced necrosis may have a more mottled appearance, but it may also show ringlike enhancement. In patients with metastatic disease treated with irradiation who then showed clinical deterioration, CT showed new lesions or the increased size of previously treated lesions more reliably than isotope scan or angiography.

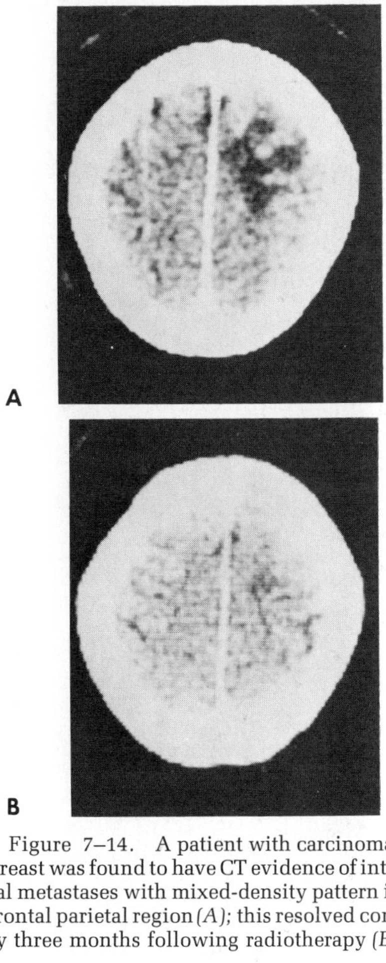

RETICULOENDOTHELIAL TUMORS

Reticulosarcomas infrequently involve the CNS primarily but may present with two clinical patterns: (1) a meningeal syndrome, manifested by cranial nerve involvement, altered mentation and truncal rigidity, in which the diagnosis is established by finding malignant cells in the CSF; (2) clinical evidence of a subacutely progressive mass causing focal neurological deficit and confusion dementia owing to tumor infiltrating widely into the frontal and temporal regions. In the latter cases, the results of EEG, isotope scan and angiography

A

B

Figure 7–14. A patient with carcinoma of the breast was found to have CT evidence of intracranial metastases with mixed-density pattern in right frontal parietal region (A); this resolved completely three months following radiotherapy (B).

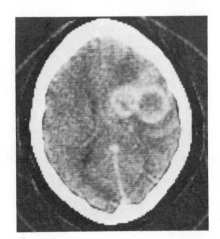

Figure 7–15. A 60-year-old woman without evidence of systemic disease developed left hemiparesis over a four-day period. EEG showed a delta pattern in right parietal region but isotope scan was negative. CT findings: two contiguous well-marginated lesions, which had high-density rims and suggested an intrinsic infiltrating lesion. Angiography showed evidence of an extra-axial lesion; operative findings consisted of a single encapsulated lesion, which was totally removed. Pathological diagnosis was primary intracranial reticulum cell sarcoma.

may be negative because these tumors are intracerebral tumors that cause diffuse infiltration, but occasionally they may be extrinsic and amenable to surgical resection.[20] CT may define the presence of these lesions, but in two cases angiography was necessary to delineate an extracerebral location, since this could not be accomplished with CT alone (Fig. 7–15).

Leukemia is not usually classified as a solid tumor of the reticular system, although, rarely, localized tumor masses may be present. An intracranial tumor mass occurs most frequently in acute myeloblastic leukemia (chloroma), and these may present when the patient is in hematological remission (Fig. 7–16). More frequently, the acute leukemias cause basal meningitis with cranial nerve root involvement and hydrocephalus. Also, coagulation disorders and inflammatory disorders due to immunosuppressive drugs, with focal expanding mass lesions, including intracerebral and subdural hematoma and abscess formation, may complicate the luekemia. Patients with leukemia may present with headache, stiff neck, fever and papilledema, and the diagnosis may be established by lumbar puncture — this may be safely performed if prior CT scan has excluded the presence of a mass lesion. In only one of 10 patients with leukemic meningitis was there evidence of enhancement suggestive of basilar arachnoiditis.

In Hodgkin's and other lymphomatous disorders, intracranial involvement is usually confined to deposits located at the base of the skull, in dura and in cranial nerves. Buckley and Warwick characterized the lesions as extradural, dural and intracerebral tumors, but emphasized their low incidence, and the presence of neurological involvement only in those cases preceded by years of illness, with generalized deposits and associated hepatosplenomegaly.[21] Since treatment of the lymphomas is de-

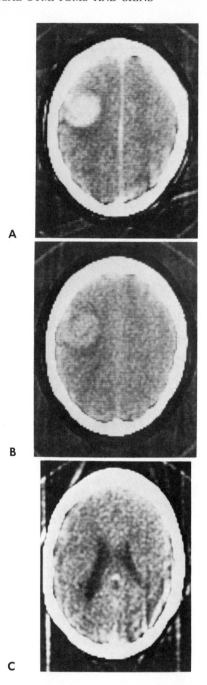

A

B

C

Figure 7–16.   A woman with acute myelocytic leukemia, treated with chemotherapy, was in complete hematological remission but developed left-sided headache. CT findings: round homogeneous high-density mass in left frontal parietal region (A); it was believed to be parenchymal leukemic infiltrate. She was treated with radiotherapy and serial scans showed a marked decrease in size and enhancement intensity (B); six months later the lesion was no longer visible (C).

pendent upon delineating the exact extent of involvement, CT may become routine in detecting any CNS involvement. The nodular granulomatous lymphomatous lesions are usually seen as infiltrating low-density areas which show a minimal enhancement pattern.

The drugs used in the treatment of these malignancies, including methotrexate and vincristine, are highly toxic to the CNS. Methotrexate may cause a chemical meningitis and a necrotizing leukoencephalopathy. In patients who are treated with these agents and later show neurological deterioration, CT may define the presence of periventricular low-density regions and also affected areas in the central white matter.

REFERENCES

1. Posner JB: Diagnosis and treatment of metastases to the brain. Clin Bull Sloan Kett Cancer Ctr 4:47, 1974.
2. Lesse S, Netsky MG: Metastasis of neoplasms to CNS and meninges. Arch Neurol Psychiatry 72:133, 1954.
3. Richards P, McKissock W: Intracranial metastases. Br Med J 1:15, 1963.
4. Vieth RG, Odom GL: Intracranial metastases and their neurosurgical treatment. J Neurosurg 23:375, 1965.
5. Paillais JE, Pellet W: Brain metastases. In: Handbook of Clinical Neurology, Vol 18. PJ Vinken, GW Bruyn (eds). North Holland Publishing Company, Amsterdam, 1975. pp 201–252.
6. Strang R, Almonc Mason C: Brain metastases. Arch Neurol 4:20, 1961.
7. Tarcon YA, Fajman W, Marc J: "Doughnut" sign in brain scanning. Am Roentgenol 126:842, 1976.
8. Boller F, Patten DH, Howes D: Correlation of brain scan results with neuropathological findings. Lancet 1:1143, 1973.
9. McCormack KR: Scanning of liver and brain in evaluation of patients with bronchogenic carcinoma. J Nucl Med 9:222, 1968.
10. Schlesinger EG, Michelsen WJ, Antunes JL: Value of sequential scanning in detection of metastatic tumors. Surg Neurol 6:239, 1976.
11. Zachrisson L: Angiography of cerebral metastases. Acta Radiol (Diagn) 1:521, 1963.
12. New PFJ, Scott WR, Schnur JA: Computed tomography in diagnosis of primary and metastatic intracranial neoplasms. Radiology, 114:75, 1975.
13. Deck MDF, Messina AV, Sackett JR: Computed tomography in metastatic disease of the brain. Radiology 119:115, 1976.
14. Haynie TP, Jhingham SF, Leavens ME: Brain scintigrams in metastatic carcinoma. Cancer 30:953, 1972.
15. Enzman DR, Norman D, Mani J, Newton TH: CT of basal granulomatous arachnoiditis. Radiology 120:341, 1976.
16. Rudermann NG, Hall TC: Use of glucocorticoids in the palliative treatment of metastatic brain tumors. Cancer18:298, 1965.
17. Fletcher JW, George EA: Brain scans, dexamethasone therapy and brain tumors. JAMA, 232:1261, 1975.
18. Marty R, Cain ML: Effect of glucocorticoid administration on the brain scan. Radiology 107:117, 1973.
19. Croker EF, Zimmerman RA: Effect of steroids on extravascular distribution of radiographic contrast material and techetium in brain tumors as determined by CT. Radiology 119:471, 1976.
20. Schaumberg HN, Plank CR, Adams RD: Reticulum cell sarcoma-microglioma group of brain tumors. Brain 95:199, 1972.
21. Buckley TF, Warwick F: Surgical management of intracranial Hodgkin's disease. J Neurol Neurosurg Psychiatry 31:612, 1968.

8 The Juxtasellar Region–Visual, Endocrine or Radiographic Abnormalities

Patients with clinical symptoms suggestive of lesions involving the juxtasellar region may present with visual, neurological or endocrine symptoms. Sixty percent of patients have symptoms of pituitary dysfunction that may be manifested as target gland failure, including amenorrhea, infertility, impotence, cold intolerance, loss of body and pubic hair, or as hypersecretion of pituitary hormones, including acromegaly (growth hormone), Cushing's syndrome (adrenocorticotrophic hormone), amenorrhea-galactorrhea syndrome (prolactin). If the symptoms are predominantly the results of endocrine dysfunction, the lesion is usually primarily intrasellar and frequently consists of a pituitary adenoma, which initially enlarges the sella and then expands to the extrasellar region. Sometimes the cause is a microadenoma less than 10 mm in size that does not compress the normal pituitary tissue or cause erosive remodeling of the sella turcica. In addition, suprasellar tumors may involve the hypothalamus, causing diabetes insipidus, precocious puberty and other symptoms of pituitary dysfunction. These tumors are usually accompanied by other neurological and visual disturbances. Less frequently, other juxtasellar lesions, including aneurysms, cysts, other tumors, and a dilated anterior third ventricle, may cause similar symptoms, clinically indistinguishable from those produced by a pituitary tumor.

The majority of patients with pituitary tumors present with visual disturbances, and a loss of visual acuity with dimming of visual brightness and color perception is noted in 58 to 88 percent. The threat to the visual apparatus is the most devastating complication of the natural history of pituitary neoplasms.[1, 2] Visual symptoms are caused by the mechanical and vascular compressive effect of the tumor upon the optic nerve and chiasm; careful tangent screen examination is necessary to detect early lesions and to document their extension. The extent of visual involvement usually defines the preferred treatment modality.[3] The typical abnormality is caused by impingement upon the crossed central fibers, resulting in a symmetrical or asymmetrical bitemporal visual disturbance, including a bitemporal quadrantanopia, hemianopia, or bitemporal scotoma in 70 to 97 percent of pituitary adenomas. At least 15 percent of patients who are found to have objective evidence of visual field defect are symptomatically unaware of any visual involvement, and this was detected by careful tangent screen examination in patients with an abnormal sella or who had symptoms of pituitary dysfunction.[1] Since the optic chiasm is located 1 cm above the diaphragma sella, the detection of early visual abnormality may indicate significant suprasellar extension. It is at this time that urgency in making the diagnosis is necessary to preserve vision.

In patients with a characteristic visual impairment suggesting the diagnosis of a juxtasellar lesion, it is important to determine the presence of any accompanying signs or symptoms that may indicate the major vector of tumor growth. Optic pallor, loss of visual acuity and pupillary nonreactivity indicate optic nerve involvement. Lateral growth may result in paresis of extraocular muscle function and trigeminal nerve involvement, with facial pain and paresthesia. If this is more pronounced, psychomotor seizures and memory impairment may result from extension into the temporal lobe. Personality change may occur with frontal extension. Rhinorrhea may result from inferior growth into the sphenoid sinus. Cerebellar, pyramidal and third nerve involvement may result from retrosellar growth. Diabetes insipidus and obstructive hydrocephalus are indicative of suprasellar growth with involvement of the hypothalamus and ventricular system.

The most frequent tumor of the juxtasellar region is the pituitary adenoma, which is usually a slow-growing tumor. More rapid progression of symptoms may be indicative of malignant transformation or a degenerative vascular change within the tumor.[4] In addition, the rapid onset of visual disturbance may be caused by nontumorous disorders, including multiple sclerosis, or vascular conditions that involve the optic chiasm; differentiation from a pituitary neoplasm may be made only with radiographic and CSF studies. In 50 to 70 percent of pituitary adenomas, headache is present, but it is the presenting symptom in only 10 to 15 percent. Certain patients have skull radiograms performed because of a headache, and the suspicion of a pituitary tumor is raised because the sella is enlarged despite the absence of endocrine, visual or neurological symptoms. Further delineation of the lesion requires radiographic analysis, including air study.

Previous clinical studies have relied heavily upon conventional plain skull radiography and tomography, followed by air study and angiography, in diagnosing parasellar lesions, whereas isotope scan, EEG and CSF examination are less helpful. DuBoulay observed positive radiographic sella abnormalities in 67 to 77 percent of sella tumors, and other studies report that in at least 90 percent of pituitary adenomas there is a radiographically abnormal sella turcica.[5]

If plain skull radiogram is negative, conventional tomography is indicated, as a normal-sized sella may harbor a pituitary microadenoma, and there may be evidence of erosive change in the floor of the sella. This is especially important in patients whose endocrine symptoms are suggestive of a hypersecretion syndrome due to a microadenoma. Hypocycloidal tomography may show evidence of a localized bulging of the anterolateral wall of one side of the sella, with a "blistering" pattern of the sella floor[6]

If the sella is enlarged, certain radiographic patterns are helpful in distinguishing intrasellar tumors from nontumorous enlargement of the sella (empty sella syndrome); symmetrical sella enlargement without bone erosion and a normal position of the clinoid processes are suggestive of a nontumorous cause, but in 25 percent of cases adequate differentiation can be made only with air study.[1, 7] In evaluation of patients with endocrine symptoms that suggest microadenoma, plain skull radiogram and tomography may have greater sensitivity than contrast radiographic procedures. In evaluating patients with a juxtasellar syndrome, additional skull radiographic views to visualize the

optic foramina and the superior orbital fissure may be necessary to indicate the presence of an optic glioma
or a carotid aneurysm.

Isotope scan has been shown to be
a poor screening procedure in the
evaluation of juxtasellar lesions, although one recent study showed 71
percent positive studies.[8, 19] Failure of
isotope scan to detect these lesions
may result from the tumor's growth
being entirely intrasellar and therefore hidden by the overlying bone.
Tumors with significant extrasellar
growth occur in a region that normally shows a high level of radioactivity,
including the carotid arteries, overlying temporalis muscle, choroid plexus,
cavernous and sphenoid sinus. Since
there is a high background activity, even if the isotope were to concentrate in the tumor, there would
be little differential from the background. In cases of pituitary adenoma, a positive isotope scan indicates
suprasellar extension of greater than
1 to 2 cm. In extrasellar lesions, detection with isotope scan is more frequent; James reported 12 of 13 positive scans in craniopharyngioma and
parasellar meningioma.[9]

EEG changes associated with juxtasellar lesions are unusual, but if there
is significant lateral extension, there
may be a spike focus in the midtem-
poral region or a bilateral frontal
delta pattern due to extension into
the deep frontal region. CSF examination shows only a nonspecific elevation of the protein content in one
third of cases, but may show bloody
fluid in pituitary apoplexy or an elevated gamma globulin content in demyelinating conditions involving the
optic chiasm and nerve.

Since many conditions may cause
an abnormal sella turcica (Table 8–1),
detection of the presence of a tumor
and definition of its pathological features require air study and angiographic analysis, but usually accurate
pathological diagnosis is not made
without surgical exploration and biopsy. In patients with a suspected pi-

TABLE 8–1. Juxtasellar Lesions

Common Lesions

Pituitary adenoma
Craniopharyngioma
Tuberculum sellae meningioma
Glioma of optic nerve and chiasm

Uncommon Lesions

Aneurysm
Atypical teratoma of anterior third ventricle
Hypothalamic glioma
Metastases to the sella
Chordoma
Dilated anterior third ventricle due to
    intracranial hypertension
Sphenoid sinus carcinoma
Mucocele
Granuloma of hypothalamus or pituitary
Intra- and suprasellar cyst
Suprasellar epidermoid tumor
Arachnoiditis involving optic chiasm
Demyelination of optic chiasm

tuitary or hypothalamic lesion, angiography or air study may precipitate a
pituitary crisis, and it is usually necessary to administer cortisone, saline,
and occasionally mannitol during
these procedures.

The most compelling reason to perform angiography is to exclude the
presence of an aneurysm, which may
mimic the clinical and radiographic
features of a pituitary adenoma. The
failure to identify an aneurysm correctly by preoperative angiography
may cause operative mortality. Lombardi reported two operative deaths
in patients diagnosed as having pituitary adenoma on the basis of skull
radiographic and air study features
without a prior angiographic study.[10]
Other studies have indicated that the
presence of an aneurysm is a rare occurrence, and in one series of 400
pituitary neoplasms only one carotid
aneurysm was identified. In this case
an internal carotid artery aneurysm
and an accompanying pituitary neoplasm were present. At surgery it appeared that the symptoms were more
likely due to the adenoma than to the
aneurysm.[4] The aneurysm may be

intrasellar in location and cause symmetrical sella enlargement and hypopituitarism, in which case radiotherapy without prior arteriography may be disastrous. The aneurysm may be more lateral, in which case the radiogram may show a unilateral sella enlargement with erosion of one anterior clinoid process, involvement of the superior orbital fissure and curvilinear calcification. There may be a unilateral temporal, nasal or visual field defect. It has been suggested that bilateral carotid angiography is indicated in all suspected juxtasellar lesions, with the only exception being those patients who present with clinical and laboratory evidence of a hypersecretion syndrome.

Angiography is more reliable in detecting lateral and anterior extension of pituitary tumors, whereas air study is more sensitive in detecting suprasellar and retrosellar extension. Lateral displacement of the posterior portion of the cavernous segment of the carotid artery is an early sign of lateral growth, but, since the tumor may encase the artery without displacing it, air study is necessary to define the position of the temporal horn and to confirm lack of lateral extension.[11]

With the introduction of magnification and subtraction techniques, the vascular supply of pituitary tumors may be identified. Powell has described extensive arterial feeding vessels derived from the dilated and hypertrophied meningo-hypophyseal trunk, supplying both the capsule and solid portion of the tumor in 80 percent of cases. Both the solid and cystic tumors had an extensive vascularity, but important differences were present; the densely cellular solid tumors more frequently showed feeding vessels to the capsule and a homogeneous stain, whereas the cystic tumors showed a less intense homogeneous stain or had a mottled appearance that was suggestive of degenerative or cystic change within the tumor.[12] This extensive vascularity was quite unexpected, as conven-

tional angiographic studies had shown these tumors to be relatively avascular, and the presence of visible feeding vessels and a stain was indicative of malignant and invasive properties. In addition, it was believed that these tumors with abnormal feeding vessels were larger, grew more rapidly, invaded and infiltrated contiguous structures, were more likely to undergo hemorrhagic necrosis and had a higher mortality.[13]

On the basis of combined plain skull radiogram and angiographic findings, other common tumors may be differentiated: (1) Parasellar meningiomas which show a hyperostotic blistering of the bone anterior to the sella. The angiogram shows early-appearing and persistent diffuse stain, with the feeding vessels derived from the enlarged meningeal and external carotid artery source. (2) Craniopharyngioma shows an enlarged sella with suprasellar calcification. The angiogram shows an avascular mass in the suprasellar region with no evidence of feeding vessels or stain pattern. (3) A glioma of the chiasm or hypothalamus, which may cause a J-shaped deformity of the sella and may be seen as a suprasellar and anterior third ventricular mass, with feeding vessels derived from the superior and premammillary arteries of the posterior cerebral artery, with early venous filling and drainage. (4) Metastatic lesions, chordoma, and carcinoma of the sphenoid sinus—all may show extensive destructive changes at the base of the skull and sella that may be better defined by tomography. Angiography may show enlargement and encasement of the carotid with an early diffuse stain pattern that disappears late in the venous phase. Despite these different patterns, preoperative differentiation of tumor pathology is not always possible.

Suprasellar extension is most sensitively detected by air study, which outlines the dome-shaped mass that bulges above the diaphragma sella and causes obliteration of the suprasellar and chiasmatic cistern with blunting of the anterior recess of the third ventricle. In many cases of pituitary adenomas with suprasellar extension defined by air study, angiography is negative, although in other cases there may be evidence of elevation of the initial segment of the anterior cerebral artery as evidence of upward growth. In patients with visual symptoms thin section polytomoencephalography is necessary to evaluate adequately the optico-chiasmatic region so as to detect minimal amounts of suprasellar extension and to define the anatomy of the optic chiasm region which is not possible with other techniques. This latter procedure permits a detailed anatomical visualization of the optic nerve and chiasm and shows distortion of the visual apparatus by tumors arising within the parasellar region, which are not detected by conventional air study.[14]

In other patients with an enlarged sella, air study is necessary to confirm the presence of an intrasellar tumor and to differentiate this from a nontumorous enlargement of the sella, in which air enters the sella to cause an air-gland interface with posterior-inferior compression of the pituitary gland. Careful analysis with thin-section laminography is necessary because a microadenoma may coexist in an otherwise "empty sella," and this small tumor may cause symptoms related to excess prolactin or growth hormone secretion.[15]

Until the introduction of CT, there was no reliable and sensitive screening procedure for evaluating lesions of the parasellar region that allowed definition of the presence of a tumor and defined its extent as well as its histopathological characteristics. Recent studies of patients with suspected sellar lesions have been directed toward determining the exact role of CT in comparison to other conventional diagnostic studies.

In 38 patients with chiasmal compressive symptoms, CT was able to define the presence of a lesion in 35 cases. Of these cases, plain skull radiogram showed a normal sella size and shape in 40 percent, but hypocycloidal tomography was not always performed; isotope scan was positive in only 46 percent. Of those 35 cases in which CT was positive, subsequent air study was performed in only six and was usually done to detect the presence of retrosellar extension. Angiography was performed in 20; in six cases, angiography failed to demonstrate suprasellar extension, which was documented by CT, whereas lateral extension was better visualized by angiography. In only one case did CT fail to detect the presence of parasellar meningioma, one that extended 1.5 cm above the sella and was clearly defined by air study. The error was due to failure to perform contrast infusion and to identify adequately the suprasellar cistern; this lesion was diagnosed in retrospective analysis. In two cases CT was entirely normal, including orbital views; subsequent CSF examination showed a markedly elevated gamma globulin, suggesting a demyelinating process involving the optic chiasm, and the subsequent clinical course confirmed the diagnosis of multiple sclerosis.

In patients with visual symptoms indicative of chiasmal involvement, skull radiogram and CT should be initially performed, but even if they are negative, polytomoencephalography should be performed, as this technique appears to be more sensitive in defining the chiasmatic cistern so that smaller tumors and inflammatory arachnoiditis may be identified.

In 15 patients with endocrine symptoms of decreased pituitary function in whom skull radiograph showed sella enlargement, the CT scan was less sensitive, and frequently air study was necessary. Five of these patients had no visual symptoms, but careful tangent screen examination performed with a small red test object detected an early bitemporal quadrant dimming effect, and in these patients CT showed a tumor distorting the suprasellar cistern. At surgery there was 8 mm to 1.5 cm suprasellar extension. Of those with endocrine symptoms, CT defined the presence of pituitary tumor in only three; and in the seven negative CT cases, subsequent air study showed a primarily intrasellar tumor in five, whereas the sella was "empty" in two.

Patients with symptoms of pituitary hypersecretion, including galactorrhea and acromegaly, had negative CT and were found to have microadenomas, which are not detected by presently available CT techniques, although thinner sections and utilization of cisternal contrast studies may outline these tumors. Since elevated prolactin may occur in more than one third of pituitary adenomas, this finding is a definite indication for CT even if sella size is normal, although if the tumor is intrasellar CT may not define the lesion.

Thirty patients with an enlarged sella without any endocrine or visual symptoms were studied, and in only one case was a pituitary adenoma defined. This is consistent with pathological findings of asymptomatic adenoma, which may rarely have significant suprasellar extension but the majority are intrasellar. If the patient has an enlarged sella and is asymptomatic or has only headache, the patient has either an "empty sella," clinically silent pituitary adenoma, or, rarely, a remote intracranial tumor that has caused longstanding intracranial hypertension. Air study with thin section laminography in both sagittal and coronal planes to detect air within the sella is necessary to diagnose nontumorous enlargement of the sella. This diagnosis is poorly established by CT and is dependent upon demonstration of an enlarged sella that contains low-density material consistent with CSF, and is defined in a tissue section which is below the suprasellar cistern. The difficulty in making this diagnosis is the partial volume effect if an 8 mm rather than a 4 mm section is utilized. In addition, reconstruction in the coronal and sagittal planes may detect herniation of cisternal spaces into intrasellar, but air study is still more sensitive in detecting this disorder as well as intrasellar cysts and nonenhancing tumors.[16]

The finding of a low-density enlarged intrasellar space may represent the necrotic core of a juxtasellar tumor.[17] Infrequently, patients with the "empty sella" syndrome present with rhinorrhea or bitemporal hemianopic defect due to depression and kinking of the optic chiasm into the sella; in these cases air study with polytomoencephalography is the most sensitive study. Since it is possible for a pituitary adenoma to occur within an "empty" sella, it is recommended that air study and hypocycloidal tomography is the most sensitive study. In addition, the normal pituitary gland may enhance slightly and this may falsely suggest the presence of an intrasellar tumor.

In summary, if visual symptoms are present, CT is entirely reliable; angiography is necessary to exclude an aneurysm, but air study is not necessary. If endocrine symptoms are present and complete visual fields are negative, air study is the more sensitive, although CT should be performed as the first study. To document the presence of an "empty sella" or to detect a pituitary microadenoma is presently beyond the resolving capability of this technique, although this may be possible with thinner sections, reconstruction in sagittal and coronal planes, and possibly intrathecal Metrizamide studies.

CT DIAGNOSIS OF SPECIFIC JUXTASELLAR LESIONS

1. Pituitary Adenoma. These are the most frequent juxtasellar lesions and may be routine necropsy findings in 30 percent of asymptomatic patients.[18] They arise initially within the sella, causing enlargement or ballooning, and then expand through the diaphragma sella, involving the suprasellar and optico-chiasmatic cistern there is early compression of the undersurface of the optic chiasm, which causes a *superior* bitemporal quadrant effect. In all patients with this visual loss, CT has been diagnostic, but even if negative it has been suggested that air study be performed, as the adenoma may cause vascular compression of the visual structure with minimal suprasellar extension. The CT diagnosis is based upon the finding of distortion of the pentagonal or hexagonal shape of the suprasellar cistern with obliteration of the normal CSF spaces by a round or irregularly shaped high-density (16 to 25 units) mass.

The tumor typically shows superior extension (90 percent), causing a deformity in the anterior portion of the cistern, and is paramedian in location. It is rare for the tumor to extend to the level of the anterior third ventricle and cause dilatation of the lateral ventricles. If the third ventricle is included in the same section as the tumor, it may appear to be obliterated because of density averaging, but in this case there is no accompanying lateral ventricular dilatation. Anterior extension into the frontal lobe may result in low-density bifrontal areas; this is presumed to be due to edema or atrophy, whereas posterior extension causes distortion and obliteration of the interpeduncular cistern. Lateral extension is determined by visualizing abnormal density in the middle fossa and by effect on suprasellar cistern, and, rarely, by lateral displacement of the supraclinoid portion of the ICA on infusion study.[19, 20]

Prior to the CT scan, there was no noninvasive technique to define pathological characteristics of juxtasellar lesions. Pituitary adenomas are multilobulated and enveloped in a well-defined fibrous envelope, which contains prominent vascular channels. The tumor is usually solid and cellular, with benign histological features. There is evidence of degenerative change, including hemorrhage, necrosis, and cyst formation, in 30 percent of tumors. This may occur in both slow-growing or more rapidly

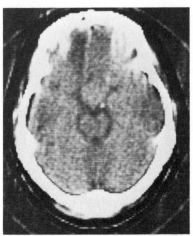

A

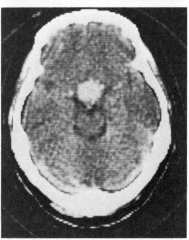

B

Figure 8–1. A 45-year-old man presented with a history of headache and visual disturbance of several months' duration. Examination showed loss of body and pubic hair, sallow, paper-thin skin and complete bitemporal hemianopia. Skull radiograph revealed a symmetrically enlarged sella. CT showed a high-density (20 to 25) area asymmetrically located in the anterior portion of the right suprasellar cistern (A), which showed marked contrast enhancement (30 to 40) (B). This was compatible with solid encapsulated pituitary adenoma, a condition that was pathologically confirmed at operation. The mass extended 16 mm above the diaphragma of the sella into the suprasellar region.

growing tumors and is most frequent in those adenomas that invade and infiltrate contiguous structures.[21]

Comparison of plain and postinfusion density values makes possible definition of certain pathological features. Most solid tumors show a diffuse homogeneous dense enhancement (25 to 40 units), but at least 30 percent have peak density as high as 40 units (Fig. 8–1). Adenomas with a large cystic component have a different pattern, in which plain scan shows a peripheral continuous high-density rim encompassing a low-density central core. Following infusion, enhancement may occur in the capsule owing to its prominent vascularity, and extravasation of contrast also occurs into the cyst in its most dependent portion (Fig. 8–2).

Hemorrhagic tumors show a round or slightly irregularly marginated high-density (20 to 40) lesion in the suprasellar region, surrounded by low-density material; following infusion, the only enhancement occurs in the low-density or isodense portion of the tumor (Fig. 8–3). Infrequently, pituitary adenomas show calcification on CT that is not appreciated with plain skull radiogram. In these cases the patient has had an episode of sudden endocrine or visual worsening consistent with pituitary apoplexy, and it is postulated that the hemorrhagic area has subsequently calcified.

Since 30 percent of pituitary adenomas show degenerative change, CT is an important diagnostic procedure to determine the appropriate treatment modality — radiotherapy or surgery via transfrontal or transsphenoidal approach. Previous indications for surgery have included an arbitrary level of visual acuity or field defect, rapid progression of visual loss, symptoms suggestive of apoplexy, large size of tumor demonstrated by contrast studies, and uncertainty as to specific tumor histopathology. Despite these criteria 25 percent of cases carefully selected for irradiation

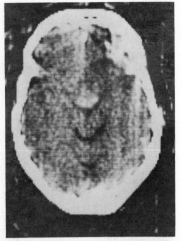

A

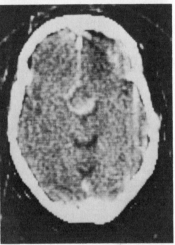

B

Figure 8–2. A 64-year-old woman with progressive visual loss and without endocrine symptoms or headache, on examination, was found to have superior bitemporal quadrantanopia and bilateral optic pallor. CT findings: on plain scan, there is an area of increased density in the region of the sella, encroaching upon the suprasellar cistern, and an area of diminished density in the right frontal region (A). Following contrast infusion, there is an increase in density of the capsule, with extravasation of contrast material in the dependent portion of the lesion, a pattern consistent with cystic pituitary adenoma (B). (Reprinted courtesy of American Journal of Medicine.)

are failures and require subsequent surgery. The radiation failure correlates with the finding of degenerative changes (cyst, hemorrhage), the presence of a thick capsular wall, and initial misdiagnosis of tumor histology.[21, 22] If CT shows a large cystic component, evacuation and drainage

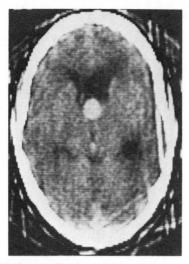

Figure 8–3. A 50-year-old man experienced sudden onset of blurring of vision and headache. The patient was lethargic and had bitemporal visual field defect and grand mal seizures. CT findings: initial scan showed a suprasellar mass which consisted of a high-density (30 units) core surrounded by a low-density area. There was no enhancement following contrast infusion. This was consistent with hemorrhagic pituitary adenoma. Operative findings confirmed the diagnosis of pituitary apoplexy.

may be indicated, whereas if a large solid tumor component is visualized, a transfrontal approach is indicated. In patients who present with rapid onset of extraocular muscle paresis and minimal visual field defect, and who show clinical stabilization and have CT evidence of hemorrhagic adenoma, conservative management with corticosteroids may be indicated; the course may be followed with serial scans.[23] CT findings of a large cystic component, calcification and hemorrhage appear to be contraindications to irradiation.

Rarely, pituitary adenomas may infiltrate to invade structures at the skull base and extend into the cavernous sinus, gasserian ganglion and brain stem cisterns. These more "malignant" adenomas cause similar symptoms, but more frequently present with facial pain, dysesthesias and extraocular muscle involvement. The progression of symptoms is more rapid, and there may be evidence of malignant transformation, with anaplastic cellular features, but this is not always true. In rare instances, these malignant features are seen following radiation, when the adenoma has undergone sarcomatous change. With CT, these invasive adenomas show lateral extension into the middle fossa by a high-density mass with markedly irregular edges (Fig. 8–4).

2. Craniopharyngioma. On the basis of clinical symptomatology, plain skull radiographic and isotope scan results, it is not always possible to differentiate accurately this lesion from pituitary adenoma. This tumor is most frequent in childhood but does occur in adults with somewhat lower incidence; 90 percent of tumors in childhood show evidence of calcification, but only 50 percent of those in adults show radiographic calcification. The majority originate in the suprasellar region, causing early compression of the superior chiasmal region and resulting in an inferior bitemporal quadrantanopia, but 20 percent originate in an intrasellar location, and in this case symptoms may be identical to those of pituitary adenoma. Endocrine symptoms reflect primary hypothalamic involvement with diabetes insipidus, growth retardation and pubescence dysfunction (delayed or precocious), whereas intracranial hypertension due to early obstruction of intraventricular foramina occurs in 60 percent.

Because of possible ventricular obstruction, ventriculography and angiography are necessary to detect the presence of usually avascular suprasellar masses, which may grow anteriorly into the frontal lobe or in a retrosellar direction into the posterior fossa. Because of the potential hazard of ventriculography in a patient with impaired pituitary function or the possible rupture of a cystic tumor by the needle, CT represents an impressive diagnostic advance in the management of these patients. In no case

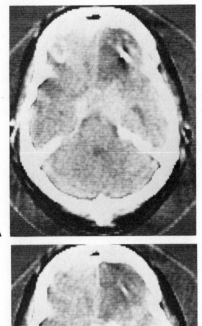

teristics are reliable indicators of the pathological features, and may show several relatively distinct patterns. The majority of tumors are calcified, and the scan may show high-density (50 to 200 units) globules or multilobulated areas in the suprasellar region. If the tumor is solid, it may appear as a calcified high-density mass or as an isodense lesion, which may

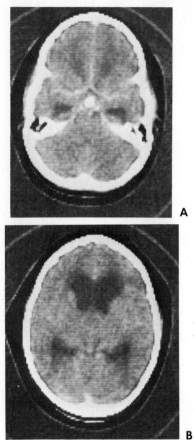

Figure 8–4. A 40-year-old man presented with headache and visual loss, and was found to have bitemporal defect. Radiograph showed an enlarged sella. Initial air study and angiogram showed suprasellar extension. Subtotal intracapsular removal of a pituitary adenoma with a benign histological appearance was followed by a complete course of radiotherapy. Three months later, visual acuity deteriorated and bitemporal field defect occurred. Plain skull radiograph showed no interval change in sella size and no bony erosion. CT showed a high-density, markedly irregular region obliterating the suprasellar cistern (A); the region enhanced and had significant lateral extension (B). Operation revealed an infiltrative and invasive pituitary adenoma without histologic criteria of malignancy or sarcomatous degeneration.

has CT failed to detect this lesion, although frequently meningiomas and aneurysms have had similar characteristics.

The location and density charac-

Figure 8–5. A 5-year-old girl of short stature was admitted because of headache, nausea and vomiting. Neurological examination was negative except for bilateral papilledema. Skull radiograph showed normal sella size but suprasellar calcification. CT revealed a dense, round, high-density area in the sella region corresponding to plain skull radiographic calcification. The lateral ventricles were markedly enlarged and obstructed by an isodense lesion at the level of the intraventricular foramina, with the mass bulging upward into the lateral ventricles (A). Following contrast infusion, there was no enhancement (B) or evidence of vascular displacement. At operation, a solid craniopharyngioma was removed.

enhance (33 percent) and cause obstruction of the intraventricular foramina, with lateral ventricular dilatation and a bulging upward of the lateral ventricle (Fig. 8–5).

Cystic tumors demonstrate round noncontinuous high-density flecks of calcification in their capsule, surrounding a low-density core (Fig. 8–6). This calcification results from degeneration of outer epithelial lining cells, and the cyst may contain thick, highly proteinaceous material with density of 6 to 18 units, or cholesterol-like material with a density as low as −40. Other cystic tumors

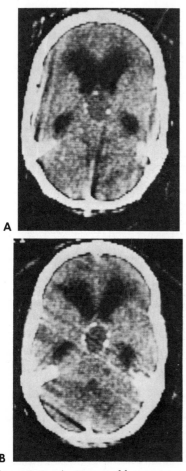

B

Figure 8–6. A 45-year-old woman experienced headache, vomiting of two weeks' duration and amenorrhea for two years. Findings included bitemporal hemianopia and early optic atrophy. Skull radiogram showed no calcification. CT findings: marked lateral ventricular enlargement with obstruction of the third ventricle by a midline lesion of decreased density surrounded by discrete globular areas of high density. On plain scan, an area of heterogeneous calcification is seen (A); following infusion, there is evidence of slight enhancement within the capsule (B). This was consistent with a diagnosis of cystic craniopharyngioma, which was confirmed at operation. Following surgical removal there is no evidence of recurrence.

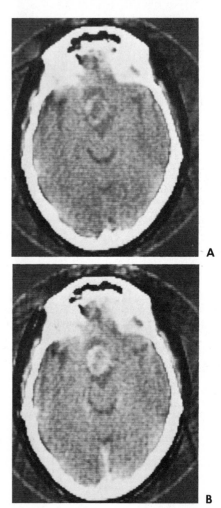

B

Figure 8–7. An elderly man developed progressive loss of vision in the left eye, which improved following prednisone therapy. One year later, vision worsened in both eyes. With prednisone it temporarily improved but subsequently deteriorated. Findings included bilaterally impaired acuity and bitemporal hemianopia. Skull radiograph and sella tomography were normal, but isotope scan showed midline uptake. CT findings: high-density capsule with low-density cyst (A); there is enhancement in the capsule and also centrally, with a peripheral low-density surrounding rim (B). Operative finding: craniopharyngioma.

show a round rim of high density, which may enhance markedly, surrounding a low-density core. Furthermore, the presence of a crescent of low density has been observed with these tumors and this has caused confusion with meningioma (Fig. 8–7).

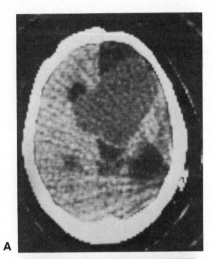

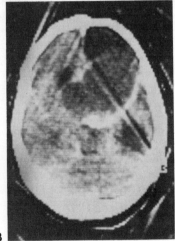

Figure 8–8. An eight-year-old child underwent surgery for craniopharyngioma. The patient developed recurrent headaches and lethargy. CT findings: a huge low-density lesion extending from the suprasellar region into the right frontal lobe (A); following contrast infusion, there is marked enhancement of the surrounding capsule (B). The right lateral ventricle is enlarged and displaced by this huge mass which, at operation, was found to be recurrent cystic craniopharyngioma filled with highly proteinaceous material. In addition, there were several areas of hemispheric porencephaly.

Other tumors reach large size, and this is indicative of a significant cystic component. There may be dense enhancement in the capsule (Fig. 8–8). Naidich found that 80 percent were densely calcified masses in the suprasellar cistern (55 to 350 units), whereas 20 percent showed a faint rim of increased density that surrounded a low-density central core, and these tumors infrequently enhanced. It is important to determine the M-values for the high-density portion of the tumor so as to differentiate calcified craniopharyngioma from hemorrhagic pituitary adenoma.[24, 25]

3. Parasellar Meningiomas. These tumors may arise from the planum sphenoidale, tuberculum, or diaphragma sella and expand into the suprasellar region, causing visual and endocrine symptoms that simulate pituitary adenoma.[26] Plain skull radiogram shows thickening of the bony cortex, with loss of distinct cortical margins and blistering of planum, but if the tumor is intrasellar the radiographic changes may be identical with those of pituitary adenoma. Isotope scan may be positive in two thirds of symptomatic parasellar meningiomas, with at least 1.0 cm extension upward. Diagnosis is best established by angiography which shows elevation and posterior displacement of the anterior cerebral artery, downward and posterior distortion of supraclinoid carotid artery, enlargement of feeding meningeal vessels, and early appearing and persistent tumor stain.

With CT, the diagnosis may be established by the demonstration of a round mass that projects into the anterior and lateral portion of the suprasellar cistern. On plain scan the appearance of density is a reflection of the degree of calcification, such that noncalcified tumor may be isodense but markedly enhance to 30 to 50 units (Fig. 8–9). If the tumor has calcification, although this is *rarely* detected by plain sella tomography, initial density may be 50 to 75, and

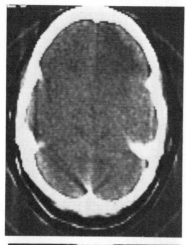

A

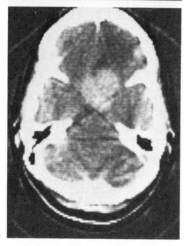

B

Figure 8–9. A 38-year-old woman experienced a six-week period of loss of visual acuity in the right eye initially, then involving the left eye. Findings included marked diminution of acuity in the right eye, mild impairment in the left eye, bitemporal superior quadrant defect and optic pallor. Skull radiograph, isotope scan and sella tomogram were negative. CT findings: plain scan shows only an extensive low-density region in the right frontal region (A), but following infusion, there is a speckled, round mass in the suprasellar region extending into the right frontal region (B). At operation a large parasellar meningioma was found.

evidence of bony hyperostosis may be detected, but this is better evaluated by plain radiograph. These tumors have always enhanced, and failure to administer contrast has led to one false negative study in which a tumor was seen by isotope scan, angiog-

raphy and air study. The ventricular system shows no evidence of distortion or enlargement. The meningiomas rarely have a cystic or hemorrhagic component, and, although well-encapsulated tumors, they show no enhancement of the capsular region, as seen with craniopharyngioma or pituitary adenoma. In some instances the CT appearance is identical to that seen in pituitary adenoma, and pre-operative diagnosis is not possible without angiography.

4. Gliomas. Optic nerve and chiasmal gliomas are hamartomatous lesions rather than true malignant infiltrative neoplasms. The symptomatology depends upon their location, as optic nerve gliomas cause proptosis, visual acuity loss and optic atrophy. The diagnosis is established by optic foramina views, which show a difference in the size of the two canals greater than 1 mm and also evidence of erosive change. Air study has been necessary to delineate the presence of the intracranial portion of the tumor, which may extend to involve the optico-chiasmatic cistern, floor of the third ventricle and hypothalamus, but occasionally small tumors involving the optic nerve and those which primarily involve the optic chiasm may be missed by skull radiograph and air study.

With CT, the orbital intracanalicular portion of the tumor causes fusiform expansion of the optic nerve, and intracranial extension may also be detected. The intracranial portion is well defined, and these tumors are well-marginated round masses, which show striking enhancement (Fig. 8–10). Gliomas of the hypothalamus are more malignant and invasive tumors and may have large cystic components that are defined by CT (Fig. 8–11). In addition, these tumors have large infiltrative solid components, which are visualized as dense, consolidated and irregularly marginated masses.

5. Chordomas. These are congen-

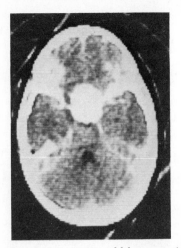

Figure 8–10. A 10-year-old boy experienced decreasing vision in the right eye. Findings included right optic atrophy and impaired acuity in both eyes. The right optic foramen was 2 mm larger than the left. CT findings: a densely enhancing round mass in the suprasellar cistern extending into the right orbital region. Operative finding: low-grade chiasmal glioma.

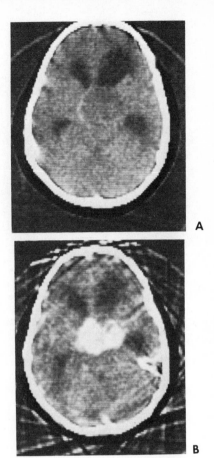

Figure 8–11. This patient had visual disturbance, headache, left-sided weakness and numbness. Findings included papilledema, left hemiparesis and hemisensory deficit. CT findings: obstruction of the interventricular foramen with lateral ventricular enlargement due to an isodense lesion with faint capsule rim (A) and dense, consolidated, irregular enhancement extending into the thalamic and hypothalamic region (B). At operation a solid hypothalamic glioma with a single large cystic component was found.

ital neoplasms that usually are located within the clivus and may grow anteriorly, destroying the sella and invading the sphenoid sinus and nasopharynx, but they may rarely arise in the sella or middle fossa. The most common early symptoms are due to involvement of the abducens nerve, and then the lower cranial nerves are involved as this extradural postclival mass enlarges, displacing the aqueduct, fourth ventricle and brain stem posteriorly.[27]

Skull radiography, including tomograms of the base of the skull, usually shows bony erosion of the clivus and posterior portion of the sella, with calcification that results from bone sequestration or tumor degenerative change. Air study and angiography are necessary to define the location of the tumor as either an extradural postclival or parasellar mass and to detect encasement, irregularity and occlusion of the displaced arteries by the chordoma. These tumors are bulky, lobulated masses that contain a gelatinous or mucoid material within a thin transparent capsule. In other cases they may be firm, containing

cartilaginous and calcified material. The microscopic appearance is cellular, and they are vacuolated, with prominent intercellular mucin.

The CT appearance may be variable and reflects the pathological characteristics. The plain scan may show a round, irregular, high-density lesion, consistent with calcification at the base of the skull, usually located posterior to the dorsum of the sella; it is contiguous with bone and shows

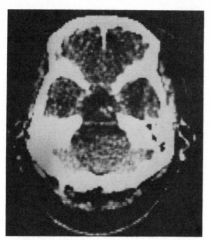

Figure 8–12. A 40-year-old man presented with clinical evidence of hypopituitarism, an enlarged sella and bitemporal hemianopia. CT findings: enlarged sella filled with low-density material with several flecks of calcification and no enhancement. Operative findings: gelatinous material within the sella consistent with chordoma.

no enhancement. In other cases, post-infusion study may show an enhancing consolidated mass that is usually located in a similar position, which may have regular or irregular edges. Lastly, plain scan may show an enlarged sella filled by speckled, low-density (-5 to $+7$) material, which is admixed with a high-density area, consistent with calcification, and there is no enhancement (Fig. 8–12). Utilizing reconstruction in the coronal and sagittal plane, the intra- and extra-axial position of the tumor may be better defined.

6. Aneurysms. These may simulate a pituitary neoplasm, and the possibility of an aneurysm constitutes the major indication for angiography, as the CT appearance may be misleading. In some cases, the wall of the aneurysm shows concentric rings of calcification, and, following infusion, there may be dense, homogeneous enhancement of the intraluminal blood pool. The size of the lesion usually does not increase, as the outer walls do not enhance. Naidich has reported that there may be conti-

nuity between the mass and adjacent vessels.[19] Differentiation from craniopharyngioma is most difficult, especially if there is calcification in the wall or enhancement in the peripheral portion only, a pattern which simulates a cystic tumor (Fig. 8–13).

7. Other Juxtasellar Lesions. Epidermoid cysts are midline in location and appear as low-density (-10 to $+4$), sharply marginated masses, which do not enhance and are usually similar in appearance to arachnoid cysts.

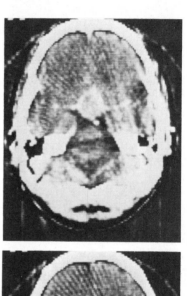

A

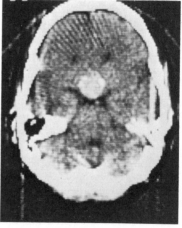

B

Figure 8–13. This patient had a bitemporal hemianopic defect and symmetrically enlarged sella. CT findings: a noncontinuous calcified wall in the central portion of the suprasellar cistern (A), with less dense core and slight central enhancement (B). Angiography and surgery demonstrated an ophthalmic-carotid aneurysm with calcified wall.

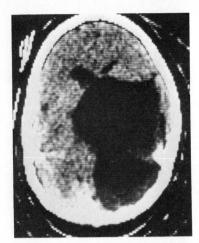

Figure 8–14. This patient was evaluated for amenorrhea and enlarged sella. CT findings: a huge, low-density, sharply marginated nonenhancing mass in the middle fossa, suprasellar cistern and posterior fossa. This was found to be an arachnoid cyst.

Arachnoid cysts may be entirely juxtasellar in location or are huge lesions originating in the middle fossa and expanding into the suprasellar region and the posterior fossa (Fig. 8–14). Recently, an epidermoid cyst was shown to be of high density, and in this case preoperative diagnosis is not possible. Atypical germinoma of the anterior third ventricle appears on plain scan as a mottled, nonhomogeneous, high-density mass, which usually obstructs the third ventricle but has density characteristics that can be distinguished from those of craniopharyngioma. Metastatic disease in the sella is best defined by plain skull radiogram, but CT may show an enhancing lesion contiguous to bone, a pattern similar to that of meningioma.

REFERENCES

1. Weisberg LA, Zimmerman EA, Frantz AG: Diagnosis and evaluation of patients with an enlarged sella turcica. Am J Med 61:590, 1976.
2. Knight CL, Hoyt WF, Wilson CB: Syndrome of incipient prechiasmal optic nerve compression. Arch Ophthal 87:1, 1972.
3. Poppen JL: Changing concepts in the treatment of pituitary adenomas. Bull NY Acad Med 39:21, 1963.
4. Weisberg LA: Pituitary apoplexy. Am J Med 63:109, 1977.
5. DuBoulay G, Trickey S: The choice of radiological investigations in the management of tumors around the sella. Clin Radiol 18:349, 1967.
6. Vezina JL, Sutton TJ: Prolactin-secreting pituitary microadenoma. Am J Roentgenol 120:46, 1974.
7. Neelon FA, Gorce JA, Lebovitz HE: The primary empty sella. Medicine 52:73, 1973.
8. Evens RG, James AE, Adatepe MH: Brain scans in pituitary tumors. Neurology 21:806, 1971.
9. James AE, DeLand FH: Radionuclide imaging in the detection and differential diagnosis of craniopharyngiomas. Am J Roentgenol 109:692, 1970.
10. Lombardi G: Radiology in Neuro-Ophthalmology. Williams and Wilkins, Baltimore, 1967. pp 182–230.
11. Bentson JR: Relative merits of pneumographic and angiographic procedures in the management of pituitary tumors. In: Diagnosis and Treatment of Pituitary Tumors, PD Kohler, GT Ross (eds). Excerpta Medica, Amsterdam, 1973. pp 86–99.
12. Powell DF, Baker HL: The primary angiographic findings in pituitary adenomas. Radiology 110:589, 1974.
13. Roth DA, Ferris EJ, Tomiyasu U: Prognosis of pituitary adenomas with arteriographic abnormal vascularization. J Neurol Neurosurg Psychiatry 34:535, 1971.
14. Johnson JC, Lubow M: The neuroradiology of the optic chiasm and adjacent structures as demonstrated by polytomoencephalography. In: Neuro-ophthalmology, Vol 5. J.S. Glaser, J.L. Smith (eds). Mosby, St. Louis, 1975. pp 72–114.
15. Ganguly A, Stanchfield T, Roberts TS: Cushing's syndrome in a patient with an empty sella and microadenoma of the adenohypophysis. Am J Med 60:30, 1976.
16. Bajraktari X, Bergstrom M: Diagnosis of intrasellar cisternal herniation by CT. J Comput Assist Tomog 1:105, 1977.
17. Rozario R, Hammerschlag SB, Post KD: Diagnosis of empty sella with CT scan. Neuroradiology 13:85, 1977.
18. Costello RT: Subclinical adenoma of the pituitary gland. Am J Pathol 12:205, 1936.

19. Naidich TP, Pinto RS: Evaluation of sellar and parasellar masses by CT. Radiology 120:99, 1976.
20. Reich NE, Zelch JV, Alfidi, RJ: CT in the detection of juxtasellar lesions. Radiology 118:333, 1976.
21. Chang CH, Pool JL: Radiotherapy in pituitary adenoma. Radiology 89:1005, 1967.
22. Kramer S: Indications for and results of treatment of pituitary tumors by irradiation. In: Diagnosis and Treatment of Pituitary Tumors, PS Kohler, GT Ross (eds). Excerpta Medica, Amsterdam, 1973. pp 217–219.
23. David NJ, Gargano FP, Glaser JS: Pituitary apoplexy in clinical perspective. Neuro-ophthalmology, Vol 8, JS Glaser, JL Smith (eds). CV Mosby, St. Louis, 1975. pp 140–165.
24. Bartlett JR: Craniopharyngioma—an analysis of symptomatology. Radiology and Histology. Brain 94:725, 1971.
25. Leeds NE, Naidich TP: CT in the diagnosis of sellar and parasellar lesions. Semin Roentgenol 12:(2):121, 1977.
26. Finn JE, Mount LA: Meningiomas of the tuberculum sellae and planum sphenoidale. Arch Ophthalmol 92:23, 1974.
27. Poppen JL, King AB: Chordoma. J Neurosurg 9:139, 1952.

Chapter 9 Increased Intracranial Pressure

Intracranial hypertension may be caused by many diverse pathological conditions including those of neoplastic, vascular, infectious, inflammatory, toxic, traumatic or metabolic etiologies. The clinical symptoms usually include headache, nausea, vomiting, diplopia, transient obscurations or blurring of vision, and there is funduscopic evidence of papilledema. If the intracranial hypertension is due to a mass lesion with cerebral edema and ventricular compression, there are usually focal neurological signs, altered mentation and frequently evidence of herniation syndrome. Although the absence of spontaneous venous retinal pulsations is usually the most reliable clinical sign of elevated CSF pressure, it is possible for intracranial hypertension to be masked by normal eye findings, either because of normal variants, the time interval required for these changes to occur or certain mechanical properties of the optic nerve. If spontaneous pulsations are absent, lumbar spinal fluid pressure is invariably elevated, and CSF examination must be performed with caution.[1]

In addition, studies with subdural continuous pressure monitors have shown that the actual intracranial pressure may not always be reflected by lumbar pressure measurement. Therefore, in patients who are clinically suspected of having an intracranial lesion, the value of diagnostic lumbar puncture must be weighed against its potential hazard.

Other neurological signs caused by intracranial hypertension are related to the direct compressive effect of the underlying pathological process, which displaces and distorts adjacent tissue, causing shifts and herniation of intracranial structures. This may produce localized neurological signs and more distant disturbances owing to the effect of the herniation syndromes. Altered mentation may result as the medially displaced temporal lobe interferes with diencephalic and upper midbrain reticular activating function or may result from the effect of generalized cerebral edema. Hemiparesis may be due to direct compressive effect or result from compression of the cerebral peduncle at the tentorial notch. In addition, compression of the dorsal midbrain at the tentorium may cause third nerve involvement (nonreactivity and dilatation of the pupil with impaired ocular motility) and paresis of upward gaze with nystagmus as a result of the involvement of the dorsal longitudinal fasciculus. Vascular compression at the tentorium may cause posterior cerebral artery infarction, which results in homonymous hemianopia or complete blindness. Tonsillar cerebellar herniation may cause marked cardiorespiratory effects, including blood pressure elevation and slowing of the heart and respiration as the medullary autonomic centers are compressed. Occasionally posterior fossa masses may cause papilledema with marked blood pressure elevation, simulating hypertensive encephalopathy (Fig. 9-1).

Other neurological disturbances are directly related to ventricular dilata-

179

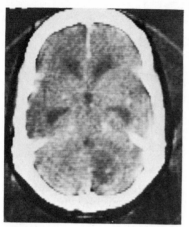

Figure 9–1.   A patient with a previous history of mild hypertension suddenly developed headache, nausea and vomiting; blood pressure was 220/140 mm Hg. Neurological examination was negative except for bilateral papilledema, with several large hemorrhages and exudates located in the periphery of the disc, and moderately advanced arteriolar narrowing. Blood pressure rapidly returned to normal with medical treatment, but severe headache persisted. Skull radiograph, isotope scan and EEG were normal. CT showed ventricular dilatation proximal to the fourth ventricle, which appeared to be obliterated by a round low-density mass in the right cerebellar hemisphere that showed ringlike enhancement. Operative findings: metastatic neoplasm with central necrotic core.

of the chiasm is compressed against the adjacent internal carotid artery. This may be associated with visual acuity impairment and optic atrophy secondary to mechanical and vascular compression of the optic nerve, and the reduced field of vision and optic atrophy may suggest a suprasellar tumor (Fig. 9–2). Endocrine symptoms consistent with hypopituitarism may also result from transmission of the pulsatile pressure of the ballooned third ventricle against the hypothalamus and pituitary with longstanding intracranial hypertension.[2] Rhinorrhea may also result from prolonged intracranial hypertension, because of the mechanical effect of the ballooned third ventricle and increased pulsations against bone in the sellar region.[3]

The diagnostic assessment of patients who present with papilledema without definite evidence of localizing or lateralizing neurological signs is an urgent and challenging problem that frequently confronts the clinician.

tion, with compression of contiguous structures without herniation. Abducens nerve paresis is manifested by lateral rectus weakness and nystagmoid jerking movements in the externally rotated eye, and this is one of the most common nonlocalizing signs of increased intracranial pressure. This is usually a unilateral finding and is due to compression of the nerve at the apex of the petrous bone. Less frequently, abducens nerve involvement is bilateral, and this may also be seen in primary intra-axial brain stem tumors, but with this lesion papilledema is a late finding. With intracranial hypertension, the anterior third ventricle may be distended and ballooned and may compress the midportion of the optic chiasm, causing bitemporal hemianopic field defect or, more rarely, binasal hemianopia, as the lateral aspect

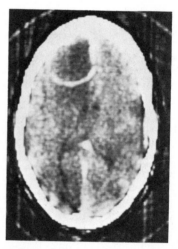

Figure 9–2.   A 25-year-old woman presented with papilledema, bitemporal hemianopic defect and enlarged sella. Isotope scan showed uptake in left frontal region extending to the midline. CT findings: large radiolucent area in left frontal lobe with surrounding thin rim of high density, which distorted the anterior portion of the lateral ventricle and showed marked enhancement. Angiograph showed abnormal filling of vessels derived from the external carotid supply. At operation an angioblastic meningioma was removed.

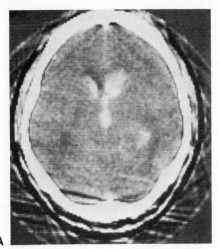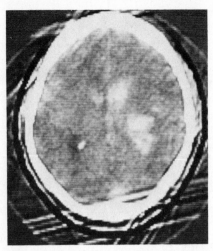

A   **B**

Figure 9–3.   A 35-year-old man suddenly developed headache and stiff neck. He had bilateral papilledema and was only slightly lethargic. EEG was diffusely slow and four-vessel angiography was negative. CT findings: mild ventricular enlargement with evidence of high-density material consistent with blood in all chambers. CSF examination showed red blood cells, xanthochromia and markedly elevated pressure. In the right thalamic region a small parenchymal hematoma was visualized as the cause of the intraventricular hemorrhage. The patient has recovered completely.

Certain ophthalmological conditions may be confused with papilledema, including optic neuritis, central retinal vein thrombosis, diabetic or hypertensive retinopathy and congenital abnormalities of the optic nerve, but these may not represent intracranial hypertension. These conditions may also cause enlargement of the blind spot as in papilledema, and exclusion of a primary intracranial lesion may require contrast radiographic procedures and lumbar puncture to demonstrate normal CSF pressure. If the papilledema is indicative of underlying cerebral edema or ventricular obstruction, preliminary neurodiagnostic studies, including EEG, isotope scan, skull radiograph and echoencephalogram, should be done prior to a diagnostic lumbar puncture. In patients with papilledema who are suspected of having an underlying infectious process or subarachnoid hemorrhage, CSF examination is mandatory to confirm this diagnosis. In cases of hemorrhage and meningitis the highest reported CSF pressures have been recorded, but unless there is a complicating condition such as intracerebral or subdural hematoma, empyema or abscess, herniation does not occur despite markedly elevated pressure (Fig. 9–3).

The method of diagnostic evaluation of patients with papilledema and no localizing signs has remained quite controversial with regard to the sequence and completeness of studies that should be performed. Several studies have described patients who presented with increased intracranial pressure without localizing neurological signs and underwent ventriculography or craniotomy with no mass lesion found.[4] Initially, it was believed that subsequent studies would detect an underlying etiology, but follow-up of these patients extending to 12 years showed no evidence of mass lesion. Despite this unusual occurrence, the prevailing belief was that papilledema alone was most likely to be caused by an intracranial neoplasm, most likely in a midline location. To support this concept, Kelly reported that of 21 patients who presented with papilledema and headache only, 10 had midline obstructive lesions, of which seven were colloid cysts of the third ventricle; but in addition, nine had lateralized supratentorial mass lesions.[5]

The finding that the syndrome of increased intracranial pressure without localizing signs was caused by lateralized mass lesion was confirmed by Berg, who reviewed the results of ventriculography or craniotomy performed in patients with this syndrome. Fifty percent had lateralized mass lesion, 27 percent had a midline obstructive process, 13 percent had subacute meningitis without evidence of mass lesion, and 10 percent had a normal ventricular system and CSF examination with follow-up of several years. In this study, EEG was localizing in 67 percent, but normal in one third of cases. The results of this study indicated that the majority of patients had a lateralized lesion, but one tenth of patients who came to contrast study or surgery had no pathological abnormality to explain intracranial hypertension.[6] Careful follow-up of these latter patients showed that the major danger was the prevention of visual loss due to the effect of increased pressure. Rarely, certain lesions were not detected with initial studies but, with the introduction of isotope scan and percutaneous angiography, the need for ventriculography or explorative craniotomy has markedly decreased (Table 9–1).

Prior to CT scan, the conventional diagnostic approach was to exclude the presence of most supratentorial or midline lesions with EEG, skull radiogram, isotope scan, and echoencephalogram, and then to proceed to angiography to determine if hydrocephalus was present. Depending on the presence or absence of ventricular enlargement, ventriculography or pneumoencephalography was then performed. EEG is believed to be an excellent procedure for supratentorial lesions and is generally reliable and sensitive in detecting 96 percent of these lesions when combined with isotope scan, but it usually does not detect midline or posterior fossa lesions.[7] In addition, if intracranial hy-

TABLE 9–1. Recognized Pathological Conditions in Increased Intracranial Pressure Without Localizing Signs

Supratentorial
  Multiple metastases
  Solitary tumors
    Glioma (temporal, frontal, parietal, thalamic, corpus callosum)
    Meningioma
  Subdural hematoma
  Arteriovenous malformation (hemispheric, dural)
  Arachnoid cyst
  Brain abscess
Midline Obstructive
  Craniopharyngioma
  Pituitary adenoma
  Intraventricular (meningioma, colloid cyst, choroid plexus papilloma, ependymal cyst)
  Pineal neoplasm (pinealoma, germinoma, metastases, glioma)
  Aqueductal stenosis
    Nontumorous
    Tumorous
  Suprasellar arachnoid cyst
Posterior Fossa
  Cerebellar neoplasm (astrocytoma, metastatic, hemangioblastoma)
  Fourth ventricular neoplasm (ependymoma, medulloblastoma, choroid plexus papilloma)
  Brain stem (glioma)
Diffuse Infiltrating Processes
  Astrocytoma
  Microglioma
  Sarcoma
  Gliomatosis cerebri
Miscellaneous
  Venous sinus thrombosis (superior sagittal, lateral)
  Communicating hydrocephalus
  Hemorrhage (subarachnoid, intraventricular)
  Cerebritis
  Lead encephalopathy
  Infectious and parainfectious diseases
  Benign intracranial hypertension
  Reye's syndrome
  Basilar meningitis (leukemic, metastatic, sarcoidosis, tuberculous, cryptococcal)

pertension is due to ventricular obstruction or cerebral edema, EEG may demonstrate a bilateral nonlocalizing frontal or posterior rhythmic delta pattern. Plain skull radiogram may show an abnormal sella with changes of a juxtasellar lesion resulting from chronic increase in intracranial pressure, including erosion of the lamina dura, enlargement with depression of the floor, and thinning and atrophy of the posterior to a greater degree than the anterior clinoid process. The shift of the pineal suggests a supratentorial lesion and usually correlates with a shift of midline echoencephalographic third ventricular pattern. With chronically increased intracranial pressure there may be decalcification of the pineal region and radiographic nonvisualization of this structure. Even if all noninvasive studies were negative, lumbar puncture was believed to be potentially dangerous and only to be attempted after angiography or ventriculography.

More recent studies have suggested an alternative approach to patients with headache and papilledema alone, an approach that emphasizes the important of lumbar puncture and possible avoidance of angiography and air study. Of 100 patients, 82 percent had no mass lesion or evidence of ventricular enlargement, and in 71 percent the final diagnosis was benign intracranial hypertension. Of those patients who had a normal level of consciousness and no localizing neurological findings associated with negative isotope scan and EEG, none had a clinically unsuspected lesion demonstrated by contrast studies. CSF examination was essential, as 7 percent had infectious or neoplastic meningitis, and in all these cases CSF pressure was elevated but herniation did not occur. In certain patients the suspicion of mass lesion or ventricular enlargement was so low, based on clinical and diagnostic evaluation, that neither air study nor angiogram was performed. CSF examination confirmed the diagnosis of benign intracranial hypertension, and in follow-up for several years the condition remained benign.[8] This approach has its dangers because in certain patients posterior fossa neoplasm may be initially undetected. Previous studies have shown that some patients with these tumors may have increased intracranial pressure but a normal-sized ventricular system, as shown by angiography or air study, and vertebral angiography is necessary to detect a shift of the posterior fossa vessels, mass effect and tumor stain.[9]

With the introduction of CT scan,

the approach to the patient who has papilledema alone or who had only abducens nerve paresis, nystagmoid jerks or minimal unsteadiness of gait has been markedly altered and the need for contrast radiographic procedures has been markedly decreased.[10] Of 50 patients with papilledema only, CT was superior to EEG, isotope scan, skull radiogram and echoencephalogram, and no lesion was missed by CT and subsequently detected by air study or angiography. The demonstration of normal CT scan may safely be followed by lumbar puncture without risk of herniation, and the presence of a normal CT scan was most consistent with the diagnosis of benign intracranial hypertension. In 15 of these patients who had benign intracranial hypertension established by CT, other diagnostic studies were abnormal, but these findings were nonspecific.

Because of our initial lack of clinical experience with CT in this condition, contrast studies were frequently carried out and were uniformly negative. Of 15 patients who had papilledema accompanied by abducens nerve paresis, nystagmoid jerks, minimal unsteadiness of gait, slight reflex asymmetry and mild pronator drift, a pattern which suggested the presence of an expanding mass, a normal CT scan obviated the need for invasive studies. In three patients, a bitemporal hemianopic defect and enlarged sella suggested a primary suprasellar tumor, but plain and contrast studies were negative. Because air study is still believed to be the most sensitive procedure to detect juxtasellar lesions, this was performed and showed an empty sella syndrome. In this case, it was postulated that the increased pulsatile force of the anterior third ventricle compressed the optic chiasm and caused remodeling of the sella region.[11] In another patient who presented with papilledema, a bitemporal visual field defect and an enlarged sella, the presence of a suprasellar lesion was suspected.

The normal results of EEG and isotope scan were consistent with this impression, but CT showed a large frontal lobe tumor that was compressing the ventricular system; the resulting intracranial hypertension caused chiasmal involvement (Fig. 9–2).

BENIGN INTRACRANIAL HYPERTENSION (BIH)

This condition occurs most frequently in young, obese and otherwise healthy patients who present with papilledema only, but occasionally these patients may present with or subsequently develop symptoms of hypopituitarism, abducens nerve paresis or bitemporal hemianopic defect. The diagnosis of this condition is established by CSF examination, which is normal except for elevated pressure, and by diagnostic studies that exclude ventricular dilatation and mass lesion.

The pathogenesis of the intracranial hypertension is not clearly established, but the role of venous sinus thrombosis in causing elevated venous pressure and impaired CSF reabsorption, as in cases of lateral sinus involvement secondary to mastoid infection or superior sagittal sinus thrombosis secondary to coagulopathy or oral contraceptives.

Other theories have postulated that intracranial hypertension is related to increased blood volume and flow of unknown cause, whereas others have implicated metabolic-endocrine disorders in causing increased intracranial pressure, as in the case of steroid use or withdrawal, obesity and menstrual disorders. Recent studies have demonstrated an increase in CSF volume with impaired reabsorption due to disturbance in flow across the microvilli of the arachnoid granulations of the subarachnoid spaces that causes distention of these spaces with normal or even small size of the ventricular system.[12]

In the majority of cases of BIH,

both EEG and isotope scan are negative. The EEG does not demonstrate the rhythmic delta slow wave pattern frequently seen in obstructive hydrocephalus, but may show nonspecific abnormalities. In 20 percent of cases plain skull radiogram shows sellar enlargement, which may raise suspicion of an intrasellar mass but is usually due to an associated "empty sella syndrome." Because this condition may be secondary to venous sinus thrombosis (lateral, sagittal, sigmoid) or underlying dural or cerebral vascular malformation, angiography or jugular venography may be necessary studies. In addition, intracranial hypertension may be the presenting symptom in systemic lupus erythematosus and angiography may document segmental arterial lesions.

In BIH, air study shows the ventricles to be of normal size and in some cases they are reported as slitlike in configuration. One report of ventricular dimensions demonstrated by air study showed normal volume in 76 percent but in 44 percent of cases the superior aspect of the lateral ventricle showed sharp acute angulation.[12, 13] The small size of the ventricular system may be obscured by an artifact, since air distends the ventricles, making the small size appear normal. The implication that the ventricles are small in size is based on a hypothesis that benign intracranial hypertension is due to a form of cerebral edema. This is supported by certain findings including cerebral biopsy specimens showing intra- or extracellular edema, the production of cerebral edema in animals by obstruction of the torcular herophili, and in humans by lateral sinus occlusion, the occurrence of cerebral edema in animals with vitamin A deficiency and abnormalities of arachnoid granulations, as well as by small-sized ventricles. The presence of a normal mental state and normal EEG findings is highly inconsistent with cerebral edema.

In BIH, CT has shown some interesting and unexpected findings. If cerebral edema were present, the scan would be expected to show a generalized, irregular, low-density pattern compressing the ventricular and cisternal spaces; and as intracranial hypertension resolves, the ventricles would be clearly visualized. In most cases this pattern is not visualized by inspection of scan, and a histogram of tissue densities on preinfusion scan showed a mean of 17 units, with the expected even distribution on both sides of the mean.[14] Hahn has demonstrated that the bifrontal ventricular dimension at the level of the head of the caudate is poorly visualized in this condition.[15] In 10 percent of cases the cisternal spaces are quite prominent and the ventricles are normal, a pattern consistent with the hypothesis that impaired CSF reabsorption is a result of abnormalities of arachnoid granulation.

In one case, CT showed a large triangular area of low density located posteriorly in the midline, without enhancement or mass effect, and this raised suspicions of cystic tumor; subsequent air study demonstrated that this was capacious cisterna magna (Fig. 9–4). This confirms the observation made at subtemporal decompression in patients with benign intracranial hypertension that subarachnoid spaces were distended and the ventricular system appeared compressed. In the remainder of cases, no abnormalities were detected on plain scan, and infusion studies were done in only 20 percent, and only at the request of the referring physician.

Huckman has suggested that, in all patients suspected of having benign intracranial hypertension, contrast infusion be done despite negative plain CT scan, so that bilateral metastatic lesions or an arteriovenous malformation, which do not cause ventricular enlargement, distortion or mass effect, may be excluded.[13] This would be a most unusual occurrence, and there have been no reports of pa-

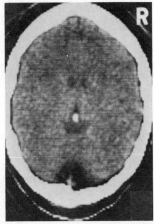

Figure 9–4. A 37-year-old woman with a six-month history of headache had bilateral papilledema only. Skull radiograph, isotope scan and EEG were negative; CSF findings included pressure at 400 mm H_2O with normal protein content. CT findings: a posterior midline area of homogeneously decreased density with normal-sized ventricular system. Air study showed capacious cisterna magna. Diagnosis: benign intracranial hypertension. (Reprinted courtesy of Radiology.)

tients who had normal plain scan but whose postinfusion scan demonstrated this abnormality[16, 17] In one patient whose symptoms reflected increased intracranial pressure and who had bilateral papilledema, the findings of CT, isotope scan and angiography confirmed the presence of an arteriovenous malformation. CT showed normal-sized ventricles without displacement and a low-density mass that did not enhance. Because the angioma was extensive, diversionary lumbar-peritoneal shunt was necessary, and the patient's symptoms disappeared, but there was no change in the appearance of the lesion size by scan.[18]

SUPRATENTORIAL LESIONS

Ten patients with papilledema only were found by CT to have supratentorial lesions. In all instances of neoplasms causing this syndrome, CT demonstrated the responsible lesion more sensitively and accurately than other conventional diagnostic studies and more reliably predicted tumor type than did angiography. In one case of chronic subdural hematoma, CT visualized only ventricular distortion and displacement of the isodense hematoma that was clearly defined by angiography. Of four cases of multiple metastatic tumors, isotope scan and EEG visualized a single lesion in two and in two others only one of these studies indicated the presence

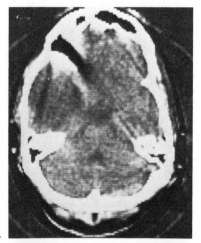

A

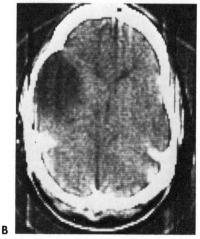

B

Figure 9–5. A 30-year-old man developed severe headache following head trauma. Neurological findings included only bilateral papilledema with normal mentation and no focal deficit. EEG isotope scan and skull radiograph were normal. CT findings: large low-density, well-marginated area in the left temporal region, which was compressing the left side of the suprasellar cistern (A) and did not enhance (B). At operation a large subarachnoid cyst was removed and a hypoplastic temporal lobe was also visualized.

of the lesion. Two patients with subarachnoid cysts had normal EEG and isotope scan, and CSF findings consistent with benign intracranial hypertension, but CT defined a well-marginated, low-density area without enhancement, consistent with non-neoplastic cyst (Fig. 9–5).

In these cases, CT showed evidence of distortion of the lateral aspect of the suprasellar cistern consistent with transtentorial herniation. Other CT signs of impending herniation include (1) displacement of the brain stem toward the contralateral side with increase in width of the subarachnoid space between the mass and the ipsilateral free tentorial edge, (2) medial stretching of the posterior cerebral and posterior communicating artery, (3) obliteration of the interpeduncular cistern, (4) occipital lobe infarction and (5) distortion of the elongated U-shaped tentorial incisura.[19] In four supratentorial gliomas, EEG lateralized the lesion in all, but isotope scan was uniformly negative, whereas in both primary callosal gliomas EEG and isotope scan were negative. In these latter cases, angiography showed tumor stain but CT accurately defined the location and tumor histology, which was confirmed by biopsy.

MIDLINE OBSTRUCTIVE LESIONS

Midline tumors may cause symmetrical hydrocephalus proximal to the site of obstruction, and initial studies of the syndrome of increased intracranial pressure without localizing signs suggested that lesions in this location were the most common cause of the syndrome. In five patients, CT clearly demonstrated the neoplastic or non-neoplastic nature of the obstructive process at the level of the third ventricle or aqueduct. In four cases, CT showed symmetrical ventricular enlargement proximal to the aqueduct, with a normal-sized fourth ventricle and no abnormal tissue density on plain and contrast infusion scan. The posterior third ventricle was directed convex posteriorly, a position most consistent with nontumorous aqueductal stenosis. If tumor is present the shape is distorted, and the ventricle is displaced anteriorly with an inversion of its shape. Ventriculography confirmed this diagnosis in all four cases, and some have suggested that positive contrast ventriculography be performed to exclude a small tumor that is not visualized by CT or air study. In two patients the presence of mild bilateral cerebellar disturbance suggested a posterior fossa tumor, but CT findings were most consistent with aqueductal stenosis; follow-up for two years has confirmed this diagnosis (Fig. 9–6).

Colloid cysts of the third ventricle may be pedunculated, causing intermittent ventricular obstruction; these patients frequently present with headache that occurs with change in head position, and they may have papilledema. If the cyst is fixed in position the symptoms may be more se-

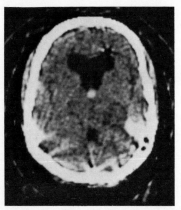

Figure 9–7. A 50-year-old woman had rhinorrhea for nine months and no other neurological findings. A skull radiogram showed an enlarged and eroded sella and air study showed an empty sella and small colloid cyst. CT findings: lateral ventricular enlargement with indentation of the anterior third ventricle by a round high-density lesion which did enhance slightly. These findings were consistent with colloid cyst of the third ventricle. (Courtesy of Dr. A. Albert Goree, Duke University Medical Center.)

vere, with dementia, gait disturbance and incontinence, mimicking the clinical presentation of normal pressure hydrocephalus.[20]

Ventriculography is the most reliable diagnostic study to demonstrate lateral ventricular dilatation and to outline the cyst, whereas pneumoencephalography is associated with greater risk and is less diagnostically accurate; angiographic diagnosis requires magnification vertebral angiotomography. The cyst usually is oval in shape, has smooth contours and may be less than one centimeter in size. The material in the cyst is highly proteinaceous and contains degenerated secretory products.

Because of their small size, CT may not always outline these cysts, and ventricular enlargement may be the only finding, but CT has been equal to ventriculography in demonstrating this lesion. The cyst appears as a smoothly contoured high-density round lesion located in the anterior third ventricular region; it may enhance slightly with infusion. The enhancement is probably intravascular,

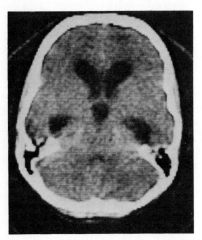

Figure 9–6. A 15-year-old boy with a six-month history of headache, nausea and vomiting had bilateral papilledema. A skull radiogram showed an enlarged sella turcica but EEG and isotope scan were negative. CT findings: marked dilatation of lateral and third ventricle with faint visualization of normal-sized fourth ventricle, a pattern consistent with aqueductal stenosis, later confirmed by ventriculogram.

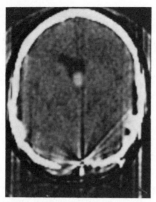

Figure 9–8. A 16-year-old girl initially presented with papilledema and headache. Following air study, a shunt was inserted, and posterior fossa exploration was negative. One year later she developed recurrence of headache and minimal gait unsteadiness. CT findings: round high-density homogeneous mass at level of anterior third ventricle with collapse of right ventricular system by shunt. This is consistent with colloid cyst. (Courtesy of Dr. A. Albert Goree, Duke University Medical Center.)

as these tumors demonstrate a choroid blush derived from the hypertrophied choroidal vessels (Figs. 9–7 and 9–8). The colloid cysts are

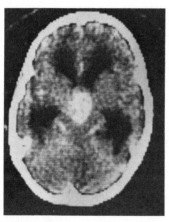

Figure 9–9. A 12-year-old boy presented with a two-week history of headache, nausea and vomiting. Findings included papilledema and all studies were negative except CSF examination, which showed elevated pressure, a cell count of 60 "atypical lymphocytes" and protein content was 60 mg per 100 ml. CT findings: marked lateral ventricular enlargement with upward displacement of posterior portion of lateral ventricles by irregularly shaped, consolidated, high-density mass obliterating entire third ventricle. Operative biopsy findings: germinoma of the third ventricle.

usually of high density and enhancement, and this differentiates them from ependymal cysts, which are usually avascular and filled with clear fluid which has density of CSF.[21] Other tumors that obstruct the third ventricle and present with papilledema only include pinealoma, glioma, craniopharyngioma and, rarely, meningioma or choroid plexus papilloma. The tumors obstruct the posterior third ventricle and quadrigeminal cistern, and symptoms may be papilledema or signs of involvement of the quadrigeminal plate region (paralysis of upward gaze, dilatation of pupils with loss of pupillary reflex to light and accommodation). Plain skull radiogram may show nonspecific sella changes of increased intracranial pressure and abnormal calcification in pineal area. Ventriculography usually shows lateral ventricular dilatation, but if obstruction is incomplete the ventricles may be normal in size. Because of the need to assess the quadrigeminal cistern, combined ventriculography and pneumoencephalography is necessary to outline the margin of the tumor, which may be widespread with direct extension along the floor of the third ventricle. With CT, it is possible to obtain a clear picture of the location and pathological characteristics of the tumor. The diagnosis may usually be made by CT alone, and this may obviate the need for air study or angiography (Fig. 9–9).

POSTERIOR FOSSA LESIONS

Ten patients with papilledema alone were diagnosed by CT as having infratentorial lesions. In six cases the tumor was midline in location, which is the most usual location for this syndrome, but in four cases the tumor was laterally located in the cerebellar hemisphere. Previous studies have found EEG to be abnormal in 82 percent of infratentorial cases if papilledema is present but in only 38 percent in the absence of papilledema. The abnormal pattern reflects a nonspecific effect of increased intracranial pressure and does not have localizing value. In two patients EEG showed definite focal delta waves, a pattern suggestive of a second supratentorial metastatic deposit, and this suspicion was confirmed by CT. Isotope scan has recently been shown to be equal to CT in the diagnosis of posterior fossa tumor, but in our experience it is much less sensitive than CT. Radionuclide scan is most reliable for metastatic lesions, but was positive in only 50 percent of other tumors and infrequently detects cystic lesions (astrocytoma, hemangioblastoma). In seven of ten cases, both EEG and isotope scan were negative in suggesting diagnosis of benign intracranial hypertension, but CT readily demonstrated the ventricular obstruction and abnormal density (Fig. 9–10).

In patients with papilledema suspected of harboring posterior fossa

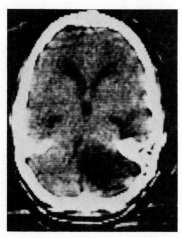

Figure 9–10. A 13-year-old girl presented with a seven-month history of intermittent headaches and multiple episodes of transient visual blurring, and showed bilateral papilledema. Skull radiograph, isotope scan, EEG and echoencephalogram were negative. CSF examination: pressure was 400 mm H_2O with protein content of 10 mg per 100 ml. CT findings: large radiolucent area in the right posterior fossa, distorting the fourth ventricle; and without enhancement, consistent was a cystic astrocytoma. This was confirmed at operation.

neoplasm, the finding of normal-sized ventricles may infrequently occur. Prior to the introduction of CT, air study was the most sensitive technique in detecting these lesions, but ventriculography may be difficult if the ventricles are of normal size because it may not be possible to accurately place the ventricular needle in the ventricle, and if air is introduced from the lumbar region, cerebellar herniation may occur. In two thirds of cases, the diagnosis was established by CT alone and no further contrast studies were necessary. In several patients who presented with papilledema, it was surprising that, although the mass lesion was clearly defined in the posterior fossa, the ventricular system was not enlarged, and the mechanism of the intracranial hypertension was not clear.

MISCELLANEOUS LESIONS

Several types of primary and secondary intracranial neoplasms seed into the meninges. This is most usually seen in leukemia and lymphoma, although medulloblastoma, ependymoma, and pinealoma may also produce CSF pleocytosis. These tumors present a confusing clinical picture if no neurological signs are present other than papilledema. The earliest symptoms may relate to increased intracranial pressure, as there is a resorptive defect involving the arachnoid granulation; this is frequently accompanied by cranial nerve involvement and gait disorder. The diagnosis is established by CSF examination with findings of pleocytosis, elevated protein and sometimes decreased sugar content. Cytological examination is necessary to establish the malignant nature of the cells. In these cases, CT is helpful in diagnosis by establishing the size of the ventricles, demonstrating evidence of parenchymatous involvement and detecting cisternal involvement, information not obtainable with other

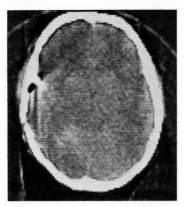

Figure 9–11. In a patient with headache and papilledema only, EEG was diffusely abnormal and isotope scan was negative. Angiography showed no mass effect or tumor stain, and air study suggested a mass in the left temporal region. CT findings: compression of lateral ventricular system with no displacement and a low-density area in the bifrontal region. Biopsy of left temporal region indicated a low-grade glioma.

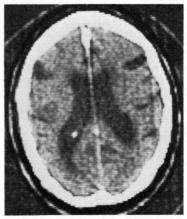

Figure 9–12. A 50-year-old man with diabetes mellitus requiring insulin presented with severe frontal headache and was found to have bilateral papilledema but no evidence of diabetic retinopathy. EEG, skull radiogram and isotope scan were negative. CT findings: ventricular, cisternal and sulcal prominence consistent with atrophic process; several wedge-shaped areas indicated multiple cerebral infarctions. Subsequent lumbar puncture showed normal CSF examination except for elevated pressure, and air study confirmed the CT findings. The headache and papilledema resolved following repeated lumbar taps.

diagnostic studies. In some cases, contrast studies demonstrate enhancement of the cisterns due to a breakdown of the blood-brain barrier. In five cases of patients who presented with intracranial hypertension with CSF findings indicative of a meningitic process, CT demonstrated the presence of a mass lesion or subependymal implant by tumor, and both EEG and isotope scan were negative.

Certain diffusely infiltrating microgliomas or sarcomas may cause obstruction of the CSF pathways and edema without exerting a significant mass effect. In these cases, the patient may not show localizing neurological signs or have seizures. If the tumor does not communicate with the ventricular or cisternal surface, the CSF examination may be normal, and angiography may show no mass effect. In this case, air study may show compression of the ventricular system, but this may be confused with small ventricles of benign intracranial hypertension; the diagnosis may be suggested by CT findings and then confirmed by biopsy (Fig. 9–11).

Two patients presented with papilledema, headache and mild unsteadiness of gait, symptoms that suggested posterior fossa tumor. CT showed only generalized ventricular and sulcal enlargement with several focal areas of low density, consistent with cerebral infarction (Fig. 9–12). Air study confirmed this impression and angiography showed multiple segmental arterial vascular occlusions. CSF study was negative except for elevated pressure. The symptoms and the papilledema responded to repeated removal of CSF.

Lead encephalopathy may present with evidence of diffuse cerebral edema and increased intracranial pressure, and less frequently there may be lateralizing neurological signs. Hungerford reported the CT findings in one documented case in which there was unilateral evidence of cerebral edema with a gyral pattern of enhancement, and in this case angiography also showed evidence of an avascular mass.[22]

REFERENCES

1. Levin BE: Spontaneous venous pulsations as an indicator of intracranial pressure. Neurology 27:346, 1977.
2. Kahana L, Lebovitz H, Lusk W, et al: Endocrine manifestations of intracranial extrasellar lesions. J Clin Endocrinol 22:304, 1962.
3. Weisberg LA, Housepian EM, Saur DP: Empty sella syndrome as complication of benign intracranial hypertension. J Neurosurg 43:177, 1975.
4. Zuidema GD, Cohen SJ: Pseudotumor cerebri. J Neurosurg 11:433–441, 1954.
5. Kelly R: Colloid cysts of the third ventricle. Brain 74:23, 1951.
6. Berg L, Rosomoff HL, Aronson N: The syndrome of increased intracranial pressure without localizing signs. Arch Neurol Psychiatry 78:498, 1955.
7. Murphy JT, Gloor P, Yamamoto YL: Comparison of EEG and brain stain in supratentorial tumors. N Engl J Med 276:309, 1967.
8. Weisberg LA: The syndrome of increased intracranial pressure without localizing signs: A reappraisal. Neurology 25:85, 1975.
9. Yashon D, White R, Croft TJ: Midline posterior fossa neoplasms without lateral ventricular enlargement. JAMA 215:89, 1971.
10. Weisberg LA, Nice CN: CT evaluation of increased intracranial pressure without localizing signs. Radiology 122:133, 1977.
11. Buckman MT, Husain M, Carlow TJ: Primary empty sella syndrome with visual field defects. AM J Med 61:124, 1976.
12. Broddie HG, Banna M, Bradley WG: Benign intracranial hypertension: survey of clinical and radiological features. Brain 97:313, 1974.
13. Johnston I, Paterson A: Benign intracranial hypertension. Brain 97:301, 1974.
14. Huckman MS, Fox JS, Ramsey RG, Penn RD: Computed tomography in the diagnosis of pseudotumor cerebri. Radiology 119:593, 1976.
15. Hahn FJY, Schapiro RL: The excessively small ventricle on CAT of the brain. Neuroradiology 12:137, 1976.
16. Delaney P, Schellinger D: CT and benign intracranial hypertension. JAMA 236:951, 1976.
17. Lightfoote WE, Pressman BD: Increased intracranial pressure; Evaluation by CT. Am J Roentgenol 124:195, 1975.
18. Weisberg LA, Pierce JA, Jabbari BD: Arterio-venous malformation presenting with intracranial hypertension. South Med J 70:624, 1977.
19. Osborn AG: Diagnosis of descending transtentorial herniation by cranial computed tomography. Radiology 123:93, 1977.
20. Little JR, MacCarty CS: Colloid cyst of the third ventricle. J Neurosurg 40:230, 1974.
21. Sackett JF, Messina AV, Petito CK: CT and magnification vertebral angiotomography in the diagnosis of colloid cysts of third ventricle. Radiology 116:95, 1975.
22. Hungerford GH, Ross P, Robertson HJK: CT in lead encephalopathy. Radiology 123:91, 1977.

10 Progressive
Mental
Deterioration
and Impaired
Consciousness

DEMENTIA

Dementia may be defined as an organic brain syndrome in which the patient demonstrates a global impairment of cognitive and intellectual function, frequently accompanied by personality changes. It usually results from extensive diffuse or multifocal cerebral pathological disturbances and less commonly is associated with a single large focal lesion. The cardinal symptoms include defects in orientation, memory, intellectual function, reasoning ability and judgment that are frequently associated with changes in behavior, personality and emotionality. This disorder accounts for 30 percent of all first admissions to psychiatric facilities.[1] In addition, patients evaluated for clinically suspected dementia compose 10 to 15 percent of admissions and represent the second or third most common admission and discharge diagnosis on the neurology service.

In certain patients with clinical evidence of dementia, there are associated neurological abnormalities that suggest the presence of a focal lesion, and in these cases complete neurodiagnostic studies, including air study and angiography, are usually indicated. In other cases the dementia is the only neurological abnormality, and it has frequently been assumed that the most likely cause was an irreversible progressive atrophic or vascular degenerative condition if no metabolic, toxic or infectious condition was detected. Because of lack of focal signs complete neurodiagnostic investigation is not always performed. In complete diagnostic studies of patients with dementia it has been reported that 20 to 30 percent of patients have a potentially reversible neurological disorder, whereas in 25 to 30 percent a definite but probably untreatable disease (multi-infarct dementia, alcoholic dementia, Huntington's disease) was defined by radiological studies; in 40 to 55 percent no specific cause was discovered.[2, 3]

Of those demented patients without focal signs in whom no specific cause was defined by neurodiagnostic procedures, almost all were judged to have a cerebral atrophic process by air study, but in several severely demented patients the ventricles and subarachnoid spaces were entirely normal. Furthermore, in one study eight of 100 patients with dementia had tumors; in three of these cases no accompanying neurological signs or evidence of intracranial hypertension was present.[2] The potential reversibility of the dementia and amenability of certain symptoms to drug treatment have been reported in many of these conditions and appear to correlate best with early diagnosis.

The findings in several studies of

the organic dementias have suggested that there is an early stage in which personality and behavioral disturbances are more prominent than is the evidence of progressive intellectual decline. In one study 23 percent of patients with presenile dementia were initially misdiagnosed as having a functional psychiatric disorder, and this may occur in other treatable conditions. These patients may present with vague memory complaints, mild episodes of disorientation, apathy, loss of interest in family and business activities, generalized slowing of mental capabilities and personality changes.[4] In these cases the diagnosis of an organic dementia may be quite difficult, despite complete examination of mental status and psychometric evaluation.

Marsden reported that 14 percent of patients with a presumptive clinical diagnosis of dementia had a clinical course and response to antidepressant drug therapy that was more consistent with a diagnosis of "depressive pseudodementia."[25] Furthermore, patients with depressive illness frequently exhibit a degree of intellectual impairment that is as severe as that seen in organic dementia, with poverty of thought, memory impairment, and flattened affect. More perplexing is the finding of neurological abnormalities in patients with clinical diagnosis of an affective disorder; one half showed intellectual decline and one third exhibited neurological abnormalities, including tremor, abnormality of tone, focal weakness and reflex asymmetries, but no further cerebral deterioration occurred over eight years.[6-8] The therapeutic response to antidepressant medication is not always conclusive evidence of primary functional psychiatric disorder, as certain patients with an organic dementia may also respond.

The performance of contrast neurodiagnostic studies in patients with psychiatric disease may be of potential hazard; but failure to detect the presence of a correctable cause of dementia at an early and reversible stage prior to the development of associated neurological signs, abnormal EEG or positive isotope scan may lead to a tragic outcome. With the utilization of CT it may now be possible to more accurately classify those patients with early symptoms of organic dementia.

If the clinical evidence of intellectual deterioration is associated with other evidence of neurological dysfunction — i.e., seizures, focal signs and intracranial hypertension — contrast radiographic procedures frequently detect a structural lesion. If there are associated disturbances of gait and posture with abnormal reflex findings, including palmomental, grasp, suck, snout and tonic foot response, and the patient shows apathy, impersistence and inability to sustain attention, a frontal lesion is suspected. Prominent memory loss is indicative of temporal lobe disorder. Disorders of spatial orientation, in which patients easily become lost in familiar surroundings and show right-left confusion is most consistent with a parietal lesion, and visual hallucinations indicate an occipital lesion.

In patients suspected of having an organic dementia, EEG has frequently been utilized as a screening procedure, as most neoplastic, vascular, inflammatory, toxic-metabolic and hydrocephalic conditions are associated with prominent EEG abnormalities. At the onset of the presenile or senile cerebral degenerative conditions there is usually slight slowing of the background activity without significant focal disturbance. In patients who present with altered mental function the finding of normal EEG constitutes good evidence against a structural lesion, whereas a diffuse or focal abnormality suggests that the mental disturbance is not due to a functional psychiatric disorder.[9] Previous studies have confirmed that EEG may be normal in patients with dementia, and one fifth of patients studied by CT and found to have hydrocephalus or an underlying structural lesion had a normal EEG, whereas EEG was normal in one third of patients with clinical evidence of a cerebral atrophic process, as defined by CT findings.

In patients with clinical evidence of dementia without focal neurological signs or intracranial hypertension, isotope scan may rarely show multiple lesions consistent with metastatic disease or a peripheral uptake consistent with subdural hematoma, or may detect a solitary tumor, in which case the dementia is usually believed due to the associated hydrocephalus. If EEG and isotope scan do not suggest a possible cause for the organic dementia, angiography is necessary to exclude a subdural hematoma, and air study to detect enlargement of the ventricles and subarachnoid spaces.

Pneumographic studies have demonstrated ventricular dilatation in subjects with intellectual impairment, and there is a rough correlation of degree of intellectual impairment with ventricular dilatation. In cases of cerebral atrophy the cerebral sulci are greater than 3 mm in width, and this is most apparent in the frontal regions but also prominent in other regions. Nielsen reported that there was a better correlation between intellectual impairment and degree of cortical atrophy than with ventricular dilatation as some patients with normal mentation had evidence of ventricular dilatation but rarely had widened sulci.[10, 11]

Several problems have occurred in evaluating the results of these air studies, as the presence of dilated ventricles may block the filling of the cortical sulci. Also, the presence or absence of widened sulci should not be equated with brain atrophy, as the width of these spaces may be influenced by the technique of air study and the condition of the patient (edematous or dehydrated state), and in other cases the spaces may be artificially widened by pressure of air

filling (pseudocortical atrophy). Because of the invasive nature of pneumography little information is available concerning normal subjects, and it has not previously been possible to evaluate serially patients with vague neuropsychiatric symptoms to determine if these patients then develop cerebral atrophy. Marsden and Harrison reported that several patients had vague memory complaints but psychometric studies indicated no evidence of organic dementia. The patients then showed more definite intellectual impairment over several years, at which time air study revealed severe and definite evidence of a cerebral atrophic process.[2] With the noninvasive technique of CT it may now be possible to follow radiographically the natural history of these dementias.

Of 30 patients with organic dementia who had no associated focal or diffuse neurological findings, CT obviated the need for contrast radiographic procedures and established the diagnosis in 26 cases. Despite the absence of neurological signs, focal lesions were present in 8 cases (subdural hematoma, 4 cases; cerebral neoplasm, 3 cases; cerebral infarction, 1 case). In the other cases, CT showed diffuse conditions (cerebral atrophy, 16 cases; communicating hydrocephalus, 2 cases; multi-infarct dementia, 1 case). In 4 cases the CT scan was negative; in 2 of these patients subsequent studies detected hypothyroidism, and in the other 2 symptomatic treatment with phenothiazine caused good results. In 14 of the 26 cases all other neurodiagnostic studies were negative, and the diagnosis was established by CT. In the patients in this series with CT evidence of cerebral atrophy, EEG demonstrated a diffuse slow wave pattern in 7, focal delta pattern in 3, and was normal in 6 cases. In 50 percent of the neoplasms and subdural hematomas both isotope scan and EEG were normal. In 2 cases of communicating hydrocephalus confirmed by isotope cisternography there was no accompanying gait disorder or incontinence.

Twenty-four patients with an organic dementia had diffuse (8 patients) or focal (16 patients) neurological signs, and CT defined the underlying pathological process in all cases. Of those with diffuse signs 2 had bilateral subdural hematoma and 2 had bifrontal gliomas. Of the 16 patients with a focal deficit having evidence of a lateralizing EEG pattern, CT defined the presence of a cerebral atrophic process in 8 cases; this was confirmed by subsequent angiography or air study (Fig. 10–1). In 8 patients, CT accurately localized and defined the pathological features of the underlying focal lesion and obviated the need for contrast studies.

Twenty middle-aged or elderly patients with clinical symptoms of an organic dementia also had prominent psychiatric symptoms. In one-half of these cases the only evidence of the organic dementia was detected by psychometric studies. The psychiatric symptoms consisted of somatic and hypochondriacal complaints, affective disorders, psychotic behavior and dramatic changes in the patient's personality and behavior. In 10 of these cases, the CT scan was abnormal, showing focal (3) and diffuse (7) abnormalities, and in the other patients the CT scan was normal.

In middle-aged and elderly patients who exhibit psychiatric symptoms with only mild or slight evidence of intellectual decline and have had a stable premorbid personality with no prior psychiatric history and a negative family history for psychiatric disorder, it is important to exclude the presence of a definable lesion by CT. In those patients who are found to have underlying cerebral atrophy, the initiation of electroconvulsive or drug therapy for symptomatic treatment may precipitate confusional states and impair memory and cognitive function. Three fourths of the patients who developed confusional episodes when treated with pheno-

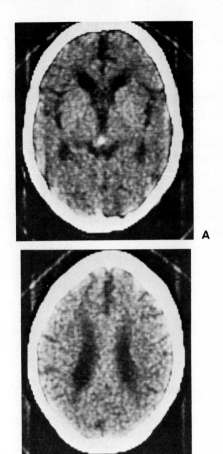

Figure 10–1. *A* and *B*, A 50-year-old woman developed memory loss, episodes of becoming lost in familiar surroundings and marked difficulty in finding the appropriate word in conversation. Neurological findings demonstrated significant nominal aphasic disturbance, constructional apraxia, recent memory impairment and concrete thought process. EEG showed a delta slow-wave pattern over the left temporal region; isotope scan was negative. CT findings: symmetrical ventricular dilatation of lateral and third ventricle, but fourth ventricle is normal in size and temporal horns are not dilated; the basal cisterns and cortical sulcal markings are quite prominent, consistent with atrophic process.

thiazines subsequently had CT scans showing significant cerebral atrophic process. Furthermore, the incidence of neuroleptic-induced dyskinesias is higher in patients who have CT evidence of a cerebral atrophic process.

In patients with predominantly psychiatric symptoms the indication for air study has been quite limited, but with the introduction of CT more patients with psychiatric symptoms have been studied, and the finding of both focal and diffuse lesions has confirmed the clinical and experimental studies of Heath and the clinical reports by Chapman and Wolff.[12, 13] The latter authors described changes in social and personality adjustment that occurred in patients with surgically induced destruction of cerebral tissue who had no neurological signs or signs of abnormal intellectual or memory function. These changes included loss of capacity to express appropriate affect and emotional response, including altered response to visceral drives, impaired capacity to employ mental mechanisms for goal achievement, and decreased capacity to initiate, organize and maintain appropriate adaptive reactions.

In patients with predominantly psychiatric symptoms, the incidence of CT scan abnormalities is approximately 2 percent, but if certain criteria are established this incidence may be as high as 20 to 25 percent. The major indications include (1) atypical clinical presentation and course for the specific psychiatric diagnosis; (2) poor response to drug or electroconvulsive therapy; (3) abnormal EEG prior to initiation of drug therapy; (4) presence of any neurological signs of focal or diffuse nature; (5) lack of any family history of psychiatric illness, a good premorbid personality and no past psychiatric history. Heath has reported the finding of focal structural leisons in patients who presented with only psychiatric symptoms and in whom EEG and isotope scan were normal. CT was performed for one of the above listed indications. In several of these cases surgical treatment was associated with a dramatic amelioration of the patient's clinical symptoms.[12]

Cerebral Atrophic Conditions

Utilizing CT it has been possible to assess ventricular and cortical sulcal size in both normal and abnormal cases, and this may be based on measurements obtained from the Polaroid pictures or from the computer printout. Huckman analyzed ventricular and subarachnoid size by measuring the distance between the most lateral portion of frontal horns of the lateral ventricle, the width of the lateral ventricles in the region of the caudate nuclei, and the width of the four widest cortical sulci.[14] The scans were then classified: (1) normal, if the scan of ventricular size is less than 15 mm with sulci less than 5 mm; (2) questionable atrophy, if ventricles are 16 to 20 mm with sulci less than 5 mm; (3) mild atrophy, if ventricles are 16 to 20 mm and sulci 6–9 mm; (4) moderate atrophy, with ventricles 16 to 20 mm with sulci 6 to 9 mm; (5) severe atrophy, with ventricles greater than 20 mm with sulci more than 9 mm or occasionally without enlarged sulci. In nondemented patients 85 percent were normal or had questionable atrophy but 15 percent had moderate or severe CT evidence of atrophy. Of those with clinical evidence of dementia, 20 percent were normal, 11 percent had mild atrophy, 60 percent had moderate to severe atrophy, and 9 percent had enlarged ventricles without enlarged sulci.

In several patients with an organic dementia but normal CT, complete medical evaluation detected reversible and treatable illness, including hypothyroidism and B_{12} deficiency. The mortality was higher in those patients with severe atrophy than in those with normal CT scan. This compared with the results of air studies, which showed ventricular and sulcal enlargement in 85 percent, and pathological studies which have shown enlarged ventricles in 95 percent but normal sulci in 40 percent of patients with clinical dementia.[15]

An alternative method to diagnose cerebral atrophy by CT scan is to use the computer printout to assess ventricular size. With this technique pixels having numerical values of less than 11 units are considered to contain CSF, and these data are used to determine ventricular dimensions. Comparison of measurements obtained by air study and CT were identical in 59 of 78 patients. In seven cases air study was incomplete because of inadequate ventricular filling and CT was necessary to exclude neoplasm as the cause of ventricular nonfilling. In six cases CT was normal and air study showed definite ventricular dilatation, and in another six both showed ventricular dilatation, but widening of the sulcal spaces was seen only on air study.[16] The higher incidence of atrophy determined by air study may be due to an occasional false positive finding of ventricular dilatation resulting from gaseous distention or because the method chosen to determine ventricular size by CT may underestimate this structure because of partial volume effect. This occurs because at the peripheral margins of the ventricle the CSF value may be included with normal brain tissue to calculate density value greater than 11 units, and this is most marked in the tips of the frontal horns and least in the measurement of the cella media.

Roberts measured ventricular size from computer printouts, utilizing a planimeter to outline the area of cells with a density less than 9 units to calculate the total ventricular area in square centimeters, whereas sulcal width was derived by counting the total number of low-density cells of the widest sulci.[17, 18] In a group of elderly patients there was a good direct correlation between ventricular dilatation and severity of intellectual impairment but a failure to correlate mentation with cortical sulcal widening.

This lack of correlation with the sulcal pattern has been described in previous air study analysis. Mann showed that one third of patients with demonstrable cortical atrophy were without clinical evidence of dementia in a 10-year follow-up.[18a] In air study the normal hemispheric sulci have a width of 1 to 3 mm, and Gyldensted and Kosteljanetz measured sulci from CT Polaroid pictures and found a mean value of 3 to 4 mm in normal subjects. In rare patients the ventricular system is not dilated but there are huge gapping sulcal spaces, consistent with cortical atrophy.[19, 20]

Other techniques to evaluate normal ventricular size include the use of a planimeter to trace the outline of the lateral ventricle to calculate area and then to compare this value to the area of the inner table of the skull.[21] This ratio was calculated for each decade of life; there was little variation up to the sixth decade but wider variation with each succeeding decade, such that assessment of cerebral atrophy was easier in younger patients with less variation, but there were wider limits of normality in the elderly. Furthermore, the planimeter is a tool more easily utilized to measure larger dimensions, and unless the scan is magnified there may be inaccuracies in the measurements.

Hahn and Rim determined a cerebroventricular index by measuring the transverse distance between the body of the frontal horn along a line drawn through the midportion of the caudate nucleus compared to the distance between the inner table of the skull at bicaudate level.[22] This was expressed as the percentage of maximum bicaudate diameter to brain width, and if the maximum bicaudate diameter was greater than 22 percent of the width of the brain, this was indicative of enlarged ventricular size.

In addition to determining the mean ventricular and sulcal size for age as a baseline for diagnosis of cerebral atrophy, recognition of certain asymmetries for men and women have been identified. Both the lateral and third ventricles are larger in men than in women. In addition, there is a definite increase with age of the size of the right anterior horn, left and right septum-caudate distance and third ventricular width, and in men the left septum-caudate distance is larger than the right.[20]

In 200 patients of all ages who were evaluated by CT because of a decline in mental capacity and in whom no specific etiology was defined, assessment of ventricular and sulcal spaces was made by multiple techniques, including the following: measurement of ventricular and sulcal spaces made by planimetric analysis of total lateral ventricular size compared to intracranial size on the same tissue section; simple measurement of the greatest lateral ventricular span of the frontal horns and cella media compared to the diameter of the skull at some level; and measurement of the five most prominent cortical sulci.

The values obtained in patients with organic dementia were compared with those of normal subjects of the same sex and decade of life. Organic dementia correlated best with the lateral ventricular span, the frontal horn–internal skull diameter ratio, and the ratio obtained by planimetric analysis, although no attempt was made to grade the severity of the organic dementia. Less reliable correlation was obtained by measurement of cortical sulci size and cella media span. If the symptoms had been present for less than three months' duration, the scan was normal in 70 percent of cases irrespective of the severity of the dementia. Of those patients who had mild impairment of recent memory, concrete thought and impaired judgment, 60 percent had enlarged ventricles and 40 percent had enlarged sulci. If confusional states and disorientation were also present, 70 percent had enlarged ventricles and 40 percent had enlarged sulci. If the patient could no longer care for himself, was incontinent of urine, and primitive reflexes were present, then 90 percent had enlarged ventricles and 55 percent had enlarged sulci.

With advancing age, there is brain atrophy, as manifested by depletion of neurons, which leads to ventricular dilatation and enlarged cortical sulci, and this may occur in the absence of intellectual impairment. Several studies have documented the slow but definite increase in ventricular size and sulcal size, as measured by CT, from the first to sixth decades, an increase which is accelerated in the seventh, eighth and ninth decades. Earnest has demonstrated that the ratio of lateral ventricular transverse width to internal diameter of the skull increases with age in patients with no evidence of intellectual decline as measured by quantitative study of orientation, memory, general information and calculation, but that ventricular area measured by planimetry did not increase with age.[23] At present, there is no entirely accurate measurement that correlates ventricular and cortical size with degree of mental impairment. The diagnosis of dementia should always be made on definitive clinical findings. It is easy to overdiagnose dementia based upon atypical clinical signs and equivocal CT findings.

Hydrocephalus

Much interest has centered on the potential reversibility of the dementia associated with communicating hydrocephalus. Associated neurological findings include gait abnormality and urinary incontinence.[24] There are no specific features that characterize the dementia of normal pressure hydrocephalus (NPH), although there is usually a slowing of mental performance, lack of emotional spontaneity and affect with generalized slowing of motor response. The gait impairment may begin with nonspecific unsteadiness and dysequilibrium and progress to apractic and spastic gait with hyperactive reflexes and Babinski sign. The diagnosis has rested upon the results of several measurements of ventricular size and CSF flow pattern, but the response to shunting procedures does not always correlate with these results. Air study shows diffuse symmetrical enlargement of all ventricles, with no visualization of cortical sulci over the convexities, even with delayed views. In cases of ventricular enlargement due to impaired CSF flow, the most striking expansion occurs in the anterior portion of the lateral ventricles, but all ventricular cavities are enlarged and there is a narrowing of the callosal angle to less than 120 degrees. The presence of large collections of air over the cortical subarachnoid space is against this diagnosis, but failure of cortical sulcal spaces to fill may be due to technical factors.

Intrathecal radiosotope cisternography provides information concerning dynamics of CSF flow and may demonstrate focal cerebral destructive and degenerative areas, as detected by retained isotope in these regions. In NPH there is early penetration of isotope into ventricles with persistent ventricular reflux and failure to show ascent over parasagittal cerebral convexities, so that no radioactivity is detected at 72 hours in the convexity region. Prolonged retention within the ventricles is considered a good prognostic sign for response to shunting. This pattern is contrasted to that seen in atrophic-degenerative disorders, in which there may be some delay in isotope circulation such that isotope may diffuse into the ventricles by 48 hours but then reflux out, and there may be pooled areas of isotope in focal cortical areas indicative of atrophy.[24, 25] EEG studies may be normal (50 percent), but the presence of high-voltage rhythmical projected activity, especially in the frontal region, is quite characteristic of active hydrocephalic disorder.[26]

Ability of the ventricular-cisternal system to reabsorb CSF may be evaluated by constant manometric infusion study, in which CSF is infused at a rate twice the normal production rate (0.72 ml/minute) over 90 minutes and CSF pressure recorded. In patients with NPH there is a sharp rise of pressure in excess of 300 mm H_2O.[27] In one study shunting gave favorable results in patients in whom (1) no etiology was detected for this condition, (2) angiogram or air study showed no evidence of cortical atrophy, (3) isotope scan showed early ventricular entry and retention within the ventricles, (4) symptoms improved after lowering CSF pressure by lumbar puncture, (5) saline infusion showed a large pressure increment and (6) duration of symptoms were less than six months.[28, 29]

Despite the multitude of diagnostic studies, the predictability of the response to therapy has not been clearly established in more than 60 percent of cases. Jacobs demonstrated that one third of patients with the pneumographic picture of NPH had evidence of cortical atrophy established by CT, and this finding was confirmed by necropsy examination.[30] This discrepancy may be explained by technical failure of air to fill cortical spaces because of impingement by the distended ventricular system; subsequent isotope cisternogram in these patients was consistent with NPH. There was no correlation with response to therapy in patients with CT scan evidence of absence of cortical sulci, but usually surgical response is most successful in patients whose CT scan shows only minimal evidence of cortical sulci. In all cases in which CT suggested NPH, a confirmatory isotope cisternogram was positive. Forty percent of patients had ventricles that remained enlarged after shunt, and there was no correlation of response clinically with CT evidence of return to normal size by operation (Fig. 10–2).

Gado described the CT pattern in NPH and compared each finding with the characteristic cisternographic pattern. The presence of fourth ventricular dilatation correlated most strongly with NPH, and dilatation of the sulci was most strongly in favor of atrophy, whereas the demonstration of normal sulci was not helpful in differentiating NPH from atrophy.[31] Our experience has indicated that dilatation of the temporal horns is most

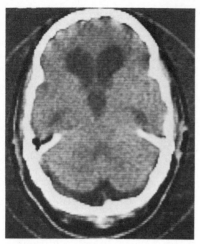

Figure 10–2. A 56-year-old man with evidence of personality change and memory impairment; neurological examination was normal except for recent memory deficit. There was no gait impairment. CT findings: massive enlargement of the ventricular system, including temporal horn, with large retrocerebellar cisternal space and no evidence of cortical sulcal markings. Air study and isotope cisternogram were consistent with communicating hydrocephalus.

consistent with NPH,[32] and the finding of a lucent collar surrounding the anterior frontal horns is believed due to transependymal resorption and is indicative of an active hydrocephalic process but is not specific, as this has been detected in other conditions.

In certain cases the etiologic basis of the NPH is believed secondary to a prior episode of meningitis or subarachnoid hemorrhage, in which there are pathological alterations in the reabsorptive surface of the CSF pathways, but in the majority of cases the etiology is not known. In rare instances cerebral cysts (porencephalic, arachnoid) may present with dementia; it has been suggested that when these cysts produce symptoms there is also an abnormality of CSF flow and ventricular enlargement. These cysts may communicate with either the ventricular system or subarachnoid spaces, and act as a space-occupying lesion to cause impaired CSF circulation. Air study shows ventricular enlargement and isotope cisternogram shows isotope collecting in

the cyst, and symptoms may respond to ventricular shunting. CT may demonstrate a low-density, sharply demarcated cystic lesion, but air study and isotope cisternogram are necessary to demonstrate dynamic aspects of the CSF flow pattern (Fig. 10–3).

Occasionally an arteriosclerotic ectatic basilar artery impinges upon the floor of the ventricular system, causing partial obstruction of CSF circulation and hydrocephalus. These patients may present with dementia, which improves following shunt procedure. Benson stated that in patients with an ectatic basilar artery who had dementia and hydrocephalus, the impairment of CSF circulation was consistent with that of NPH, and patients with such findings benefited from surgery.[25] In several cases the patients presented with a clinical triad characteristic of NPH, but CT detected hydrocephalus and evidence of a posterior fossa mass that was believed to be vascular in nature. The

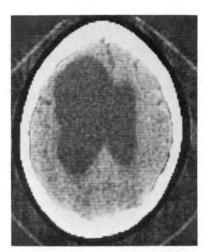

Figure 10–3. A 45-year-old woman had been involved in an automobile accident several months previously, and her family noted that her behavior was markedly changed; she had several episodes of agitated confusional states. She had mild memory impairment and concreteness of thought, but EEG, skull radiogram and isotope scan were negative. CT findings: enlargement of the entire ventricular system, with a low-density cystic lesion in the left frontal region that appears to communicate with the lateral ventricle; the communication was confirmed by air study.

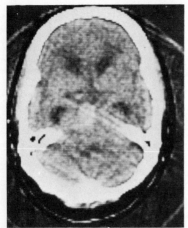

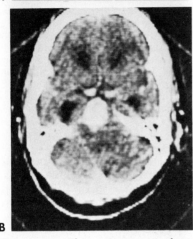

Figure 10–4. This patient was evaluated for dementia, urinary incontinence and mild gait disturbance. CT findings: preinfusion study showed lateral and third ventricular enlargement with normal-size fourth ventricle; immediately posterior to dorsum sella was a round high-density (40 units) mass (A), which markedly enhanced (B). Angiography showed ectatic tortuous basilar artery but no angioma or neoplasm. The patient was treated with shunt.

presence of an ectatic basilar artery was confirmed by angiography, and the clinical symptoms improved following shunt therapy.[33] If air study alone had been performed, the nature of the obstruction may not have been defined (Fig. 10–4).

Chronic Subdural Hematoma

In patients with an organic dementia this is a not uncommon and frequently a remediable disorder. Prior to

the introduction of CT, diagnosis required angiography or air study. Of patients with chronic subdural hematoma (SDH) the presence of a space-occupying mass lesion was frequently not considered as the initial primary diagnosis. These patients frequently present with diffuse mental changes (memory loss, intellectual decline, personality and behavioral changes), gait disorders, increased tone and deep tendon reflexes, pathological reflexes (suck, grasp, snout and palmomental) and diffuse paratonia.[34]

The presence of these nonlocalizing findings and the absence of intracranial hypertension suggest a diffuse or multifocal process rather than a structural lesion. Fluctuations in the severity of the clinical symptoms in patients with chronic SDH is believed due to shifts in intracranial pressure, intermittent vascular compression or paroxysmal bursts in cortical electrical activity. This course is not diagnostic, as it may be seen also in vascular and degenerative disorders. In one series symptoms included headache (85 percent), alteration in consciousness (48 percent) and confusion (38 percent), and over one half of patients lacked signs of intracranial hypertension and pupillary, motor or reflex abnormalities.[35]

Conventional neurodiagnostic studies may be inconclusive: CSF may be clear or xanthochromic, with elevated pressure or protein content (50 percent); skull radiogram may not detect fracture, pineal shift or sella abnormality; and echoencephalography may show no significant pineal shift. EEG may show a focal delta pattern of low voltage, diffuse slow pattern or may be entirely normal. Isotope scan has been reported to be accurate in 91 percent of chronic SDH, and the characteristic finding is a peripheral crescent of increased radioactivity seen most clearly on anterior-posterior view, but this pattern has also been reported in cerebral infarction, skull lesions and metastatic carcinoma.[34, 36] It is not clearly established if the peripheral uptake is due to the well-organized and developed membrane or to the presence of subdural fluid. In one series the operative finding of a well-organized membrane correlated with a positive scan, and its absence correlated with negative isotope scan.[36]

Occasionally, the SDH causes vascular compression and the scan may show a pattern of cerebral infarction. Because of the lack of definitive noninvasive study, angiography is required if SDH is clinically suspected. Since this procedure carries a definite risk many patients are incompletely studied and these lesions are discovered only at necropsy.

With CT the diagnosis of subdural hematoma has been greatly facilitated, and the diagnosis has been readily made in many patients who presented with dementia alone and in whom all other neurodiagnostic studies were negative. Ambrose reported the diagnostic accuracy of CT in seven cases in which there was ventricular compression, but in only one case was the hematoma actually visualized because the fluid collection was usually isodense with the surrounding parenchyma. The CT scan characteristics of chronic SDH include: (1) evidence of mass effect with compression distortion and displacement of the ventricular system; (2) failure to visualize the ventricular system, especially in elderly patients; (3) asymmetry or absence of the cortical sulcal markings ipsilateral to the lesion (Fig. 10–5); (4) presence of a semilunar concave low-density lesion, which may be admixed or appear speckled with high-density material and which is clearly separated from the normal brain structure; (5) contrast enhancement may be seen in the medially located capsule or within the subdural collection, with progressive increase in density in a six hour delayed scan owing to extravascular diffusion.[37, 38] In 10 to 20 percent of cases the fluid collection may be bilateral and, if approximately

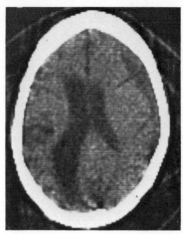

Figure 10–5. An elderly patient was evaluated for a one-year history of headache and progressive dementia. EEG, isotope scan and skull radiogram were negative. CT findings: a low-density, smoothly contoured, medially convex area, which compressed and displaced the lateral ventricle to the left side with obliteration of the sylvian cistern and cortical sulcal markings. At operation, a chronic subdural hematoma was evacuated.

equal in size, there may be no shift of midline structures. Because of associated cerebral edema there is compression of ventricles and nonvisualization of the cortical sulcal pattern (Fig. 10–6). Rarely, CT may be negative with isodense or bilateral SDH, and the presence of normal or small ventricles in these patients should suggest the need for angiography.

Certain patients with an organic dementia present more unusual CT scan findings in which differentiation of SDH from enlarged extracerebral spaces may be difficult.[39] In these cases differentiation may require angiography, isotope scan or air study, but can usually be made on the basis of several characteristic CT findings. Firstly, in SDH there are smooth medial borders as contrasted to the interdigitations caused by the cortical gyral and sulcal pattern in cerebral atrophic conditions. Secondly, SDH causes a mass effect ipsilaterally, with contralateral ventricular dilatation, as compared to symmetrical ventricular dilatation in cortical atrophy

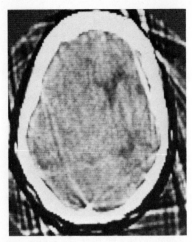

Figure 10–6. A 40-year-old man had intermittent headaches and fluctuations in the level of consciousness, EEG was diffusely slow and isotope scan was negative. CT findings: marked compression and displacement of the ventricular system to the right side, with contralateral ventricular dilatation by an isodense subdural hematoma over the left hemisphere. This was confirmed surgically. (Courtesy of Dr. Roger Tutton, Ochsner Foundation Hospital.)

usually accompanied by widening of the interhemispheric fissure. In pa-

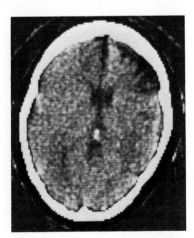

Figure 10–7. This patient developed progressive mental impairment but had no neurological signs. EEG showed delta slow-wave pattern over the left hemisphere, and isotope scan showed crescent-shaped uptake over the left hemisphere. CT findings: irregularly shaped low-density area over the right hemisphere with no evidence of ventricular shift, consistent with widened extracerebral space. Following treatment with corticosteroids, the patient's headache and mentation cleared. An isodense SDH with obliteration of subarachnoid space in left hemisphere was presumptive diagnosis.

tients with dementia the CT pattern has been 100 percent reliable in differentiating an atrophic process from SDH, based on these criteria, with subsequent angiography and necropsy confirmation. In one instance both conditions were present, and the CT scan findings are nicely contrasted (Fig. 10–7).

Arteriosclerotic Dementia

The diagnosis of "generalized arteriosclerotic cerebrovascular disease" is frequently implicated as the cause of dementia, but recent studies have suggested that this is not as common as believed and have limited the syndrome of dementia resulting from vascular disorder to those patients who have clinicopathological verification of multiple cerebral infarctions.[40] It was commonly believed that cerebral arteriosclerosis caused decreased cerebral perfusion with resultant ischemia and neuronal depletion in diffuse or multifocal distribution. The varied clinical pattern of intellectual decline and behavioral changes that occurred in patients who were believed to have suffered multiple "little strokes," which may be reversed by vasodilation and anticoagulant therapy, was popularized by Alvarez, but in these cases there was no angiographic or pathological documentation.[41] There have been reports of patients with clinical evidence of an organic dementia characterized by confusion, hallucinations and waxing and waning of symptoms, without focal neurological abnormalities, who were found to have bilateral carotid stenosis; their symptoms resolved following carotid endarterectomy. This suggested that mental aberrations in these cases were caused by decreased perfusion rather than by multiple infarctions.

The clinical picture of multi-infarct dementia differs from that of Alzheimer's disease and a positive diagnosis should be made only if the following criteria are fulfilled: a significant history of elevated blood pressure, multiple sudden and discrete episodes of focal neurological signs that develop in stepwise progression, and evidence on neurological examination consistent with bilateral stroke syndromes. In certain cases there may be definite evidence of prior stroke syndromes, but in others there may be no definite history; this may be due to multiple lacunar infarctions, which are too small individually to produce a major clinical event but may in series act to impair mentation. Multiple hypotensive episodes may impair the perfusion of the arterial boundary zones, which are most vulnerable to decreased perfusion.

Forty consecutive patients with the initial diagnosis of "arteriosclerotic dementia" were evaluated by CT. In 15 cases a potentially reversible lesion was identified that had not been detected by other diagnostic studies. In the other cases 16 had CT evidence of generalized cerebral atrophy indicative of Alzheimer's disease, and in four there was evidence of only cortical atrophy without ventricular enlargement. In five cases the clinical history was that of stepwise neurological deterioration, and CT showed evidence of multiple cerebral infarction (Fig. 10–8). In one case, the clinical history was that of progressive clinical deterioration and CT showed evidence of a generalized atrophic process, but necropsy showed multiple bilateral infarctions 2 to 3 mm in size, which were not detected by CT.

Acute confusional states without evidence of focal neurological signs are usually not due to focal pathological lesions and are most often associated with toxic, metabolic, postictal, infectious, postconcussive or cerebral atrophic conditions. Occasionally these episodes represent the initial clinical presentation of cerebral infarctions involving the territory of the posterior or anterior cerebral arteries. With infarction of

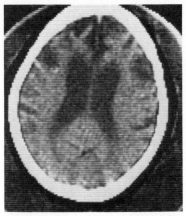

Figure 10–8. A hypertensive man had previously had several episodes of sudden onset of hemiparesis, initially involving the left arm and six months later the right arm and leg. Three months after the last episode the patient's family noted that he suffered periods of confusion that cleared over 24 hours and that he could not attend to his financial affairs. Neurological findings showed evidence of dementia, bilateral pyramidal tract signs, and cogwheel rigidity. CT findings: symmetrical ventricular dilatation and sulci with several large focal areas of low density. Necropsy showed that these represented old cerebral infarctions.

the medial temporo-occipital region, the patients present with agitation, visual impairment (hemianopia or cortical blindness) and dementia. In cases of infarction of the medial frontal region due to anterior cerebral artery occlusion, the patient appears confused and may also show sexually inappropriate, markedly irrational behavior or catatonic-like posturing, frequently associated with the presence of primitive reflex changes. Rarely, right middle cerebral artery syndrome unassociated with any motor, visual or sensory disturbance may be the cause of an acute confusional state. The acute confusional state may then resolve into a clinical picture of dementia with inattention, memory impairment, cognitive defects, concrete thought and disorders of high cortical function.[42] Because of the lack of focal neurological deficit the underlying lesion is frequently not identified, as EEG also shows diffuse slow pattern indicative of diffuse en-

A   **B**

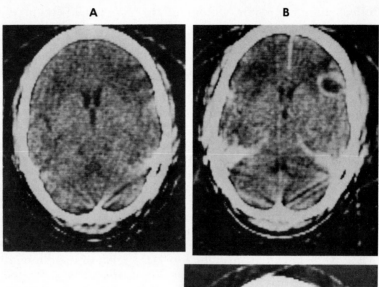

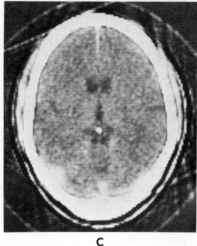

C

Figure 10–9. A 55-year-old man was evaluated because of sudden onset of confusional episodes. Neurological examination showed a confused and agitated patient without any focal motor, sensory or visual field abnormalities. EEG showed a delta pattern in the right frontal parietal region and isotope scan was negative. CT findings: plain scan showed irregularly shaped, low-density lesion without mass effect (A); marked ringlike enhancement was confined to the arterial territory of the middle cerebral artery (B). Angiogram was entirely negative and the patient's mentation cleared completely within two weeks. Repeat scan six months later was entirely negative (C), and this was most consistent with an enhancing infarction.

cephalopathy. With CT we have identified three patients with acute confusional states in whom the initial diagnosis was diffuse encephalopathy. In one case CT showed a low-density area in the right inferior frontal region, but in two others the CT scan initially was thought to indicate tumor or abscess. Subsequent clinical resolution of symptoms and serial CT scan were indicative of infarction (Fig. 10–9).

Neoplasms

The incidence of finding a neoplasm or cyst in patients with dementia may be as high as 10 percent, and many are found to be benign lesions.[2] In these cases other neurological signs may be present but occasionally no associated signs are present. Neoplasms involving the midline frontal region produce disorders of attention and memory function, apathy and impersistence. Tumors of the anterior third ventricle, subfrontal and parasellar region may also produce dementia, and because of the mental disturbances it may be difficult to demonstrate the anosmia of subfrontal and bitemporal visual impairment of chiasmal involvement or hearing impairment of cerebellopontine angle lesions.[43-45] Dementia alone may be caused by diffuse and infiltrating tumor, including the reticulum cell sarcoma-microglioma. These patients present initially with generalized intellectual and motor deterioration, and all diagnostic studies may be negative, a pattern that may suggest a degenerative disorder.

In patients with dementia associated with neurological findings including evidence of hydrocephalus, EEG, isotope scan and skull radiogram usually indicate the presence of the lesion but, even if negative, contrast studies are indicated. Of 20 patients with dementia and neurological signs who had tumor, the diagnosis was established by CT in all cases, and in 10 no further contrast studies were necessary. Despite the presence of neurological signs, isotope scan and EEG were negative in eight but CT clearly defined the location of the tumor, which was consistent with the clinical findings. In 10 patients who had dementia alone, isotope scan and EEG were not sensitive enough to detect the presence of tumor in seven cases, whereas CT was 100 percent accurate. Previous studies have shown that 2 to 3 percent of patients with dementia have benign lesions, which are frequently cystic; these have required air study or angiography but may be readily detected by CT and do not require further contrast studies.

Huntington's Disease

This disorder involves patients who develop abnormal adventitious movements (chorea) and associated mental deterioration, in which psychiatric symptoms including psychotic episodes, affective disorders, paranoid states and personality disorders, may be most prominent. It is familial and inherited as an autosomal dominant condition. Pathologically there is early degeneration and atrophy of the caudate nucleus and also of the frontal-temporal cortex. The diagnosis of Huntington's disease is established clinically, and air study may be confirmatory, with evidence of "squaring out" of the anterior horn of the lateral

ventricle and prominence of the cortical sulci in the frontal region. Sax determined that, in patients with clinical evidence of this disorder, CT shows that the ratio of maximum distance between frontal horns compared to intercaudate distance becomes smaller (less than 2.0), a state which probably results from a relatively selective pattern of atrophy.[46]

The cortical atrophy is most prominent in the frontal-temporal-basal cisterns and these findings correlate with air study findings. This frontal horn/caudate ratio is frequently normal in the early clinical stages, as well as for those patients who are at risk of developing this clinical condition, but in several patients in whom mental disturbances were the most prominent feature of the disorder, with minimal chorea or tic-like movements, the characteristic CT scan appearance helped to establish the diagnosis, later confirmed by the development of more full-blown chorei-

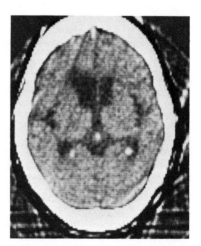

Figure 10–10. A 40-year-old woman was initially evaluated because of her inability to function as an accountant and her unusual behavior. On examination, she showed evidence of mild dementia but no choreiform movements. CT findings: enlargement of the lateral ventricles in the anterior frontal region, most specifically in the region of the caudate, with frontal horn/caudate ratio of less than 1:5. Several months later she was noted to have an intermittent shoulder tic and facial grimacing, consistent with Huntington's disease.

form manifestations (Fig. 10–10). This pattern of atrophy is quite specific for Huntington's disease and was not present in any patient with Alzheimer's disease. One problem involves the pathological evidence that in 10 percent of cases there is minimal pathological evidence of caudate atrophy. Further studies will be necessary to determine the CT findings in these cases.

Parkinsonism

The cardinal symptoms include disorders of tone (rigidity) and movement (tremor bradykinesia), but frequently mental changes are present, including dementia. Previous air study evidence demonstrated that cerebral atrophy was present in up to three fourths of patients, and this correlated with the necropsy findings, but the presence or degree of atrophy did not correlate with the clinical severity of the disorder. With CT, cerebral atrophy and calcification of the basal ganglia have been detected. Further studies are necessary to determine if these CT abnormalities correlate with the severity of the disease, clinical response to drug treatment or development of psychiatric disorders following treatment with L-dopa.[47]

Progressive Multifocal Leukoencephalopathy

This condition occurs in patients with an altered immune response, and clinically there is evidence of involvement of the CNS in an asymmetric pattern at multiple sites, with predominant involvement of the white matter. The clinical symptoms include confusional states with prominent visual hallucinations, progressive dementia, cranial nerve and corticospinal tract involvement. There are no specific neurodiagnostic studies and the diagnosis is frequently established only by necropsy exam-

ination. This diagnosis may be established from the CT finding of prominent patchy low-density irregular areas in the periventricular region and corona radiata.[48] Conomy reported that a large low-density region that extends to the ventricular surface represents a confluent demyelinating lesion in the centrum semiovale; this may be differentiated from tumors by lack of mass effect and failure to enhance. In addition, a low-density oval-shaped lesion in this region may mimic nonhemorrhagic infarction, and the sparing of the cortex is not

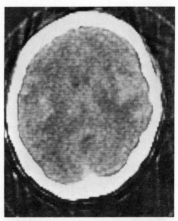

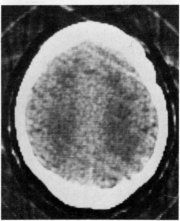

Figure 10–11. CT scan in two patients who had progressive dementia and confusional states with visual hallucination. *A*, diffuse symmetrical, speckled, low-density pattern throughout both hemispheres, involving the white matter, a pattern consistent with leukoencephalopathy. *B*, symmetrical, oval, low-density regions in centrum semiovale, consistent with confluent regions of demyelination (pathologically verified).

accurately visualized by CT. Differentiation must rely on clinical findings (Fig. 10–11).

DISTURBANCES OF CONSCIOUSNESS

Of patients admitted to the hospital with a diagnosis of "coma of unknown etiology," two thirds were subsequently found to have a metabolic or diffuse cerebral disorder, and in only one third was an underlying structural lesion detected.[49] In those patients with a supra- or infratentorial lesion, focal neurological signs appropriate to the lesion were invariably present, but rarely did these lesions cause alterations in intracranial dynamics, resulting in impaired consciousness without focal findings. Structural intracranial lesions most likely to cause coma with signs of only diffuse motor dysfunction and without lateralizing EEG abnormalities include deeply located intracerebral or intraventricular hemorrhage, whereas this is most unusual with even massive nonhemorrhagic cerebral infarction.

CT in comatose patients without localizing neurological signs has confirmed the results of previous studies indicating that 90 percent do not have underlying structural lesions, but it has occasionally identified several clinically unsuspected conditions. This has surprisingly included patients with nonhemorrhagic supratentorial infarction who presented with coma, bilateral spasticity and Babinski signs, and whose neurological condition rapidly improved with corticosteroids. Other nontrauma-related conditions that may present with diffuse disturbance of consciousness include fat embolism, endocarditis and hypertensive encephalopathy. The neuropsychiatric manifestations of endocarditis include a diffuse encephalopathy (20 percent), which is believed to result from microembolization or multiple small miliary brain

abscesses but may also occur in the absence of any pathological change, in which case the pathophysiological mechanism is the toxemia. Coma is a rare presenting feature of endocarditis but may be caused by infarction from embolus or by hemorrhage from a mycotic aneurysm.[50] These conditions are usually detected by isotope scan and EEG, and the exact pathophysiological disturbance may be defined by CT. In the multiple small lesions there may be only diffuse EEG abnormality and negative isotope scan, but CT may detect multiple cerebral lesions.

Fat embolism is most frequent following trauma and may result in neurological symptoms; this may be secondary to hypoxia due to multiple pulmonary microemboli or may directly result from fat emboli that lodge in the cerebral vessels, causing infarction. In these cases CT may detect infarction or possibly the presence of very low-density fat embolic deposits. Hypertensive encephalopathy usually causes disturbed consciousness and seizures and is the direct consequence of elevated blood pressure, leading to cerebral edema which may be visualized by CT.

Conversely, patients with metabolic or diffuse cerebral disturbance may demonstrate focal neurological signs, suggesting the diagnosis of a structural lesion, and CT may be of value in obviating the need for angiography. The pathophysiological basis for these lateralizing findings is not definitely known, but if the patient has had an old cerebral injury, even if he is presently asymptomatic, this previously damaged region may be most vulnerable to the effects of metabolic disturbances. In patients who have abnormalities of glucose metabolism (hypoglycemia, nonketotic hyperosmolar coma), sodium (hypo- or hypernatremia), renal and liver impairment or chronic alcoholism, the presence of focal signs may present difficult diagnostic problems.

In one series, one third of patients

with nonketotic hyperosmolar coma were initially admitted with a diagnosis of "acute stroke." There is experimental evidence that insulin may precipitate cerebral edema, which may worsen the neurological condition.[51] Patients with "water intoxication" (hyponatremia) usually have disturbed consciousness, and this condition may be associated with basilar skull fracture, chronic meningitis, hypothalamic tumor or an occult metastatic lesion, all of which may cause characteristic CT findings.

Uremic encephalopathy results from the metabolic consequences of renal failure and may be reversed by dialysis; there are usually no associated neuropathological changes. Following dialysis patients may develop a confusional state that may be caused by transient metabolic dysequilibrium; this occurs most often in newly dialyzed patients and is not associated with lateralizing neurological signs. Transient but no persistent headache may be present. Furthermore, 3.3 percent of dialyzed patients have been found to have subdural hematoma. In patients who are being dialyzed and in whom mentation deteriorates CT may define this lesion.[52] In other patients who have been on long-term maintenance hemodialysis, a progressive neurological disorder resembling cerebral degeneration occurs (dialysis dementia), and this may be reliably differentiated from hematoma by CT, and early in vivo neuropathological changes may be defined by CT.[53]

The chronic alcoholic patient who presents with coma poses a problem in differentiating those conditions directly related to alcohol (withdrawal state, seizures with post-ictal depression of consciousness) and progressive liver impairment with resultant hepatic encephalopathy from those due to an occult structural lesion, which may frequently occur in alcoholic patients. These patients are especially susceptible to inflammatory lesions because of an impaired im-

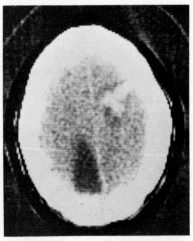

Figure 10–12. A 34-year-old chronic alcoholic fell and hit her head and was admitted to the hospital following generalized motor seizure. The patient was agitatedly confused, with auditory and tactile hallucinations, but no neurological signs were present. EEG showed diffusely slowed background activity, and CSF examination showed xanthocrhomic fluid. Liver function studies were markedly abnormal, with prolonged bleeding and prothrombin time. CT scan was performed with Amytal sedation and showed a wedge-shaped nonenhancing, high-density lesion in the right frontal region, extending deeply, with a low-density porencephalic cyst in the left parieto-occipital region.

mune system in addition to intracerebral or subdural hematoma related to impaired hematological and hepatic function (Fig. 10–12). In addition, certain clinical features of Wernicke's syndrome, including third and sixth nerve involvement with Babinski sign, may suggest the presence of increased intracranial pressure. CT may be of crucial diagnostic value in these patients but may present problems of sedation if the patient is confused or combative. Because these patients may be dehydrated and hypotensive, they are vulnerable to cardiovascular collapse precipitated by sedative drugs.

CEREBRAL ANOXIA

If blood flow to the brain is suddenly interrupted and restored several minutes later, the presence and development of a neurological deficit is dependent upon whether the circulation has been adequately restored to all areas of the brain or whether decreased perfusion persists because of cerebral edema and irreversible vascular changes (no-reflow phenom-

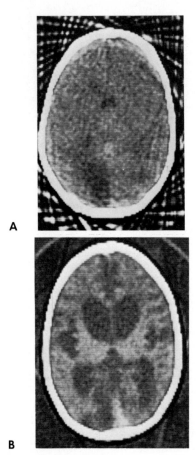

A

B

Figure 10–13. Patient complained of headache and then suddenly became obtunded. Examination showed early papilledema but no lateralizing neurological findings. EEG showed symmetrical monorhythmic delta pattern, but isotope scan was negative. CT findings: nonvisualization of the ventricular system, but no shift was detected. There was a low-density lesion in the left occipital region, consistent with infarction of the posterior cerebral artery, presumably secondary to cerebral edema (A). Despite treatment with corticosteroids, the patient suffered a cardiac arrest, from which there was successful resuscitation. Unfortunately, the patient recovered slowly and incompletely, and repeat CT scan one year later showed massive ventricular and sulcal enlargement (B). (Courtesy of Dr. Roger Tutton, Ochsner Foundation Hospital.)

ena).[54] Rapid cessation of cerebral circulation, as follows a cardiac arrest, results in coma, convulsions, Babinski sign, and pupillary dilatation. If circulation is restored, consciousness frequently returns, although there may be a prolonged confusional state. The prognosis for complete recovery may be difficult to determine. Some patients recover completely although initial arousal was delayed, whereas other patients may recover consciousness rapidly and then lapse into coma.[55] This latter condition is believed caused by delayed demyelination. In some cases the acute onset of coma is associated with electrocardiographic features consistent with primary cardiac disease, but these changes may also be associated with neurological disorders (hemorrhage, encephalitis), and this etiologic basis may be detected by CT. In addition, CT may demonstrate the temporal evolution of pathophysiological changes following cardiac arrest and may correlate with prognosis for recovery (Fig. 10–13).

IRREVERSIBLE COMA AND BRAIN DEATH

If the patient presents in deep coma but retains some evidence of neurological function, the prognosis for potential recovery may better be predicted if the nature of the underlying condition is known. The pathological lesions may be limited to laminar necrosis of the cortex, subcortical demyelination and focal contusions in the brain stem, and the presence of some of these changes may be visualized by CT.[55] Cerebral death implies irreversible loss of brain function in which there is a lack of spontaneous respiration and all neurological function, the absence of cerebral electrical activity, and radioisotope and angiographic studies indicating absence of brain circulation and metabolism. The most common cause of these conditions is an intracranial catastrophe but it may result from extracranial conditions including potentially reversible conditions — drug overdose, hypothermia, and encephalitis. CT may reliably demonstrate the nature of the intracranial pathologic condition, an achievement not possible with other diagnostic studies.

Following severe brain anoxia, edema occurs and a decrease in cerebral circulation as perivascular astrocytes enlarge, compressing the capillary lumina and reducing cerebral perfusion. When intracranial pressure exceeds systemic arterial pressure, cerebral circulation stops. In cases of cerebral death, recent CT studies have demonstrated that the ventricles and subarachnoid spaces are not completely compressed; this suggests that obstruction of intracranial vessels occurs before severe edema has occurred. Furthermore, there was no characteristic change in the attenuation value of the brain, but in one case there was a decrease in gray matter values, which may represent a decrease in blood flow rather than a pathological change.[56] In these cases, CT was more reliable in establishing the brain lesion than other diagnostic studies. CT may also detect quantitative changes of attenuation values for cerebral parenchyma and white matter characteristic of cerebral death, and obviate the need for angiography.

REFERENCES

1. Malzberg B: Important statistical data about mental illness. In: Handbook of Psychiatry, Vol 1. Basic Books, New York, 1959. pp 161–174.
2. Marsden CD, Harrison MJG: Outcome of investigation of patients with presenile dementia. Br Med J 2:249, 1972.
3. Freeman F: Evaluation of patients with progressive intellectual deterioration. Arch Neurol 33:658, 1976.
4. Malamud N, Wagoner RW: Genealogic and clinicopathologic study of Pick's disease. Arch Neurol Psychiatry 50:288, 1943.
5. Kiloh LG: Pseudo-dementia. Acta Psychiat Scand 37:336, 1961.
6. Post F: The development and progress of senile dementia in relationship to the functional psychiatric disorders of later life. In: Senile Dementia, C Muller, L Ciomi (eds). Bern, Hans Huber, 1968. pp 84–100.
7. Post F: Dementia, Depression and Pseudo-dementia. In: Psychiatric Aspects of Neurologic Disease. DF Benson, D Blumer (eds). Grune and Stratton, New York, 1975, pp. 99–120.
8. Post F: Diagnosis of Depression in Geriatric Patients and Treatment Modalities Appropriate for the Population. In: Depression, DM Gallant, GM Simpson (eds), Spectrum Publications, 1976. pp 205–231.
9. Harner RN: EEG evaluation of the patient with dementia. In: Psychiatric Aspects of Neurologic Disease. DF Benson, D Blumer (eds). Grune and Stratton, New York, 1975. pp 63–81.
10. Nielsen R, Petersen D, Thygessen P: Encephalographic ventricular atrophy. Acta Radiol Diagn 4:240, 1966.
11. Nielsen R, Petersen O, Thygessen P: Encephalographic cortical atrophy. Acta Radiol Diagn 4:437, 1966.
12. Heath R. Personal communication.
13. Chapman LF, Wolff HG: The cerebral hemispheres and the highest integrative functions of man. Arch Neurol 1:357, 1959.
14. Huckman MS, Fox JH, Topel JL: Criteria for the diagnosis of brain atrophy by computerized tomography. Radiology 116:85, 1975.
15. Fox JH, Topel JL, Huckman MS: Use of computerized tomography in senile dementia. J Neurol Neurosurg Psychiatry 38:948, 1975.
16. Gawler J, DuBoulay GH, Bull JWD, Marshall J: CT: comparison with PEG and ventriculography. J. Neurol Neurosurg Psychiatry. 39:203, 1976.
17. Roberts MA, Caird FI: CT and intellectual impairment in the elderly. J Neurol Neurosurg Psychiatry 39:986, 1976.

18. Roberts MA, Caird FI, Glossart KW: CT in the diagnosis of cerebral atrophy. J Neurol Neurosurg Psychiatry 39:909, 1976.

18a. Mann AH: Cortical atrophy and air encephalography: clinical and radiological study. Psycholog Med 3:374, 1973.

19. Gyldensted C, Kosteljanetz M: Measurement of the normal hemispheric sulci with CT. Neuroradiology 10:147, 1975.

20. Gyldensted C, Kosteljanetz M: Measurements of the normal ventricular system with CT. Neuroradiology 10:205, 1976.

21. Barron SA: Changes in size of normal lateral ventricles during age determined by CT. Neurology 26:1011, 1976.

22. Hahn FJY, Rim K: Frontal ventricular dimensions on normal CT. Am J Roentgenol 126:593, 1976.

23. Earnest MP, Manke W, Wilkenson WE: Cortical atrophy, ventricular enlargement and mental impairments in the aging. Neurology 27:351, 1977.

24. Benson DF, LeMay M, Patten DH, Rubens AB: Diagnosis of normal pressure hydrocephalus. N Engl J Med 283:609, 1970.

25. Benson DF: The hydrocephalic dementias. In: Psychiatric Aspects of Neurologic Disease, DF Benson, D Blumer (eds). Grune and Stratton, New York, 1975. pp 83–98.

26. Brown DG, Goldensohn, ES: The EEG in NPH. Arch Neurol 29:70, 1973.

27. Trotter JL, Lugecky M, Siegel B: CSF infusion test. Neurology 24:181, 1974.

28. Wood JHM, Detlet B, James AE: Normal pressure hydrocephalus. Diagnosis and patient selection for shunt surgery. Neurology 24:517, 1974.

29. Messert B, Wannamaker BB: Reappraisal of the occult hydrocephalus syndrome. Neurology 24:224, 1974.

30. Jacobs L, Kinkel W: CT in normal pressure hydrocephalus. Neurology 26:501, 1976.

31. Gado MH, Coleman RE, Lee KS, et al: Correlation between CT and radionuclide cisternography in dementia. Neurology 26:555, 1976.

32. Sjaastad D, Skalpe ID, Engeset A: The width of the temporal horn in the differential diagnosis between pressure hydrocephalus and hydrocephalus ex vacuo. Neurology 19:1087, 1969.

33. Peterson NT, Duchesnau PM, Westbrook EL, et al: Basilar artery ectasia demonstrated by CT. Radiology 122:713, 1977.

34. Plum F, Posner JB: Diagnosis of Stupor and Coma, 2nd ed. F.A. Davis, Philadelphia, 1972. pp 102–105.

35. McKissock W, Richardson A, Bloom WH: Subdural hematoma, a review of 389 cases. Lancet 1:1365, 1960.

36. Cowen RJ, Maynard DC, Lassiter KR: Isotope brain scan in the detection of subdural hematoma. J Neurosurg 32:30, 1974.

37. Manning EJ, Kinkel WR: CT in subdural hematoma. Neurology 26:392, 1976.

38. Ambrose J: Computerized transverse axial scanning (tomography). Clinical application. Br J Radiol 46:1023, 1973.

39. Davis KR, Taveras JM, Roberson GH, et al: CT in head trauma. Semin Roentgenol 12:53, 1977.

40. Hachinski VC, Lassen NA, Marshall J: Multi-infarct dementia. Lancet 2:207, 1974.

41. Alvarez WC: Little Strokes. JB Lippincott, Philadelphia, 1966. pp 10–40.

42. Mesulam MM, Waxman SG, Geschwind N, Sabin TD: Acute confusional states with right middle cerebral artery infarctions. J Neurol Neurosurg Psychiatry 39:84, 1977.

43. Remington FB, Rubert SL: Why patients with brain tumors come to a psychiatric hospital. Am J Psychiatry 119:256, 1962.

44. Malamud N: Psychiatric disorder with intracranial tumors of the limbic system. Arch Neurol 17:113, 1967.

45. Malamud N: Organic Brain Disease Mistaken for Psychiatric Disorder. In: Psychiatric Aspects of Neurological Diseases. Grune and Stratton, New York, 1975. pp 287–305.

46. Sax DS, Menzer L: CT in Huntington's disease. Neurology 27:388, 1977.

47. Gath I, Jorgensen A, Sjaastad D, et al: PEG findings in Parkinsonism. Arch Neurol 32:769, 1975.

48. Huckman MS, Fox JS, Ramsey RG: CT in the diagnosis of degenerative diseases of the brain. Semin Roentgenol 12:63, 1977.

49. Plum F, Posner JB: Diagnosis of Stupor and Coma, 2nd ed. FA Davis, Philadelphia, 1972. pp 2–4.

50. Jones HR, Siekert RG, Geraci JE: Neurologic manifestations of bacterial endocarditis. Ann Intern Med 71:28, 1969.

51. Arieff AI, Carroll HJ: Nonketotic hyperosmolar coma with hyperglycemia. Medicine 51:73, 1972.

52. Leonard A, Shapiro FL: Subdural hematoma in regularly hemodialyzed patients. Ann Intern Med 82:650, 1975.
53. Mahurkor SD, Salta R, Smith EC: Dialysis dementia. Lancet 1:1412, 1973.
54. Ames A, Wright RL, Kowada M, et al: Cerebral ischemia. 2. The no-reflow phenomenon. Am J Clin Pathol. 52:437, 1968.
55. Plum F, Posner JB: Diagnosis of Stupor and Coma, 2nd ed. FA Davis, Philadelphia, 1972. pp 166–170.
56. Radberg C, Soderlundh S: CT in cerebral death. Acta Radiol (suppl) 346:119, 1975.

Early detection of acoustic neurinomas represents an important and challenging diagnostic problem because at least 10 percent of unilateral hearing loss is caused by these tumors, and they account for 8 to 10 percent of primary intracranial tumors. In the majority of cases they arise from the peripheral portion of either the acoustic or vestibular division of the eighth nerve within the internal acoustic meatus, and later expand in size to extend into the posterior fossa in the cerebellopontine angle (CPA) region. Less frequently, they originate in the posterior fossa and may reach much larger size in this location (2 to 3 cm) before becoming symptomatic and may mimic primary brain stem or cerebellar tumors. In exceptional cases of von Recklinghausen's disease bilateral acoustic neurinomas may be present and these may be associated with neurinomas involving multiple cranial nerves.

The most common early symptoms of tumors in this location are caused by compression of the acoustic and vestibular nerve in the internal acoustic meatus, and 50 percent of patients do not have any objective neurological findings except those related to eighth nerve dysfunction. Eighty percent of patients with acoustic neurinoma have symptoms of disturbed vestibular function as manifested by systematized dizziness or vertigo. An early and characteristic symptom of vestibular involvement is a feeling of unsteadiness, which is described as dysequilibrium and occurs following rapid changes in body position or sudden head movement; this is most severe early in the day, becomes less noticeable later in the day and is not necessarily associated with vertigo. These symptoms have been reported in patients with intracanalicular tumors and are most likely due to labyrinthine and not cerebellar dysfunction.

Headache may also be a prominent symptom and occurs with small tumors in the absence of intracranial hypertension; in this case it may be caused by impaired vestibulo-spinal reflexes, causing contraction of cervical paraspinal muscles in an attempt to accommodate the barrage of aberrant vestibular reflexes. Vestibular dysfunction may be documented by objective methods by the use of electronystagmography and reduced response to caloric stimulation. The latter study was most specific and correlated with tumor size; 50 percent of patients with intracanalicular small tumors have impaired response on the involved side; 78 percent with tumors extending into the CPA but without other signs of cranial nerve dysfunction have an abnormal response, whereas 93 to 98 percent with signs of posterior fossa involvement have an abnormal caloric response.

Other early symptoms include dysesthesias or pain in the involved ear, which may be caused by compression of the nervus intermedius and does not always indicate extension into the posterior fossa.[1-3]

As the tumor expands into the

CPA, the earliest symptoms are referable to involvement of the sensory portion of the trigeminal nerve and include painful facial "tic," numbness or paresthesias; this is accompanied by early loss of the corneal reflex. In patients with a diagnosis of trigeminal neuralgia (tic douloureux) who have accompanying neurological findings — most usually impaired corneal response — diagnostic studies for an underlying tumor of trigeminal, facial or acoustic nerve origin should be undertaken, but the diagnostic yield for evaluating patients with trigeminal neuralgia without any neurological findings is quite low. As the tumor in the CPA enlarges there may be facial palsy, nystagmus, extraocular muscle involvement and ataxia with other cerebellar signs and evidence of intracranial hypertension resulting from compression of the fourth ventricle.

In the majority of CPA tumors the clinical findings are predominantly unilateral; whereas in intrinsic brain stem, fourth ventricular and cerebellar midline lesions they are bilateral. Less frequently, extrinsic CPA tumors may present with bilateral findings while other intrinsic posterior fossa tumors may expand exophytically, growing into the laterally located angle cistern, mimicking a CPA lesion.

The diagnostic evaluation of patients whose symptoms are confined to the eighth nerve alone may differ from that of patients whose symptoms indicate posterior fossa involvement, although some patients with only eighth nerve symptoms have lesions that extend 1 to 2 cm into the posterior fossa. The smaller, primarily intracanalicular, tumors are most reliably detected by plain skull radiogram, and this may detect 70 to 95 percent of lesions. Reidy reported positive studies in 70 percent and also 5 percent false positive studies. This study emphasized the importance of obtaining multiple views, including Stenver and Towne antero-

posterior views of orbit and basal sections to detect any asymmetry or erosive change in petrous bone structure; these multiple views were slightly more sensitive than Stenver views alone.

The characteristic radiographic finding consists of widening of the internal auditory canal with an asymmetry greater than 2 mm; this is usually associated with porosis and erosion, and in 4 percent of cases porosis and erosion were seen without widening of the canal. In addition, in 29 percent of acoustic neurinomas there were radiographic sella abnormalities consistent with increased intracranial pressure, and in 3 percent the sella was abnormal but the canal size was normal. This latter pattern suggests that in rare instances acoustic tumors in the posterior fossa may cause early ventricular obstruction with eighth nerve involvement and without any widening or erosive change in the internal auditory canal.[4, 5]

In patients with unilateral hearing impairment or vestibular symptoms tomography of the internal auditory canal and iophendylate (Pantopaque) cisternography are the most sensitive studies to detect the presence of an intracanalicular tumor. Tomography has greater sensitivity (78 percent) than multiple plain skull radiograms, and cisternography may detect 98 percent of tumors. Pantopaque cisternography involves performance of lumbar puncture with the instillation of a small amount of iodized oil into the subarachnoid space to outline the structure of the internal auditory canal and CPA cistern. This may detect tumors as small as 4 mm in diameter. Utilizing this technique, tumors have been detected that were too small to enlarge the canal radiographically. Positive contrast material is more sensitive than air study because the small amount of air that may be delivered to the cistern and canal does not provide sufficient contrast to detect small intracanalicular tumors.[6,7] In addition, when lumbar puncture is performed, CSF should be examined for protein content analysis, as small tumors may cause elevation (66 percent), but normal value does not exclude the presence of a small acoustic neurinoma.

If the tumor extends into the posterior fossa, isotope scan may detect those larger than 2 cm in diameter. Baum reported detecting uptake in 18 of 22 surgically proved CPA tumors with diameters of 2 to 6 cm, and the scan estimate of size correlated with the actual size of tumor. If the initial scan performed one hour after injection was negative, the scan was repeated at three hours; this improved the diagnostic yield by 25 percent. Of the false negative studies, two were scanned only at one hour, and these had diameters of 1.5 and 3.5 cm; both petrous bone tomography and Pantopaque cisternography were positive, consistent with the greater sensitivity of these techniques. Isotope uptake was greater in those tumors characterized by spindle-shaped closely packed cells (Antoni A) than with rounded cells (Antoni B), which frequently undergo microcystic degeneration.

Isotope scan is also of help in evaluating completeness of tumor removal or recurrence if the patient develops neurological deficit postoperatively (immediate or delayed). This technique is more reliable than skull radiography, which usually shows no evidence of recurrence, or Pantopaque cisternography, which shows poor filling of the involved area due to postoperative change that may be difficult to differentiate from tumor recurrence. Following craniotomy, superficial areas of increased uptake may be due to surgically induced change, but with delayed scan it may be possible to distinguish this from tumor recurrence.[8]

Since tomography and cisternography are more sensitive if the lesion originates in the internal auditory canal, they are almost always positive if isotope scan detects a lesion. If the tumor originates in the posterior fossa, the patient may present with unilateral deafness and negative radiographic study but a positive isotope scan. If the patient has clinical symptoms suspicious of a CPA lesion, cisternography may detect an intracanalicular lesion even if isotope scan and tomography are negative.

If a lesion causing dizziness or hearing impairment originates in the auditory canal, the pathological entity is almost always in acoustic neurinoma. If a mass is detected in the CPA, 80 percent are acoustic neurinomas; the remaining 20 percent consist of other lesions, of which one half are meningiomas and less common lesions, including metastatic tumors, chordoma, cholesteatoma, arachnoid cyst, arachnoiditis, granuloma (sarcoid, tuberculoma), posterior fossa angioma and aneurysm. In addition, tumors originating in the fourth ventricle (ependymoma, medulloblastoma, choroid plexus papilloma), cerebellum or brain stem may grow eccentrically and exophytically into the CPA, simulating the clinical presentation of an acoustic neurinoma.[9]

Vertebral angiography is usually reserved for special situations, including the suspicion of a vascular lesion (angioma or aneurysm), the presence of intracranial hypertension contraindicating lumbar puncture that is necessary to perform air study or cisternography, and the suspicion of the presence of a large tumor, in which case information concerning tumor blood supply, degree of distortion and compression of blood vessels in the posterior fossa is vital to the surgical procedure. In approaching certain acoustic neurinomas, it is crucial to demonstrate the course of vessels traversing the tumor by preoperative angiography to avoid the complication of brain stem hemorrhage or infarction due to surgical damage to the anterior inferior cerebellar arterial branches or draining petrosal veins.

The angiographic diagnosis of an extra-axial CPA tumor is based upon characteristic vascular displacements, including posterior displacement of the basilar and superior cerebellar arteries and anterior pontomesencephalic vein, stretching and vertical displacement of the anterior cerebellar artery, elevation of the petrosal vein, posterior displacement of the posterior inferior cerebellar artery with lateral displacement of the hemispheric branches.[10] In addition, a transient faint tumor stain may be seen in all CPA tumors, but the presence of markedly enlarged supplying and draining vessels with an intense prolonged stain is more characteristic of meningioma or metastases than an acoustic neurinoma. If the tumor originates in the fourth ventricle, cerebellum or brain stem and secondarily extends into the CPA, the angiographic findings may be confusing, owing to the opposing vector forces, and will be determined by the portion of the tumor that causes the most significant mass effect. In those cases in which tumor is located in both locations, angiography may most accurately reflect the resultant summation of these changes and not the individual vector forces.[11]

With the availability of CT, several studies have reported their experience in assessing the sensitivity and accuracy of CT in distinguishing specific pathological conditions as compared with other diagnostic procedures. Ambrose reported 100 percent accuracy in 12 surgically documented lesions and found that 10 were high- and two were low-density in preinfusion study, and all showed striking contrast enhancement. Other studies have reported 95 percent accuracy in detecting acoustic neurinomas that were greater than 2.0 cm in diameter and projected further than 1.5 cm into the CPA.[12] Of 53 patients in whom there was clinical suspicion of CPA tumor, Gyldensted reported that 17 (32 percent) had a tumor detected by CT. Of these, 12 were surgically proved to be acoustic neurinoma, whereas three others were meningioma, metastatic melanoma and calcified epidermoid, and one patient was found to have a supratentorial tumor with no lesion in the posterior fossa. The smallest lesion detected by CT extended 7 mm out of the porus acusticus. In these patients CT was more reliable than petrous tomography and compared favorably with angiography but was inferior to Pantopaque cisternography, which defined predominantly intracanalicular tumors. In addition, there was one false positive CT scan that was due to movement artifact, but there were also false positives for petrous tomography, Pantopaque cisternography and air study.[13]

The CT scan diagnosis of the presence of CPA tumor is dependent

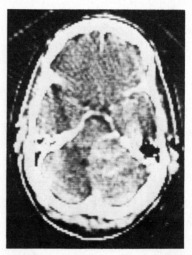

Figure 11–1. A 47-year-old man presented with progressive hearing loss in his right ear and sudden development of right facial paralysis two weeks previously. Findings included right side fifth, sixth, seventh and eighth nerve involvement with bilateral cerebellar signs. CT findings: a patchy, lamellated, nonhomogeneous high-density lesion with peripheral medial dense enhancement, compressing the fourth ventricle laterally to the left side. Vertebral angiography showed slight mass effect in the right cerebellopontine angle (CPA), with an abnormal venous pattern. Operative findings: extra-axial hematoma in right CPA with evidence of dilated tortuous veins, consistent with an angioma.

upon finding lesions of abnormal density in the posterior fossa, enhancement with contrast infusion, displacement of the midline fourth ventricle to the contralateral side, and narrowing or widening of adjacent cisternal spaces. The density characteristics, enhancement pattern, location and shape may frequently permit differentiation of the multiple pathological conditions. Of the acoustic neurinomas, the preinfusion scan may show no abnormal density (60 percent), as the lesion is initially isodense compared to the tissue densities in the opposite CPA. In 40 percent a low-density lesion was detected but in no case did the plain scan show a high-density lesion. Although these tumors may contain hemorrhagic foci, they do not usually show high-density characteristics prior to contrast infusion, and this finding should suggest an alternative pathological diagnosis (Fig. 11–1).

Following contrast infusion, the acoustic neurinoma appears as a

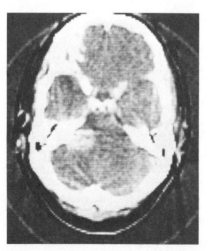

Figure 11–2. This 35-year-old man had an eight-month history of hearing impairment in his left ear. Petrous tomograms showed asymmetrical enlargement of the left auditory canal with erosive change. CT findings: plain scan showed no definite abnormality, but following contrast infusion a large, round, irregular high-density area was visualized in the left cerebellopontine angle that appeared contiguous with the petrous pyramid. Operative findings confirmed the diagnosis of acoustic neurinoma.

sharply marginated, homogeneous high-density area, which may appear to be contiguous with the posterior portion of the petrous pyramid (Fig. 11–2). The postinfusion density is usually 25 to 40 units, and occasionally the peripheral edges may appear less well-defined, owing to the partial volume effect (Fig. 11–3). Less commonly, there is a thick peripheral high-density rim that encompasses a low-density lucent core, but this is more suggestive of a metastatic lesion. In other cases the central region may be of very low density with negative values, which is suggestive of cyst formation containing xanthomatous lipid material (Fig. 11–4). Immediately following contrast infusion, these tumors show striking enhancement, which is maximal immediately after infusion and then shows striking decrement when repeated at 15-minute intervals to one hour, at which time subsequent 2- or 3-hour scans show little further decrement; the enhancement is believed due to an intravascular component. This is to be contrasted with meningioma, in which maximal enhancement may occur at 60 minutes following infusion (Fig. 11–5). Acoustic neurinomas cause distortion and displacement of the fourth ventricle in two thirds of cases. The tumor usually causes a flattening of the side of the ventricle with contralateral displacement, and in one third of cases displacement occurs without compression.[14]

With larger tumors the fourth ventricle may be compressed and decreased in volume, such that it is poorly visualized. Larger tumors may cause obliteration of the CPA cistern, whereas in other cases there may be widening of the cistern, which is believed to result from compression of normal parenchyma in the posterior fossa. The presence of widening of the CPA or ambient cistern is the most reliable CT sign of an extra-axial position of the tumor (Fig. 11–5). Acoustic tumors usually are round in shape (80 percent), but less frequently are roughly triangular, with

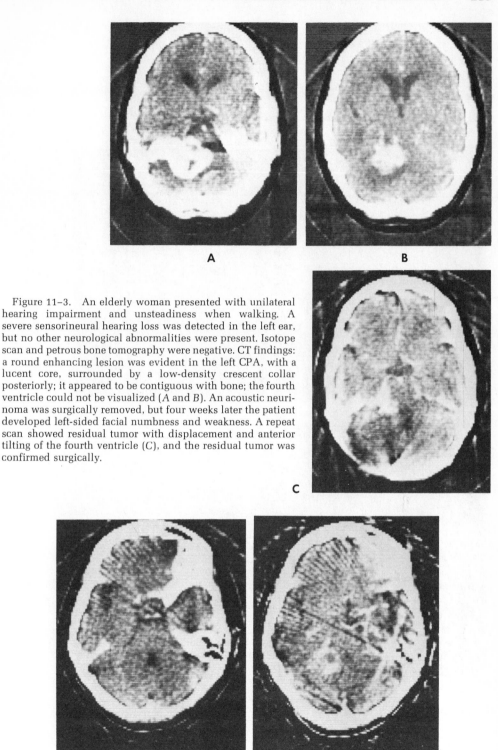

A   B

Figure 11-3.   An elderly woman presented with unilateral hearing impairment and unsteadiness when walking. A severe sensorineural hearing loss was detected in the left ear, but no other neurological abnormalities were present. Isotope scan and petrous bone tomography were negative. CT findings: a round enhancing lesion was evident in the left CPA, with a lucent core, surrounded by a low-density crescent collar posteriorly; it appeared to be contiguous with bone; the fourth ventricle could not be visualized (A and B). An acoustic neurinoma was surgically removed, but four weeks later the patient developed left-sided facial numbness and weakness. A repeat scan showed residual tumor with displacement and anterior tilting of the fourth ventricle (C), and the residual tumor was confirmed surgically.

C

A   B

Figure 11-4.   This patient had severe vertigo and left-sided hearing loss. CT findings: plain scan shows only lateral displacement of the fourth ventricle (A); following contrast infusion, a high-density peripheral rim of enhancement with a low-density central region was evident (B). Operative findings demonstrated an acoustic neurinoma with cystic component.

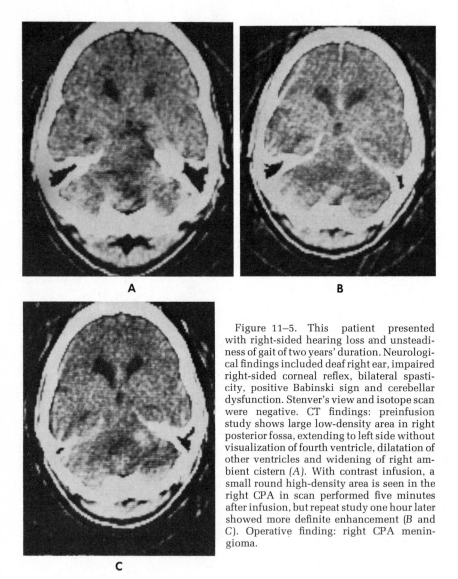

Figure 11–5. This patient presented with right-sided hearing loss and unsteadiness of gait of two years' duration. Neurological findings included deaf right ear, impaired right-sided corneal reflex, bilateral spasticity, positive Babinski sign and cerebellar dysfunction. Stenver's view and isotope scan were negative. CT findings: preinfusion study shows large low-density area in right posterior fossa, extending to left side without visualization of fourth ventricle, dilatation of other ventricles and widening of right ambient cistern (A). With contrast infusion, a small round high-density area is seen in the right CPA in scan performed five minutes after infusion, but repeat study one hour later showed more definite enhancement (B and C). Operative finding: right CPA meningioma.

the base toward the petrous bone (Fig. 11–6). Extension of the tumor into the ambient cistern and transincisural extension of the tumor into the ipsilateral portion of the quadrigeminal cistern, with distortion of the posterior third ventricle, may be visualized by CT. The high-density tumor may be surrounded by a low-density lucent collar, which is consistent with surrounding focal edema or atrophy. Since it may be present in

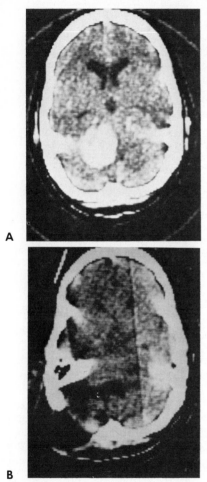

Figure 11–6. A 27-year-old woman developed left-sided sensorineural hearing loss. Tomograms of petrous bone showed enlargement and erosion of internal auditory canal. CT findings: plain scan showed no abnormal density but displacement of flattened fourth ventricle with lateral and third ventricular dilatation. Following infusion, a large round homogeneous density was detected in the left CPA (A). At operation an encapsulated acoustic neurinoma was removed. Six months later, the patient developed a left peripheral facial paresis and recurrent tumor was suspected. Repeat CT showed low-density area in the left CPA, with a dilated midline fourth ventricle but no enhancing lesion (B). The lack of recurrence was confirmed by air study.

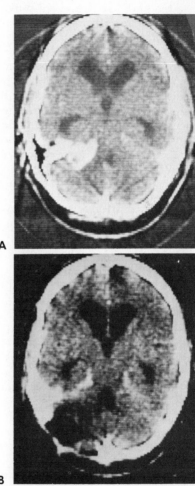

Figure 11–7. A 53-year-old man developed vertigo, unsteadiness of gait and headache. Neurological findings included gait ataxia, increased tone and reflexes in legs and bilateral papilledema. Plain skull radiogram showed an enlarged eroded sella turcica, but Stenver's views were negative. CT findings: dilated lateral and third ventricle with compression and displacement of fourth ventricle to the right side, and an enhancing irregularly shaped high-density lesion in the left CPA that was separate from the petrous pyramid (A). At operation, a 2.5 cm acoustic neurinoma was removed. Seven weeks later the patient became lethargic and was found to have bilateral Babinski sign. Repeat scan showed craniotomy defect with low-density region in left CPA, with enlarged midline fourth ventricle, consistent with communicating hydrocephalus (B).

the absence of shift of the fourth ventricle, it is more likely to be a result of atrophy; this is more frequently seen with meningioma but occurred in 25 percent of acoustic neurinomas.

In one third of cases, the acoustic tumor appeared to be contiguous with bone, but this is more consistent with meningioma. An unexpected finding was that in two thirds of cases, ventricular dilatation with compression of the fourth ventricle was visualized, although these patients only rarely present with or have radiographic evidence of intracranial hypertension (Fig. 11–7). Schwannomas (neurinomas) that arise from the trigeminal nerve have similar features but may be distinguished by the finding that they are confluent with the posterior region of the petrous pyramid close to its apex, and usually extend through the tentorial region, distorting the quadrigeminal cistern and posterior third ventricle.

It may frequently be difficult to differentiate certain CPA extra-axial tumors from intra-axial posterior fossa tumors, but certain signs are consistent with extra-axial location: (1) widening of the cistern due to displacement of parenchyma away from bone; (2) hyperostosis, erosion or destruction of bone or contiguity of tumor with bone; (3) sharp peripheral edges of the tumor; (4) presence of normal size and position of the fourth ventricle; (5) presence of a lucent peripheral collar.[14] No other spatial or density characteristics were of help in defining the presence of extra-axial lesions, although all acoustic neurinomas and meningiomas have shown evidence of enhancement, whereas certain low-grade cerebellar and brain stem gliomas do not enhance (Fig. 11–8).

Other pathological conditions may simulate acoustic neurinomas, but certain CT scan characteristics make preoperative diagnosis possible. Meningiomas originate from the arachnoid villi of the venous sinus in the petrous portion of the temporal bone, and dif-

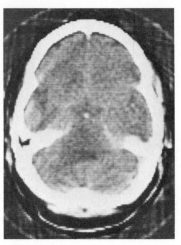

Figure 11–8. This patient developed numbness over the left side of her face and became deaf in her left ear. The only other neurological abnormality was a decreased corneal reflex on the left side. Petrous tomography, CSF examination and isotope scan were negative. CT findings: low-density region in left CPA extending medially and upward to ambient and interpeduncular cistern, but no abnormality of quadrigeminal cistern, with the fourth ventricle displaced slightly to the right side; there was no enhancement. Vertebral angiography was consistent with an extra-axial CPA lesion; at operation, a primary cerebellar neoplasm (gemistocytic astrocytoma) projected prominently into the left CPA.

ferentiation from acoustic tumor may be based on the type of bony radiographic abnormalities (hyperostosis and calcification) and the angiographic stain pattern of supply from dural vessels. The CT scan shows a round irregular high-density lesion with broad base, contiguous with bone. Frequently the plain scan shows high density (25 to 40) owing to presence of psammomatous calcification, and most meningiomas show dense, homogeneous, consolidated enhancement (Fig. 11–9). The meningioma is less frequently round in shape and may be comma-shaped as it grows upward through the tentorial notch (Fig. 11–10). Meningiomas of the tentorial region may grow to enormous size (Fig. 11–11) and occupy almost the entire posterior fossa. Smaller meningiomas are surrounded by a lucent low-density collar and displace the fourth ventricle and CPA cisterns, and they enhance with contrast infusion;

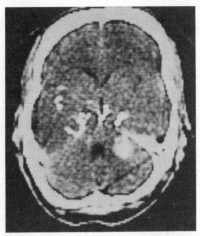

Figure 11–9.   This patient experienced a six-month history of right-sided hearing impairment, especially affecting the ability to understand conversation on the telephone and to judge the direction of sound. There were associated paroxysms of vertigo. Petrous tomography was negative, but Pantopaque cisternogram showed a lesion in the right CPA. CT findings: round, slightly nonhomogeneous, enhancing lesion 2.5 cm in diameter in the right CPA. The lesion is contiguous with bone and is not displacing the fourth ventricle. There also appears to be some thickening of the right petrous bone. In addition, there are multiple high-density Pantopaque droplets in the basal cisterns. Operative findings: a 2.5 cm meningioma in the right CPA.

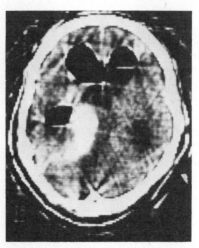

Figure 11–10.   This patient had had a meningioma resected from the left CPA several years previously and recently developed unsteadiness of gait but no new cranial nerve involvement. CT findings: marked lateral and third ventricular enlargement and nonvisualization of the fourth ventricle due to a high-density, homogeneous and consolidated enhancing comma-shaped mass extending from the left CPA through the tentorium. In addition, the ventricles show residual air.

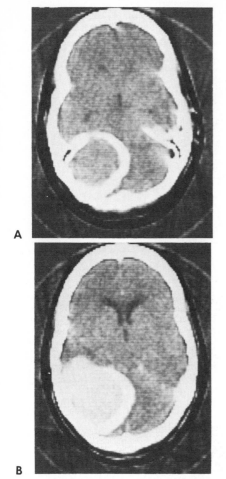

A

B

Figure 11–11. Patient with cerebellar dysfunction, vertigo and left-sided auditory loss. CT findings: plain scan shows round thick rim of high density (40 to 55) in left side of posterior fossa contiguous with bone (A); there is striking enhancement of isodense central portion (B). In addition, the fourth ventricle is not visualized and on right side of capsule there is a low-density rim. Operative findings: CPA and lateral tentorial meningioma.

but CT differentiation from acoustic neurinoma is not reliably established preoperatively.

Primary cholesteatomas arise from congenital epithelial rests and may present as a CPA mass but more frequently have a midline location in the posterior fossa. Pathologically the tumor is multilobulated and contains lipid material, and with air or Pantopaque study a very distinctive scalloped margination is observed. With

CT it appears as a homogeneously low-density (−5 to 5 units) sharply marginated lesion with no enhancement. One clinical point of distinction is that these tumors frequently involve the facial rather than the acoustic nerve initially.

Epidermoid and dermoid tumors are also congenital tumors, which usually occur in midline but may involve the CPA. These are usually large tumors, which invariably compress the fourth ventricle, causing obstructive hydro-

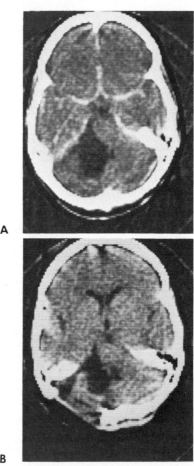

A

B

Figure 11–12. Patient with left-sided hearing loss and facial pain syndrome. CT findings: low-density, sharply marginated region contiguous with CPA cistern; the lesion is displacing the fourth ventricle to the right side and does not enhance (A). At operation, an epidermoid cyst was removed. Repeat study three months later showed decreased size but persistence of lesion, with continued contralateral displacement of the fourth ventricle (B).

cephalus. They usually appear as lucent round lesions with intermixed high-density calcified regions with no enhancement, but may be homogeneously dense or have a high-density calcified capsule with a lucent core, produced by low-density cholesterol and desquamated epithelial cells (Fig. 11–12).

Subarachnoid cysts of the posterior fossa are readily detected by CT, and failure to detect any contrast enhancement and their extension through the tentorium and into the supratentorial component differentiate them from cystic cerebellar astrocytomas (Fig. 11–13). Metastatic lesions usually show a dense thick enhanced rim with a low-density core due to necrotic material and may show multiple lesions. Aneurysms of the posterior fossa rarely present as CPA lesions, and CT usually shows calcification in the walls of the aneurysm. Primary intra-axial lesions may have extrinsic exophytic extension that may grow into the CPA, and the differentiation from acoustic neurinoma may not be established by CT, air study or angiography.[15] This occurrence is most frequent with ependymoma, medulloblastoma and brain stem glioma (Fig. 11–14). Bilateral acoustic neurinomas or multiple neurofibromas in patients with von Recklinghausen's disease are readily defined by CT (Fig. 11–15).

The limitations of CT in evaluating

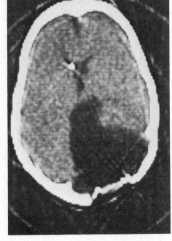

A

B

Figure 11–13. A ten-year-old child presented with loss of balance and dysequilibrium. Findings included right-sided cerebellar dysfunction and horizontal nystagmus. Skull radiogram and isotope scan were negative. CT findings: huge right-sided posterior fossa subarachnoid cyst, which extends through the tentorium into the occipital region and has sharp margins and density of CSF (A). The cyst was marsupialized with the cerebellum split, and repeat study showed a slight decrease in the size of the cyst (B).

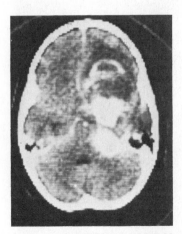

Figure 11–14. An eight-year-old girl had had an intramedullary cervical astrocytoma surgically decompressed and irradiated three years previously. Recently, she developed right-sided hearing loss, facial pain and paresis. CT findings: an enhancing lesion in the right CPA displacing the fourth ventricle to the left side; it is contiguous with bone and extends to the apex of the petrous pyramid. In addition, there are other lesions in the right middle and floor of the anterior fossa, consistent with cisternal spread of the glioma.

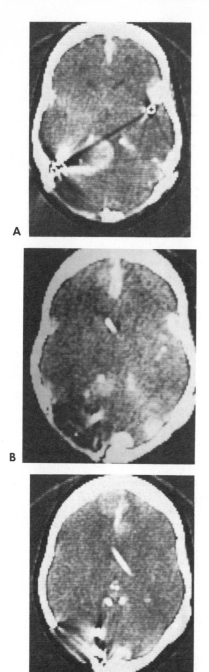

Figure 11–15. A patient with von Recklinghausen disease had had several intracranial neurofibromas removed surgically. She was deaf bilaterally and had severe cerebellar deficit. CT findings: enhancing lesions in left CPA (A), posterior to fourth ventricle in midline, and in the frontal region (B and C). In addition, there is a postoperative defect in the left posterior fossa; a shunt tube appears in the lateral ventricle.

CPA tumors include the fact that lesions with less than 8 mm extension through the porus acusticus are usually not detected and require Pantopaque cisternography. CT is superior to isotope scan, as only 40 percent of CPA lesions detected by CT were visualized by isotope scan. Evaluation of the CPA by CT may be difficult because of its proximity to dense bone, and false positive results may occur if there is even a slight motion artifact. False negatives have resulted from failure to administer contrast. By increasing the degree of angulation to 20 or 25 degrees, it is possible to avoid bony interference. To detect smaller lesions it is necessary to use 8 mm collimators. Consistently excellent results are possible if a single scan sequence (two sections) of the posterior fossa is obtained at 15-degree angulation with an 8 mm collimator, although others have advocated a 20-degree angulation to obtain two scan sequences (four sections) with eight to 12 overlapping 13 mm tissue sections.

Postoperatively, serial CT affords the most reliable technique to assess the pathophysiological basis for any clinical deterioration. If tumor removal has been complete, CT shows only a nonenhancing low-density region, which is usually associated with midline or ipsilateral shift of the fourth ventricle and CPA cisternal expansion toward the side of the tumor removal (Fig. 11–6). The most definitive sign of residual or recurrent tumor is contrast enhancement (Fig. 11–3). Following surgical removal, the development of facial paralysis or paresthesia may result from residual tumor or operative complication, and this may be best assessed by CT. Failure to improve or sudden clinical worsening in the immediate postoperative period may have multiple causes, including development of CSF circulatory impairment, edema, posterior fossa hemorrhage or infarction due to occlusion of the anterior inferior cerebellar artery (Fig. 11–7).

References

1. Johnson EW, House WF: Auditory findings in 53 cases of acoustic neuromas. Arch Otolaryngol 80:667, 1964.
2. Pulec J, House WF, Hughes RL: Vestibular involvement and testing in acoustic neuromas. Arch Otolaryngol 80:677, 1964.
3. Austin D: Modern diagnosis and treatment of acoustic neurinoma. Am J Med Sci 251:468, 1966.
4. Valvassori GE: The abnormal internal auditory canal in the diagnosis of acoustic neuroma. Radiology 92:449–459, 1969.
5. Reidy J, DeLacey GJ, Wignall BK: The accuracy of plain radiographs in the diagnosis of acoustic neurinomas. Neuroradiology 10:31, 1975.
6. Scanlan RL: Positive contrast medium (iophendylate) in the diagnosis of acoustic neuroma. Arch Otolaryngol 80:698–705, 1964.
7. Britton BH, Hitselberger, Hurley BJ: Iophendylate examination of posterior fossa. Arch Otolaryngol 88:608, 1968.
8. Baum S, Rothballer AB, Shiffman F: Brain scanning in the diagnosis of acoustic neurinomas. J Neurosurg 36:141, 1972.
9. Hambley WM, House WF: The differential diagnosis of acoustic neuroma. Arch Otolaryngol 80:708, 1964.
10. Takahashi M, Okudera T, Tomanaga M, Kitamura K: Angiographic diagnosis of acoustic neurinomas. Neuroradiology 2:191, 1971.
11. Wolpert SM, Hammerschlag SB: Extra-axial growth of fourth ventricular tumors — angiographic changes. Neuroradiology 12:191, 1977.
12. Davis KR, Parker SW, New PFJ: Computed tomography of acoustic neuroma. Radiology 124:81, 1977.
13. Gyldensted C, Lester J, Thomsen J: CT in the diagnosis of cerebellopontine angle tumors. Neuroradiology 11:191, 1976.
14. Naidich TP, Lin JP, Leeds NE: CT in the diagnosis of extra-axial posterior fossa masses. Radiology 120:333, 1976.
15. Kendall B, Symon L: Investigation of patients presenting with CPA syndromes. Neuroradiology 13:65, 1977.

Chapter 12

Intracranial Inflammatory Disease

Intracranial inflammatory conditions may present with a bewildering array of neurological signs and symptoms without any accompanying evidence to suggest an infectious origin. If the patient presents with headache, nuchal rigidity, confusion and fever, the clinical impression of infectious meningo-encephalitis is confirmed by CSF cell count, abnormal sugar and protein content and bacteriological studies. On the basis of results of these studies treatment with appropriate antibiotics is initiated and the outcome is usually favorable. In other patients there is a resolution of the CSF formula, but the patient's clinical condition deteriorates, and neurodiagnostic studies are necessary to determine the underlying complicating pathophysiological disorder. In cases of uncomplicated acute meningitis, CT is usually normal, but occasionally in basilar granulomatous meningitis, there is diffuse cisternal enhancement, and early CT study may be indicated to detect this pattern and to define the baseline size of the ventricular system (Fig. 12–1).

Less frequently patients who have laboratory evidence of infectious meningo-encephalitis present initially with seizures, focal neurological signs or papilledema, and these symptoms raise the clinical suspicion of a complicating localized pathological process which may include suppurative cerebritis, cerebral abscess, epidural or subdural empyema, arteritis, thrombophlebitis, mycotic aneurysm or hydrocephalus. In patients with bacterial meningitis, the finding of markedly elevated CSF pressure is

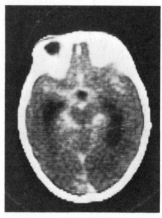

Figure 12–1. A patient who was currently being treated for tuberculous meningitis had intermittent periods of confusion. CT findings: following contrast infusion, there is dense enhancement which outlines the brain stem cisterns.

not uncommonly seen, but the presence of papilledema is most unusual.[1] Its infrequent occurrence in uncomplicated infectious meningitis may be related to the brief duration of the disorder, with normalization of CSF pressure within 48 hours. In patients with meningitis papilledema should suggest the possibility of associated lateral sinus thrombosis, cerebral abscess or subdural empyema, and other radiological studies are indicated to exclude these conditions. If seizures, focal neurological deficit or cranial nerve involvement are present, a focal lesion should be suspected. The performance of lumbar puncture may then be potentially dangerous, as deaths in meningitis temporally related to lumbar puncture are not uncommon if complicating conditions are present.[2]

In these clinical situations, CT may

be performed and if it is normal CSF examination may be safely performed. Recent experience has shown several cases in which the CT scan demonstrated a focal lesion that was clinically unsuspected and required emergency angiography; prior lumbar puncture would have been a dangerous procedure. With antibiotic therapy, the incidence of hydrocephalus complicating meningitis is low, but it occurs in 17 to 33 percent of cases of neonatal meningitis. This complication is most likely to develop insidiously over several years. In addition the mortality rate of neonatal meningitis is 40 to 60 percent and a significant number of survivors develop serious sequelae. Both the severity and frequency may be reduced by early diagnosis utilizing CT.[3]

In fungal and tuberculous meningitis, there is a coexisting ependymitis and ventriculitis, which may result in subependymal gliosis, causing intraventricular obstruction. More frequently the basilar meningitis causes arachnoiditis with reactive gliosis in the basal cisterns, and communicating hydrocephalus results. This may also occur in inadequate or late treatment of bacterial meningitis when there is a proliferation of fibroblasts and dense collagenous adhesions in the meninges. This diagnosis may be established by CT; this will localize the site of the CSF obstruction. Contrast infusion may show a diffuse enhancement pattern in the basal cisterns, reflecting the presence of contrast material in richly vascularized fibroblasts, which also have a poorly formed endothelial junction. In addition, the fibroblast proliferation may cause development of encysted loculation of CSF over the cerebral convexities. Focal or generalized cerebral atrophy may develop and is most frequent with nonbacterial infection; this is quite characteristic as a sequela to herpes encephalitis. These conditions may be well documented with CT and serial studies may show their progression. In all patients with incomplete recovery from CNS inflammatory disorder, who are left with neurological sequelae, CT is indicated.

Inflammatory intracranial disorders may also cause vascular disorders and clinically these patients may present with strokelike syndromes. There may be an arteritis with swelling and proliferation of endothelial cells and infiltration of vessel walls with inflammatory cells and fibrinoid deposits. This may occur with purulent bacterial meningitis but is more frequent with granulomatous meningitis. It may be angiographically defined by alternating focal constriction and dilation of both proximal large caliber and distal smaller caliber vessels.[4, 5] The vascular changes are not detected by CT but pathological changes resulting from this vasculitis may be defined as multiple low-density areas of cerebral infarction (Fig. 12–2).

In bacterial endocarditis, infected cardiac vegetations may embolize to the brain and lodge in the blood vessel walls, causing an inflammatory process with subsequent weakening and production of mycotic aneurysms. These aneurysms are usually less

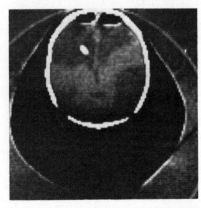

Figure 12–2. A neonate developed Gramnegative meningitis, which required treatment with intraventricular antibiotics. The CSF formula cleared as the child became increasingly obtunded, with generalized seizures. CT findings: multiple wedge-shaped low-density lesions without mass effect, consistent with multiple infarctions (confirmed by necropsy findings). Shunt tube is located in left lateral ventricle.

than 2 cm in diameter and are located in the distal branches of intracranial vessels. They are soft and friable and contain necrotic material and may cause intracerebral hemorrhage (Fig. 12–3). Because of their size, the aneurysms are not usually defined by

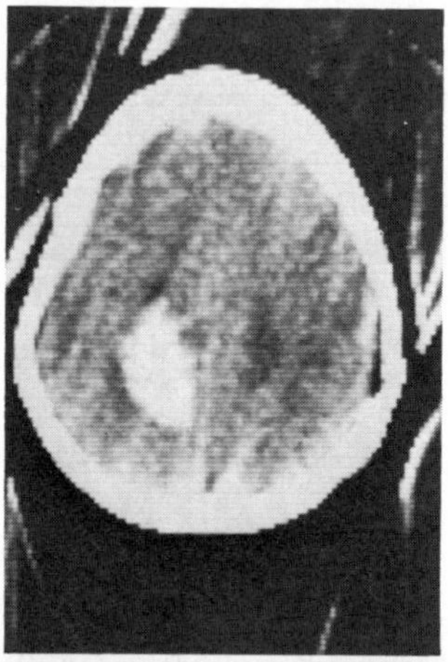

A

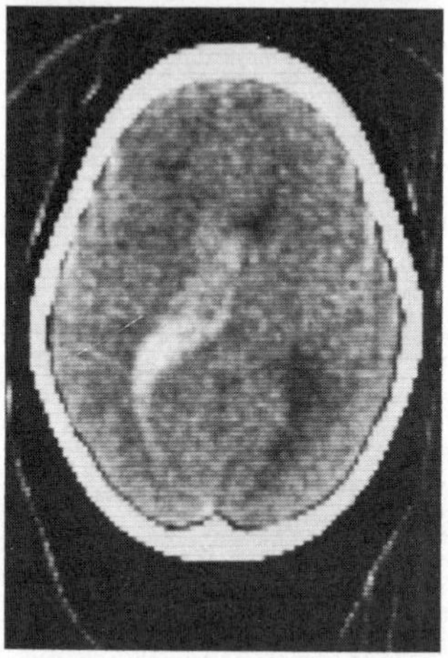

B

Figure 12–3. A six-year-old girl with a two-week history of fever and chills suddenly developed headache and neck pain. Examination showed a lethargic patient with bilateral retinal hemorrhages and right-sided hemiparesis, and a systolic basilar murmur consistent with aortic stenosis. CSF contained a half-million red cells and was xanthochromic. CT findings: a high-density area in the left temporo-parietal region; it extends superficially to the cortex (A) and has a significant intraventricular component (B) but no evidence of an aneurysm. Necropsy findings were small mycotic aneurysm of the left middle cerebral artery, which had ruptured to cause an intracerebral hematoma.

CT, even with enhancement, but the site of the hemorrhage is well defined. Operative intervention is dependent upon the clinical status of the patient, and the resolution of the hematoma or intraventricular extension may be followed by serial scans.[5] In addition, the most frequent neurological manifestation of bacterial endocarditis is a toxic encephalopathy without focal signs due to multiple small emboli to the brain, and in this case CT is normal or may show evidence of multiple areas of infarction.

Ventriculitis may complicate meningitis and may impair response to antibiotics as the loculated pockets of infection within the ventricles cause progressive ventricular enlargement, acting as an intraventricular abscess. A ventriculogram may define the extent of ventricular dilatation and provide fluid for culture and antibiotic sensitivity determination but may not show the loculated area in the ventricle. CT may define ventricular size and delineate the presence of high-density thick loculated pus, usually in the dependent portion of the ventricle (occipital regions), or may define the presence of stringlike gliotic bands which encapsulate the necrotic material (Fig. 12–4). This occurs most frequently in young children, especially those with myelomeningocele, but in adults ependymitis may also occur in fungal and bacterial meningitis.[7]

Cerebral abscess may present with meningitic syndrome, and early recognition of the focal pathological lesion should contraindicate lumbar puncture. The following should suggest a high probability of brain abscess: evidence of an active inflammatory process involving a contiguous or distant site, or serial CSF examinations containing inflammatory cells with borderline sugar content and negative gram stain and culture. The most common source is pleuropulmonary in origin, with septic emboli causing tissue infarction and rendering the brain parenchyma

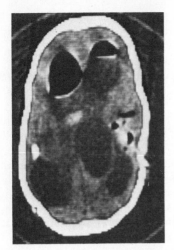

Figure 12–4. A child who had required multiple shunt revisions for congenital hydrocephalus was now evaluated because of fever and stiff neck. CSF examination showed pleocytosis with negative culture. CT findings: markedly enlarged ventricles with high-density material contained by fibrous band loculations in the right body and occipital horns, consistent with ventriculitis. Air from previous ventriculogram is also visualized in the ventricles.

more vulnerable to necrosis by other microorganisms. More direct local sources — nose, ear or eye infection introduced by a penetrating wound or skull fracture — may lead to osteomyelitis with perforation through the dura and leptomeninges, establishing suppuration intracranially. In one fifth of cases of brain abscess, the source of the infection is not established, and in these cases differentiation from other intracranial mass lesions may not be possible preoperatively.[8] Because of the hematogenous source, these metastatic abscesses occur in the territory of the middle cerebral artery, but not infrequently they may be deep-seated (thalamus, brain stem, cerebellum, basal ganglion, pituitary) or have a paraventricular location.[9]

Clinically, there are two distinct patterns of presentation. In one group, the patients present with fever, altered mentation and generalized seizures without clinical evidence of focal neurological deficit or intracranial hypertension. Despite the lack of focal findings, there may be laboratory studies which are consistent with a focal lesion, including EEG and isotope scan, and CSF pressure may be elevated.[10] Other patients present with a rapidly evolving clinical picture of focal neurological deficit and intracranial hypertension in the absence of fever and signs of meningeal irritation.

The specific clinical symptoms in an individual case are dependent upon multiple factors, including the following:

1. The presence of an active unrecognized septic focus and meningitic reaction, causing a febrile response; in the absence of these findings the patient may be afebrile.

2. Hematogenous dissemination may lead to multiple abscesses; these patients appear toxemic and febrile and may have confusional states and seizures, whereas a single lesion may simulate a primary intracranial neoplasm, with signs of progressive neurological deterioration.

An understanding of the pathogenesis of brain abscess is important in defining the value of diagnostic studies at different stages of the temporal evolution. If there is direct local extension, plain skull radiography and tomography may demonstrate sinusitis, fracture or osteomyelitis as the probable cause of intracranial infection, whereas if there is hematogenous spread, these studies are normal. In addition, the radiographic demonstration of intracranial air is indicative of gas within the abscess cavity.[11]

In both hematogenous and local extension of infection the earliest pathological change is that of focal septic encephalitis, characterized by tissue necrosis, polymorphonuclear cellular response, and petechial hemorrhages in multiple areas, which may then coalesce to form a large macroscopic area of cerebritis. This is surrounded by edema in white matter and astrocytic-microglial proliferation with endothelial hyperplasia and lymphocytic venous cuffing surrounding the focal encephalitis. At this stage the focal cerebritis is not clearly delineated from the normal brain parenchyma. Early symptoms include headache, fever and meningitic syndrome, and with cerebritis CSF findings are similar to those of aseptic meningitis, including mixed pleocytosis, elevated protein and borderline or normal sugar content with sterile fluid. If there is a predominantly polymorphonuclear response, the sugar content may be low. The EEG will invariably show evidence of a focal slow-wave pattern but may not be differentiated from that of encapsulated abscess.

Because of the inflammatory changes, the blood-brain barrier is no longer intact and isotope scan shows accumulation of isotope. The abnormal uptake may occur with focal cerebritis prior to the accumulation of pus within a walled-off capsule; the sensitivity of isotope scan at this stage appears lower than that of EEG. The uptake pattern usually indicates a spherical homogeneous lesion or appears as an annular doughnut-shaped lesion.[12] The latter pattern was initially believed specific for brain abscess and was consistent with a lesion containing an avascular and necrotic core, but it may also be seen in intracranial neoplasms, infarctions or hematomas. Angiography may show an avascular space-occupying lesion, but not infrequently the cerebritis is not focal or large enough to displace or distort blood vessels.

In rare patients, surgical biopsy may even be negative, and patients may recover completely with antibiotic therapy alone. Heineman reported six cases in which clinical isotope scan and CSF findings were consistent with intracranial suppurative disease and antibiotic therapy was successful, with biopsy documentation of angiographic evidence of a mass lesion, although it was not always possible to differentiate cerebritis from cerebral vasculitis, septic emboli or thrombophlebitis.[10]

Initially in focal suppurative cerebritis, the separation from surrounding parenchyma and definition of the wall of the abscess capsule is poorly defined, but later the abscess capsule becomes thicker and more complete. The capsule may vary from 1 to 3 mm in thickness and is usually thicker on its lateral than on its medial surface, a characteristic which explains its propensity to rupture into the ventricular system. It may take two weeks or more for capsule formation to occur, and before becoming contained the infection may spread more deeply into the white matter toward the ventricular surface and produce secondary daughter abscesses.[13] The center of the abscess contains necrotic material and microorganisms (pus), and edema is present at the periphery, with compression and atrophy of the underlying normal brain tissue. In the acute phase the wall of the abscess contains a thin irregular layer of granulation tissue, whereas in more chronic lesions the granulation layer is surrounded by a thicker collagenous wall.[14]

Isotope brain scan will detect all abscesses greater than 1 cm in diameter. With lesions this size, EEG demonstrates a focal slow-wave abnormality indicative of a space-occupying lesion.[15, 16] Since 20 percent of intracranial abscesses are multiple, isotope scan has been more reliable than EEG or angiography in delineating this occurrence.

When the abscess becomes encapsulated, it is almost always defined by angiography as an avascular lesion.[17] Less frequently, certain vascular patterns may be seen that are typical but not diagnostic of brain abscess. In 20 to 50 percent of cases a vascular rim of hyperemia is visualized in the capsular wall in the early venous phase, and this surrounds the radiolucent core.[4, 18, 19] In addition, there may be alternating concentric bands with radiolucent areas at the periphery of the lesion, which are believed to represent bowing of the vascular gyral pattern that is separated from compressed or edematous intervening parenchyma.[20] The vascular rim is postulated to be due to vascular proliferation from fibroblasts within the capsule or reactive hyperemia. The sensitivity of angiographic diagnosis is limited in the phase of focal cerebritis prior to any mass effect or vascular alterations. Samson reported that in 25 abscesses, 80 percent showed a focal avascular mass, 16 percent had only a shift of midline structures compatible with edema or cerebritis, and in one case (4 percent) angiography was entirely normal; this compared with only 80 percent accuracy for isotope scan.[15]

CT has become the most reliable procedure for defining the presence of an intracranial inflammatory process, differentiating it from other pathological conditions, defining the temporal pattern of evolution, delineating accompanying pathological changes, identifying multiple lesions, and serially following response to therapy.[21] In the stage of focal cerebritis preceding capsule formation the pre-infusion scan usually shows the following characteristics:

1. Irregular poorly defined areas of low density, consistent with edema fluid, which causes marked mass effect.

2. The density characteristics are nonhomogeneous and mixed owing to the relative contribution of edema fluid, tissue necrosis and petechial hemorrhage.

3. Following contrast infusion there is usually an irregular speckled or gyral pattern of enhancement, which does not give the appearance of a peripheral rim of capsular enhancement, or less commonly there may be no evidence of enhancement. This scan pattern correlates with the pathological finding of inflammatory change, and treatment should include corticosteroids and antibiotics. Sur-

gery should be delayed until the abscess shows better defined and more regular encapsulation. Occasionally, if surgery is performed at this stage, herniation may occur into the surgically decompressed area, causing further tissue necrosis.

The demonstration of the capsule wall is usually possible two to four weeks after the neurological symptoms begin to develop, and this temporal evolution is consistent with capsule formation that is experimentally produced.[22] At this stage the abscess is becoming walled off from the surrounding parenchyma and the CT characteristics, reflecting these pathological changes, include the following:

1. A central low-density core, with density values ranging from 6 to −15 units and occasionally lower values if the abscess contains air.

2. A less pronounced mass effect than with cerebritis.

3. With contrast infusion there is enhancement in the capsule that is usually regular but may be irregular, with a thicker segment on the surface adjacent to deep nuclear masses and cortex. This may occur because the vascularity of the superficial gray matter is more extensive than that of the deeper white matter such that capsule formation is slower and weaker on the inner or white matter side.

CT is better able to define accompanying smaller satellite or daughter abscesses frequently not detected as separate lesions by isotope scan.[22] In addition CT may define mass effect (ventricular distortion or dilation), hemorrhage into the abscess cavity or vasculitis with infarction. In patients who have been treated with corticosteroids there may be marked reduction in contrast enhancement in the abscess capsule as a result of the effect of the medication in reducing extravascular diffusion as the capillary endothelial membrane junction is stabilized.[23] In addition, the enhancement in the falx may show marked bowing owing to diffuse edema of the septic cerebritis (Fig. 12–5).

If the gradual evolution of cerebritis to a well-encapsulated area is observed, this is pathognomonic for cerebral abscess, but if the CT scan shows only a low-density core surrounded by a high-density capsule, this pattern is less specific and may occur with glioblastoma, metastases, cerebral infarction, intracerebral hematoma, and postoperative changes[24] (Figs. 12–6 and 12–7). Although dif-

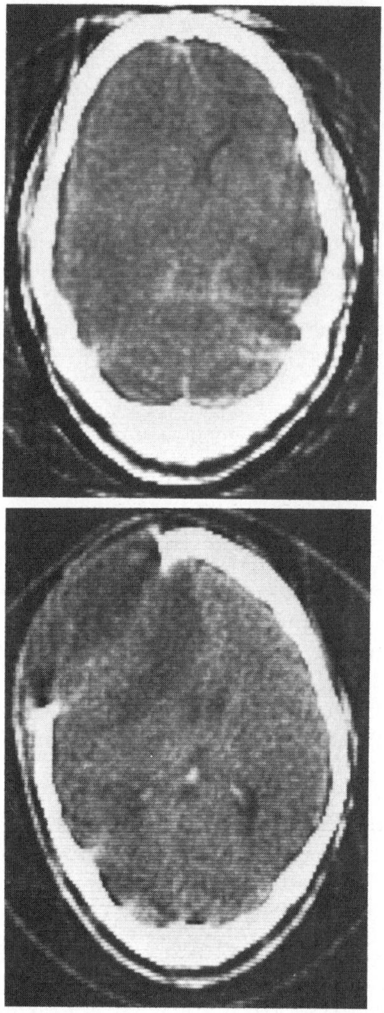

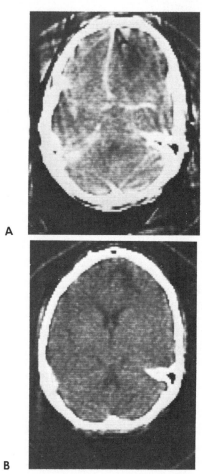

Figure 12–5. An 18-year-old youth was evaluated because of fever, confusion and right-sided weakness. The patient had nuchal rigidity but CSF was sterile and acellular. EEG showed a slow wave pattern over the left hemisphere, and isotope scan was negative. Angiography showed vascular displacement and mass effect in the left hemisphere. CT findings: Marked mass effect in left hemisphere, with compression of lateral ventricle, shift of pineal body, bowing of falx but no enhancement (A). Operative decompression revealed diffuse cerebritis. Despite administration of corticosteroids, the patient's condition worsened. Repeat scan showed marked bulging at the operative decompressive site, with continued compression of the ventricular system (B).

Figure 12–6. A 15-year-old child with a history of frontal sinusitis became febrile and confused. Neurological findings included mild left hemiparesis and mild confusion. EEG and isotope scan were consistent with abnormality in right frontal region. CT findings: Large area of low density in right frontal region with compression of the ventricular system with incomplete capsule formation. There is also bowing of falx to the left side (A). Following removal and drainage of abscess, the patient's clinical condition continued to deteriorate; repeat scan showed slight postoperative low-density area but no enhancement or mass effect (B).

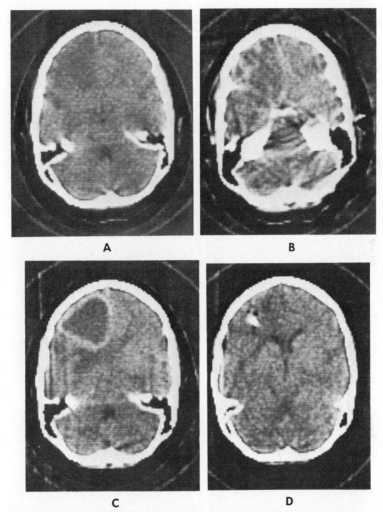

Figure 12–7.   A ten-year-old girl had periorbital cellulitis, which was treated with antibiotics. She then suffered right focal motor seizure. When initially examined she was febrile and confused and had early papilledema but no localizing neurological findings. Skull radiogram showed no evidence of osteomyelitis. Isotope scan was negative, and EEG showed slow wave pattern in the left frontal region. Because of suspicion of intracranial abscess or empyema, lumbar puncture was omitted. CT findings: large low-density nonhomogeneous area in left frontal region extending into inferior and midfrontal region; this was causing significant mass effect with compression of left ventricular system (A). With contrast infusion, the falx appeared bowed and stretched, and there was diffuse contrast enhancement without capsule pattern, consistent with focal cerebritis (B). The patient was treated with intravenous antibiotics and corticosteroids and studies were repeated one month later. Isotope scan was now positive in the left frontal region. CT findings: a thick rim of peripheral enhancement, less well formed on the medial aspect (C). Because of CT evidence that necrotic focus had now localized, surgical intervention was performed with drainage and excision. Two weeks later, CT showed residual low-density region with no mass effect or enhancement; indwelling catheter and air are visualized (D).

ferentiation is not always possible, certain points of differentiation have been observed:

1. Glioblastomas have more bizarre and irregular contours, with focal thickening of the capsule wall, especially on the medial surface, although in cases of ganglionic-thalamic or posterior fossa abscess formation differentiation is not possible.

2. Infarction may appear normal on preinfusion study and show prominent enhancement with minimal mass effect.

3. Intracerebral hematoma usually shows high density on plain scan with contrast enhancement in the periphery.

4. Postsurgical changes show a thinner rim of enhancement.

5. Metastatic neoplasms may mimic cerebral abscesses, and differentiation rests upon the clinical history (Fig. 12–8). In patients with a previously treated abscess who have been asymptomatic, the development of sudden neurological symptoms may be unrelated to the previous in-

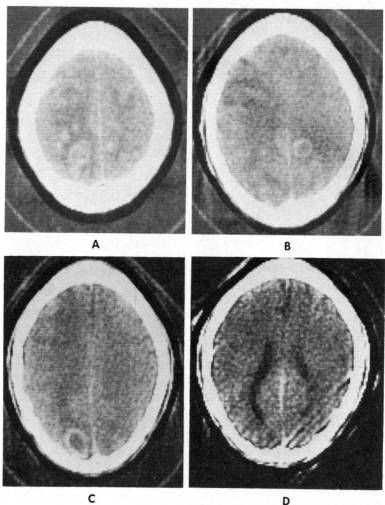

A

B

C

D

Figure 12–8.   A 35-year-old heroin user who had had recent dental work was admitted to the hospital confused and disoriented but without focal neurological findings. EEG was diffusely slow and isotope scan was negative. CSF showed pleocytosis and decreased sugar content, and culture was positive for *Staph. aureus*. Patient was febrile and had loud basal systolic murmur of aortic stenosis. CT scan showed multiple (total of 8) round, high-density areas, consistent with diagnosis of multiple brain abscesses (*A, B* and *C*). Patient was treated with antibiotics and there was clearing of mental state associated with clearing of abscesses, as evident in CT scan (*D*).

fection — for example, hemorrhage into an old abscess cavity may be clearly defined by CT, although the angiographic finding of an avascular mass may not be differentiated from recurrent abscess.

The CT scan pattern does not always correlate with the clinical picture, the duration of symptoms and results of conventional diagnostic studies. Seven patients presented with fever, altered mentation and generalized seizures. EEG was diffusely abnormal in five and two had a focal abnormality. Isotope scan was positive in only two cases, and in all cases CSF examination showed sterile pleocytosis. In four cases, CT showed a focal low-density area with marked mass effect and a diffuse enhancement pattern consistent with cerebritis, whereas three showed well-encapsulated abscess formation. Angiography was negative in two of four cases of diffuse cerebritis and was not performed in the other three cases because of a characteristic CT finding. Five other patients presented with progressive focal neurological deficit that developed over a one-month interval; in all isotope scan and EEG showed a focal abnormality. In two cases CT delineated a pattern consistent with cerebritis and angiography showed an avascular mass; three others showed a pattern of encapsulated abscess.

CT is the only nonsurgical procedure that can differentiate focal cerebritis from abscess formation. Since the operative mortality has remained 30 to 40 percent and the diagnosis is dependent upon the nature and extent of intracranial focal suppuration, it is possible that lower mortality may result from more appropriate timing for surgical intervention. In certain cases, based on a CT scan pattern showing focal cerebritis, the need for craniotomy may be obviated.[24] In the stage of edema and hyperemia with minimal frank tissue necrosis, treatment with antibiotics and corticosteroids is indicated, and complete clinical recovery without abscess formation may result; this may be defined by a characteristic CT appearance. At this stage, infarction secondary to infectious arteritis may

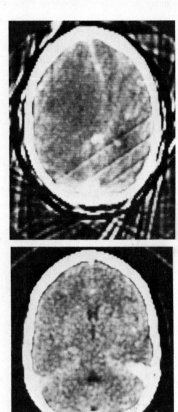

A

B

Figure 12–9. A 31-year-old woman with ventricular septal defect but no cardiovascular symptoms developed headache, stiff neck and fever, and two days later was noted to have right hemiparesis–sensory syndrome. EEG showed a delta pattern, and isotope scan was positive in left fronto-parietal region; CSF examination was normal. CT findings: Large nonhomogeneous low-density area in left frontal temporal region which compressed the ventricular system. Following contrast infusion, bowing of anterior portion of falx without any definite enhancement were visualized (A). Angiography showed an avascular mass without abnormal vascularity. On basis of scan, with clinical history of sudden neurological deficit, differentiation of cerebritis from vasculitis with edema and necrosis is not always possible, even with angiography. Following administration of antibiotics and corticosteroids, the clinical and scan abnormalities resolved (B).

not be differentiated from cerebritis, except that in the latter condition the margins of the lesion are confined to the boundaries of the arterial tree. The rationale for surgical intervention is to remove necrotic tissue and to relieve intracranial pressure and prevent herniation. The CT scan finding of a well-encapsulated rim surrounding a low-density necrotic core defines the need for operative intervention.

In those patients who are treated nonsurgically, CT is superior to isotope scan and clinical status as a monitor of therapeutic response. With CT the resolution of the cerebritis and mass effect may be detected (Fig. 12–9). If the isotope scan abnormality becomes more prominent, there is usually corresponding clinical deterioration, and it is more difficult to evaluate the finding of a positive scan in the immediate postoperative stage. In several cases isotope scan findings have increased in size and number and the underlying pathophysiological disturbance has been defined by CT.

In cases of multiple contiguous abscesses, it appears that resolution may follow antibiotic therapy (Fig. 12–10). Furthermore, experience has shown that patients with a well-formed and complete ring capsule are good operative candidates. Studies are necessary to correlate the thickness of the wall with risk of ventricular rupture or response to treatment. CT is a most reliable and

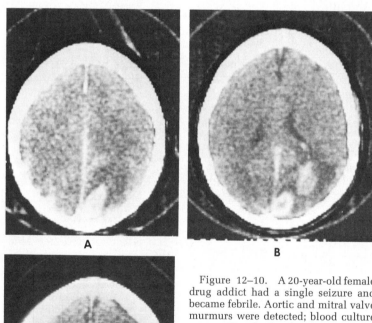

A

B

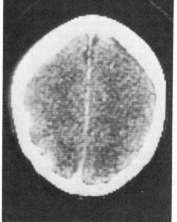

C

Figure 12–10. A 20-year-old female drug addict had a single seizure and became febrile. Aortic and mitral valve murmurs were detected; blood culture was positive for *Staph. aureus.* Isotope scan showed single uptake in right occipital region, and CT initially showed mixed-density pattern in this region (*A*). She was treated with multiple antibiotics and was neurologically asymptomatic but isotope scan now showed several lesions. CT revealed two definite right occipital lesions (*B*). Two months later isotope scan was still positive but CT showed complete resolution (*C*).

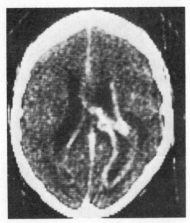

Figure 12–11. A 60-year-old man presented with headache and stiff neck. CSF findings included 1700 white blood cells, of which 70 percent were polymorphonuclear, with elevated protein but negative culture. Despite antibiotic therapy, patient became confused. CSF showed 14,000 white blood cells, of which 80 percent were polymorphonuclear. Isotope scan and EEG were negative. CT findings: Enlarged ventricles with ependymal enhancement and high-density speckled material in right lateral ventricle, consistent with intraventricular inflammatory process.

sensitive procedure to detect multiple abscesses and has detected some less than 8 mm in size.

The most unusual CT pattern seen with brain abscess is that of ependymal enhancement, with evidence of high-density material within the ventricle. This correlates with a finding of pus in the CSF examination. Despite antibiotic therapy the outcome has been unfavorable (Fig. 12–11). Despite advances in surgical and antibiotic therapy, the morbidity and mortality rates of brain abscesses have remained high, but preliminary studies since the advent of CT have indicated that there appears to be a definite decrease in these figures.[16, 25]

FOCAL NONSUPPURATIVE ENCEPHALITIS

Herpes simplex may cause an acute necrotizing and hemorrhagic encephalitis that has a predilection for involving the temporal, insular and or-bital surface of the frontal lobe; the involvement may be so predominantly unilateral as to simulate an intracranial neoplasm. The majority of patients present with rapid onset, but in 20 percent the onset is more insidious. Patients develop symptoms suggestive of an infectious inflammatory disorder. This is followed by a focal neurological deficit and intracranial hypertension caused by focal edema, hemorrhage and necrosis, which may be severe enough to cause a herniation syndrome and accounts for high mortality. In rare instances psychiatric symptoms (hallucinations, psychoses, catatonia) may be the initial manifestation and precede seizures or focal neurological findings.[26]

The diagnosis can be definitively established only by obtaining a brain biopsy specimen for specific cytopathological and viral studies but may be suggested by certain neurodiagnostic findings. EEG abnormalities include a marked and characteristic periodic delta pattern in the frontal-temporal region, and isotope scan is frequently positive.[27] The CSF findings are nonspecific and include pleocytosis, presence of red blood cells, elevated protein and reduced sugar content; rarely, CSF findings may be negative. Angiography shows a marked mass effect in temporal and frontal opercular regions owing to edema and hemorrhage. In addition there is a localized vascular stain, which results from arterial vasodilatation, and early venous opacification without abnormal vessels. The demonstration of tumor stain without significant mass effect is seen in focal encephalitis and is not specific for herpes simplex.[28]

Since there is evidence that herpes simplex encephalitis is responsive to certain antiviral agents, it is important to establish this diagnosis, but this has required brain biopsy. In several cases, the CT pattern has permitted an accurate diagnostic assessment that has been confirmed by necropsy findings. The abnormal re-

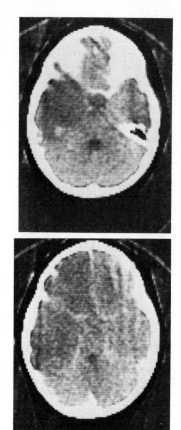

A

B

Figure 12–12. A three-year-old girl began to "act strangely" and then developed right focal motor seizures and became progressively more obtunded. When initially examined she was comatose, had right hemiparesis and showed decerebrate posturing. CSF examination showed pleocytosis and elevated pressure. EEG showed bitemporal spike and slow wave pattern but isotope scan was negative. CT findings: large low-density region in left fronto-temporal region which distorted and compressed ipsilateral ventricular system (A) and impinged upon lateral aspect of suprasellar cistern, consistent with temporal lobe herniation (B). There was a high-density area consistent with hemorrhage, and there was no enhancement pattern. Despite high dosage corticosteroids, mannitol and surgical decompression, the patient died. Necropsy findings showed a swollen and necrotic temporal region with a single hemorrhage area; microscopic analysis showed inclusion bodies typical of herpes simplex and this virus was subsequently cultured from the brain.

gion is located in the frontal-temporal area, is of low density, causes significant mass effect, does not enhance and has scattered large or small high-density hemorrhage areas. If the patient survives the acute episode, there may be large cystic areas in the temporal region (Fig. 12–12).

EXTRACEREBRAL INFLAMMATORY COLLECTIONS

In infants and children subdural loculation of fluid may complicate purulent meningitis, and this is most frequent following *Hemophilus influenzae* infection. The exact incidence of this complication is not known because subdural taps are not routinely performed if the child is asymptomatic, but in several large series it has been reported to occur in 10 to 43 percent of cases of meningitis[29] The presence of subdural effusion is suspected in patients whose fever and positive CSF cultures persist significantly longer than 48 hours after initiation of appropriate antibiotic therapy. Other signs are convulsions or focal neurological symptoms developing as CSF abnormalities resolve, the presence of a tense or bulging fontanelle, an abnormal pattern of transillumination, and radiographic evidence of progressive suture separation.[3] The fluid collection may vary from 2 to 150 ml, may be xanthochromic and may be present bilaterally.

Diagnosis is established by subdural taps and treatment consists of continued taps until the volume is less than 5 ml. With CT, it is possible to demonstrate the presence, location and size of these fluid collections in patients with meningitis prior to the development of focal neurological deficit. The sensitivity of subdural taps is much greater than that of CT, as collections of up to 20 ml have occasionally gone undetected by CT. In children with meningitis who respond to antibiotics and become neurologically asymptomatic but with evidence by scan of ventricular dilatation or infarction, the subsequent

development of symptomatic subdural effusion has been noted in several patients (Figs. 12–13 and 12–14).

The majority of these effusions
have been drained with repeated
taps, but occasionally craniotomy or a
shunt procedure is required if a densely adherent membrane has formed.
In utilizing CT, the finding of en-

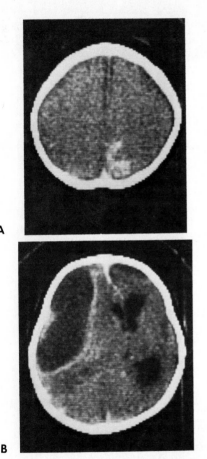

A

B

Figure 12–13.   This child had recovered completely from bacterial meningitis, but initial CT
scan showed serpentine areas of enhancement in
the right occipital region consistent with infarction (A). Four weeks later the patient became
increasingly lethargic, with right hemiparesis. CT
showed a large subdural collection over the left
hemisphere which showed enhancement in the
medial capsule and marked mass effect (B). Surgical drainage removed over 100 ml of highly
proteinaceous sterile fluid, but this collection
recurred and required craniotomy to remove
dense adherent membranes surrounding the effusion.

hancement in the medially located
capsule may be helpful in predicting
the presence of a thick membrane.
Further studies are necessary to determine if there are any prognostic
signs that may suggest which patients
are most likely to develop subsequent complications, and in whom
early CT should be performed. In all
patients who developed delayed subdural effusion, initial CT study
showed an intraparenchymal abnormality.

Collections of pus may form in either the epidural or subdural space
and may occur without an underlying
intracerebral abscess. Epidural abscess frequently follows craniotomy
or results from infection in the frontal
sinus or frontal bone osteomyelitis.
The inflammatory mass is well localized and flattened between the dura
and bone. CT usually shows a well-
localized extracerebral low-density
mass, which compresses the underlying brain and is directly convex in-
wardly. Lott has reported that epidural lesions extend across the frontal
midline, whereas subdural empyema
is localized to one side, and there is
posterior compression and bowing of
the falx[30] (Fig. 12–15).

Subdural empyema may result from
penetration of the dura by frontal sinusitis or from septic thrombophlebitis
involving emissary veins, allowing or-
ganisms to enter dural space. Rarely,
this may result if sterile effusion becomes infected. Clinical findings may
be directly related to meningeal involvement or the effect of an expanding extracerebral lesion. Since patients with subdural empyema may
also have septic dural venous thrombosis or brain abscess, as has been
reported in up to one fourth of cases,
clinical differentiation of the presence of these several conditions is
not always possible. Important diagnostic studies include the following:
(1) plain skull radiogram demonstrating osteomyelitis or clouding of
paranasal sinuses; (2) EEG showing a
unilateral focal delta pattern but more

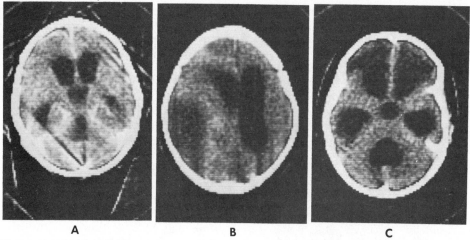

A   **B**   **C**

Figure 12–14.   This child was treated for bacterial meningitis with ampicillin, with resolution of CSF abnormalities. Initial CT scan showed ventricular dilatation including fourth ventricle *(A)*. She developed right hemiparesis with focal seizures, and three weeks later CT showed large loculated subdural collection in the left parieto-occipital region, displacing and distorting the left lateral ventricle to the right *(B)*. Following drainage, CT showed more extensive ventricular dilatation with low-density, periventricular, crescent-shaped areas, consistent with active hydrocephalus; a shunt was required *(C)*.

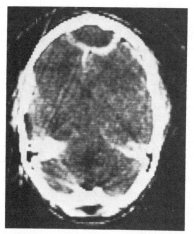

Figure 12–15.   CT shows a large low-density lesion in the frontal midline region; it is convex posteriorly and has a high-density capsule, which does not enhance and causes posterior displacement of the falx, which does not extend to the inner skull table. Operative finding: epidural abscess.

frequently a bilateral slow pattern; (3) isotope scan showing peripheral uptake, but this may blend with normal peripheral uptake and may be falsely negative in bilateral collections; (4) CSF findings may simulate partially treated meningitis and are almost always abnormal.

Angiography is the definitive diagnostic procedure but occasionally may be negative. The characteristic angiographic findings include a scalloped appearance of terminal branches of the middle cerebral artery with irregular displacement from the inner table by an avascular mass seen on anteroposterior view and a vascular stain surrounding an avascular area seen in the early venous phase, caused by neovascularization in granulation tissue. The pus collection may spread diffusely and bilaterally over both hemispheres (25 percent of cases), or it may become loculated by the formation of surrounding granulation tissue over the convexity or in the parafalcial region.[31, 32, 33]

The high mortality in this condition has been related to diagnostic error and late surgical intervention after focal neurological deficit and intracranial hypertension have developed. The clinical presentation may be predominantly meningitic, but lumbar puncture may precipitate a herniation syndrome. Results with CT indicate that it is highly accurate; CT defined the presence of ten consecutive empyemas, was more sensitive than angiography, and was positive in patients without lateralizing neurological signs.

The characteristic CT findings include an extensive poorly localized, low-density, extracerebral lesion, which causes compression, distortion and displacement of the ventricular system. If the collection is highly proteinaceous it usually has low density, but if it is thicker with more puslike material it may be isodense (Fig. 12–16). Empyemas that are isodense may be missed unless contrast infusion is performed to detect the presence of enhancing membrane. If the subdural empyema is bilateral there may be no shift of midline

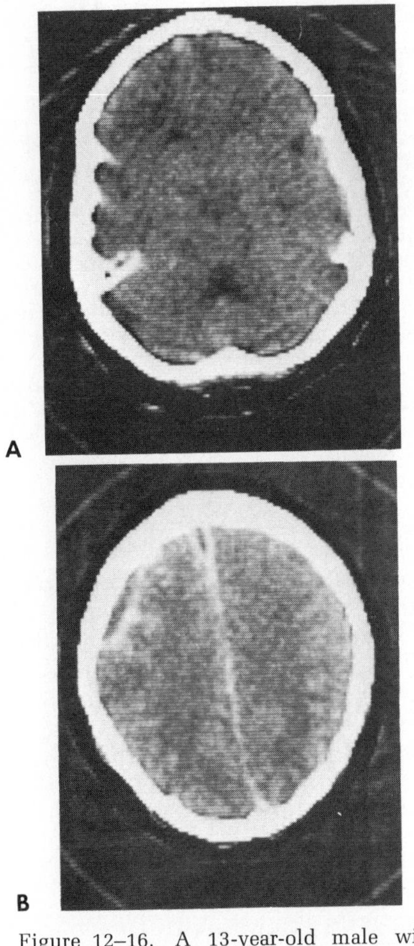

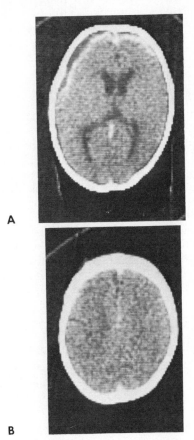

Figure 12–16. A 13-year-old male with a history of frontal sinusitis, fever and headache of two weeks' duration developed right-sided focal motor seizures. Neurological abnormalities included bilateral papilledema, right hemiparesis and oppressive aphosia. EEG showed bilateral frontal spike discharge with delta pattern in left frontal parietal area. Isotope scan was positive in that area. CSF pressure was elevated but fluid was acellular. CT showed nonhomogeneous low-density area in left hemisphere (A) and high-density convex area in left posterior frontal area, visualized with contrast enhancement (B). Angiographic findings were compatible with left subdural collection, but no mass effect was detected. Evacuation through bilateral burr holes revealed 20 ml collection of purulent exudate in the left posterior frontal region.

Figure 12–17. An eight-month-old child with bacterial meningitis developed right hemiparesis; angiography demonstrated left frontal subdural empyema, which was surgically drained. Three weeks later her symptoms recurred and CT showed a low-density crescent-shaped region with enhancing membrane, which extends to the right frontal region (A). This was surgically drained, and follow-up scan one month later was normal (B).

structures, but there is usually compression and collapse of the ventricles. The scan may detect the presence of an underlying cerebritis or, less frequently, an intracranial abscess.

Following complete surgical evaluation by either repeated taps or craniotomy, the evidence of an extracerebral lesion usually disappears, and there is no evidence of an enhancing membrane (Fig. 12–17). In other cases after surgical treatment blood under the craniotomy site may appear on the CT scan as a high-density area with irregular edges; the position of the ventricles is normal. This pattern should not be confused with recurrence.

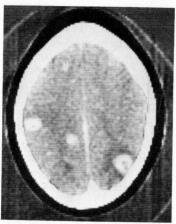

Figure 12–18. A 15-year-old boy with juvenile rheumatoid arthritis had been treated with prednisone for 10 years. He developed a febrile illness, and biopsy of his knee showed granuloma. CSF examination showed pleocytosis with elevated protein and negative culture. CT scan: multiple high-density (30–35) lesion in both hemispheres, with surrounding low-density edema. Biopsy showed evidence of vasculitis but no granuloma.

GRANULOMA

In the absence of a known history of tuberculosis, the preoperative radiographic diagnosis is difficult to establish, as these infectious lesions mimic either a solitary or multiple tumors. In the majority of cases the isotope scan is positive and angiography reveals an avascular mass. CT experience with these lesions has been limited, but the scan may detect a high-density (35 to 39) lesion with surrounding edema and no enhancement.[34] Since vasculitis is commonly seen in association with tuberculous infection, it may not be possible to differentiate tuberculoma from the pathological sequelae of arteritis (Fig. 12–18). In multiple sclerosis enhancing lesions are usually found in periventricular locations, and other diagnostic entities should include abscesses and metastases.

REFERENCES

1. Swartz MN, Dodge PR: Bacterial meningitis — a review of selected aspects. II. Special neurological problems, post-meningitic complications, and clinico-pathological correlations. N Engl J Med 272:954, 1003, 1965.
2. Duffy GP: Lumbar puncture in the presence of raised intracranial pressure. Br J Med 1:407, 1969.
3. Menkes JH: Textbook of Child Neurology. Lea and Febiger, Philadelphia, 1974. pp 213–221.
4. Ferris EJ, Rudikoff JC, Shapiro JH: Cerebral angiography of bacterial infection. Radiology 90:727, 1968.
5. Wise GR, Farmer TW: Bacterial cerebral vasculitis. Neurology 21:195, 1971.
6. Suwanwela C, Suwanwela N: Intracranial mycotic aneurysms of extravascular origin. J Neurosurg 36:552, 1972.
7. Salmon JH: Ventriculitis complicating meningitis. Am J Dis Child 124:35, 1972.
8. Banker BQ, Victor M: Brain Abscess. Med Clin North Am 47:1335, 1963.
9. Law JD, Lehman RAW: Diagnosis and treatment of abscess of the central ganglia. J Neurosurg 44:226, 1976.

10. Heineman HS, Braude AI, Osterholm JL: Intracranial suppurative disease. J A M A 218:1542, 1971.
11. Norrell H, Howieson J: Gas-containing brain abscesses. Am J Roentgenol 109:273, 1970.
12. Crooker EF, McLaughlin AF, Morris JG, et al: Technetium brain scanning in the diagnosis and management of cerebral abscess. Am J Med 65:192, 1974.
13. Falconer MA, McFarlan AM, Russell DS: Experimental brain abscess in the rabbit. Br J Surg 30:245, 1943.
14. Waggener JD: The pathophysiology of bacterial meningitis and cerebral abscesses. Adv Neurol 6:1, 1974.
15. Samson DS, Clark K: Current review of brain abscess. Am J Med 54:201, 1973.
16. Garfield J: Management of supratentorial abscess. Br Med J 2:7, 1969.
17. Jordan CE, James AE, Hodgess FJ: Comparison of angiogram and radionuclide image in brain abscess. Radiology 104:327, 1972.
18. Davis DD, Taveras JM: Radiological aspects of inflammatory conditions affecting the CNS. Clin Neurosurg 14:192, 1966.
19. Altemus LR, Taveras JM: Current concepts in the neuroradiologic diagnosis of intracranial infection. Adv Neurol 6:229, 1974.
20. Heinz ER, Cooper RD: Several early angiographic findings in brain abscess including the "ripple sign." Radiology 90:735, 1968.
21. Nielsen H, Gyldensted C: CT in the diagnosis of cerebral abscess. Neuroradiology 12:207, 1977.
22. Zimmerman RA, Patel S, Bilaniuk LT: Demonstration of purulent bacterial intracranial infections by computed tomography. Am J Roentgenol 127:155, 1976.
23. New PFJ, Davis KR, Ballantine HT: CT in cerebral abscess. Radiology 121:641, 1976.
24. Zimmerman RA, Bilaniuk LT, Shipkin PM: Evolution of cerebral abscess: correlation of clinical features with CT. Neurology 27:14, 1977.
25. Shaw MDM, Russell JA: Value of CT in diagnosis of intracranial abscess. J Neurol Neurosurg Psychiatry 40:214, 1977.
26. Adams JH, Jennett WB: Acute necrotizing encephalitis: a problem in diagnosis. J Neurol Neurosurg Psychiatry 30:248, 1967.
27. Bligh AS, Weaver CM, Wells CEC: Isotope encephalography in the management of acute herpesvirus encephalitis. J Neurol Neurosurg Psychiatry 35:569, 1972.
28. Radcliffe WB, Guinto FL, Adcock DF: Herpes simplex encephalitis: radiologic-pathologic study. Am J Roentgenol 112:263, 1971.
29. Rabe EF, Flynn RE, Dodge PR: Subdural collections of fluids in infants and children. Neurology 18:559, 1968.
30. Lott T, Gammal ELT, Dasilva R, et al: Evaluation of brain and epidural abscesses by CT. Radiology 122:371, 1977.
31. Galbraith JG, Barr VW: Epidural abscess and subdural empyema. Adv Neurol 6:257, 1974.
32. Hitchcock E, Andreadis A: Subdural empyema. J Neurol Neurosurg Psychiatry 27:422, 1964.
33. Kaufman DM, Miller MH, Steigbigel NH: Subdural empyema: Analysis of 17 recent cases and review of the literature. Medicine 54:485, 1975.
34. Leibrook L, Epstein MH, Rybock JD: Cerebral tuberculoma localized by EMI scan. Surg Neurol 5:305, 1976.

Chapter 13 Head Trauma

As CT becomes more readily available, it is assuming an increasingly important role in demonstrating the type and severity of head trauma by identifying underlying brain pathology in a direct manner that has not previously been possible. At present it appears of greatest value in closed head injury and is of less value in penetrating head injuries because of the associated artifacts from high-density objects, including shrapnel, bullets and bone fragments. Because of limitations in resolving capability it is less sensitive than plain skull radiograph in detecting the presence of skull fracture. In addition, because many patients who suffer head trauma cannot remain completely motionless for the several minutes required to complete the scan sequence, there may be significant degradation of scan quality, although this is becoming much less of a problem with newer models with markedly reduced scanning time.

This problem may be avoided if sedation is employed but there are several contraindications to this, including loss of the level of mentation as the earliest and most reliable clinical sign of deterioration and the sedative effect, which depresses the respiratory drive, with carbon dioxide retention causing vasodilatation, increased intracranial pressure and herniation syndrome. An alternative approach is to perform CT with sedation, and if the scan is normal and there is no need for angiography, to use pupillary and motor signs as evidence of subsequent neurological deterioration. In the acute stage of head trauma, the indications for subsequent angiography are becoming very limited if CT is normal.[1]

Based upon the severity and type of clinical neurological abnormality, the differentiation of cerebral concussion and contusion has been arbitrarily established. Immediately following a blow to the head the patient may become unconscious or dazed and suffer a primary generalized convulsion. Unless focal neurological findings (hemiparesis, pupillary abnormalities) are present, it may not be possible to determine if these changes in brain function are due to the circulatory or metabolic effect of the trauma or to the presence of a localized pathological lesion. In those patients who show complete recovery within 24 hours without subsequent worsening and have no further attacks after the initial impact seizure with residua of only mild retrograde or anterograde amnesia, it is believed that no gross pathological changes have occurred and the diagnosis of concussion is made. Because of the good clinical recovery of such patients, clinicopathological studies are few, but necropsy studies of patients with a diagnosis of "concussion" who died of other causes demonstrate definite pathological changes, both supratentorially and in the brain stem.[2]

Confirmatory diagnostic studies include normal CSF examination (free of blood cells) and normal EEG pattern, but if the patient has no neurological sequelae, this diagnosis may be made even if some red cells are present in CSF or EEG is diffusely slow. The diagnosis is therefore made by exclusion of other pathological conditions and cannot be made in the immediate post-traumatic period. With CT it is now possible to exclude many other pathological disorders and to assess the prognosis for recovery. Of 30 patients with a diagnosis of "concussion" on the basis of rapidly clearing clinical status who were studied in the 24 hours post-injury, CT was abnormal in seven and was normal in the remaining 23, who then had complete recovery. In those with abnormal study clinical worsening occurred within hours after the scan and surgery was frequently necessary.

If the scan is performed immediately after trauma, it may appear normal despite the presence of pathological evidence of focal or diffuse cerebral edema. In several cases the patient has been unconscious and has had a negative scan, which showed the ventricles clearly visualized, midline in position and of normal size. The patient subsequently deteriorated and died, and necropsy showed evidence of cerebral edema and herniation, which had not been detected by CT. Furthermore, more severely impaired patients who were believed to have contusion of the brain stem, in which CT scan would be normal, were found to have other potentially surgically remediable lesions in 45 percent of cases.[1] Of 300 patients with a diagnosis of "concussion" who were studied up to six months after the episode of head trauma either because of headache or dizziness indicative of "postconcussive symptoms," in only three cases did CT demonstrate an abnormality including a cyst or chronic subdural hematoma. In these cases the presence of normal CT is reassuring and usually obviates the need for further studies, although in very rare instances a structural lesion may be missed.

Following the episode of trauma, patients may not recover immediately or completely; this is indicative of gross pathological change, which usually consists of contusion or hematoma. The clinical course of these disorders may take one of the following patterns: (1) an initial short period of unconsciousness followed by a lucid interval before a secondary period of unconsciousness supervenes, usually associated with pupillary and motor signs; the presence of this lucid interval has been characteristically described in epidural hematoma; (2) no initial period of unconsciousness but a progressively deteriorating mental state evident several hours or days later, a pattern more characteristic of subacute subdural or delayed intracerebral hematoma; (3) initial and then progressive unconsciousness and focal deficit, which is typically seen in intracerebral hematoma or contusions; (4) alternating periods of mental confusion and normal consciousness, most often seen in subacute or chronic subdural hematoma. Although these clinical patterns are quite characteristic in the majority of cases, there are exceptions in 30 to 40 percent of cases; in 25 percent of cases of intracerebral hematoma, consciousness is preserved throughout the entire course of the disorder, and in one third of cases of epidural hematoma, there is no lucid interval.[3]

Since the clinical course of the level of consciousness is such a crucial factor in prognosis and diagnosis of severity of head injury, it is unfortunate that it may be clouded by multiple factors. The patient may have had a seizure and the post-ictal confusional state may continue. The patient may have been drinking or using drugs prior to the trauma. Details of the accident may not be available, and there may be no external stigmata of trauma. In these cases clinical diagnosis may not be possible.

Prior to the CT scan it was not possible on a clinical basis to distinguish the effects of edema, contusion and hemorrhage without contrast studies or trephination. In these cases CSF, skull radiogram and EEG findings may be nondiagnostic, and lumbar puncture is usually contraindicated because of the possibility of intracranial shifts and increased intracranial pressure. In patients with head trauma and multiple other injuries utilization of hypertonic contrast material in angiography may be toxic to the kidney and may precipitate shock and worsen CNS function as blood vessel and brain-blood barrier permeability are impaired. In severe emergencies trephination may be necessary, but burr hole placement close to the lesion may occasionally fail to detect a lesion and angiography is required for definitive diagnosis of extracerebral hematoma.

CT is superior to other diagnostic studies in that it is noninvasive and permits serial studies as clinical findings change and cerebral edema or delayed intracerebral hematoma develop. Its limitations involve the requirement of complete head immobilization for several minutes and an extended position of the neck, which may be dangerous if there is accompanying cervical spinal cord injury. Sedation is usually contraindicated and, if utilized, should be accomplished with Amytal or general anaesthesia to guarantee high quality of the scan, as the physician is sacrificing an important parameter of clinical change.

PATHOLOGICAL CONDITIONS

EDEMA

There may be cerebral edema in experimentally induced concussion but it is usually not of a degree sufficient to cause distortion and displacement of brain structures.[2] In cases of more severe trauma in which contusion, laceration and hemorrhage occur, accompanying focal or generalized edema are present. In other experimentally induced traumatic lesions, fluid extravasates from injured blood vessels in focally injured tissue and penetrates into the white matter, and there may be no other evidence of contusive or hemorrhagic injury. If the edema is well localized then focal neurological signs may be present, or if generalized it may cause a depressed level of consciousness associated with bilateral EEG disturbances. This is a serious complication

of head trauma, as it may cause mechanical compression with displacement and distortion of intracranial structures and herniation as the most lethal complications.

With angiography the diagnosis of cerebral edema cannot usually be established except in its more severe form, but the effect of edema may be visualized by CT when angiography is negative. These findings may include a focal low-density area, which may be irregular or wedge-shaped in

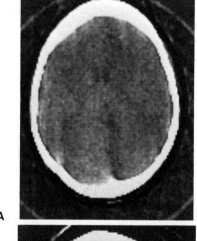

A

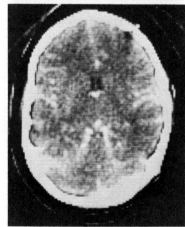

B

Figure 13–1. A 50-year-old man was involved in an automobile accident and became poorly responsive without other neurological findings. CT findings: poor visualization of ventricles with vague low density regions in both hemispheres, a pattern consistent with diffuse cerebral edema (A). The patient clinically improved following treatment with dexamethasone. Compare with similar pattern of diffuse low-density area with compression of ventricles and patchy enhancement pattern in biopsy-proved post-traumatic edema (B).

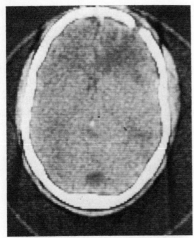

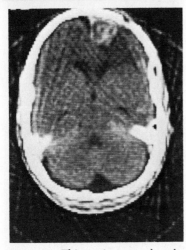

appearance, or a homogeneous or speckled low-density area that causes slight distortion and compression of the contiguous ventricular structure but no midline shift of nonadjacent midline structures and usually no enhancement with contrast. More marked edema shows displacement and shift of midline structures by a low-density area that is more widespread or bilateral.[4] In most severe bilateral cerebral edema, the entire ventricular system is collapsed by swelling in adjacent white matter, but the actual edema fluid has the density of normal brain and may not be detected by CT (Fig. 13-1). In several cases of diffuse cerebral edema without other pathological lesions demonstrated by necropsy, CT was normal but the suprasellar cistern was not detected; this may be an early clue to the presence of cerebral edema. If the ventricles are poorly visualized serial scans following treatment may then show better visualization, providing indirect evidence of cerebral edema (Fig. 13-2).

CONTUSION

This is related to rotational injuries and occurs following a sudden blow to the head, most frequently in regions at which the skull moulds to underlying convolutions; the brain is bruised by its being crushed against the bony structures at the base of the skull. In addition, this injury may occur at a site distant from the blow, including the anterior temporal tip, the inferior surface of the frontal lobe or the inferior and lateral temporal surface as a result of a negative pressure vector (contra-coup injury), or it may occur directly contralateral to the point of impact.

The predominant pathological changes occur in the superficial cortical surfaces; they consist of multiple petechial hemorrhages, tissue necrosis and surrounding edema. These hemorrhagic foci result from extravasation of blood from the cortical ves-

A

B

Figure 13-2. This patient was knocked unconscious in an automobile accident and then regained consciousness. Several hours later he became increasingly lethargic without focal neurological signs. Skull radiogram showed a right frontal depressed skull fracture and this was elevated surgically. Following surgery the patient regained consciousness but then became increasingly lethargic over 48 hours. Initial CT scan showed a low-density area in the right frontal region, distorting and displacing the right ventricular system and causing generalized ventricular cular system and causing generalized ventricular compression consistent with focal edema (A). The patient was treated with dexamethasone but his clinical condition did not improve. A repeat scan showed a low-density lesion and a diffuse pattern of enhancement but less ventricular compression (B). Angiography showed a right frontal diffuse mass effect. Operative findings included a focal edematous and contused area in the right frontal region, which was debrided. Following clinical recovery, CT showed no ventricular mass effect and only a low-density area in the region of previous surgery.

sels and may be confluent, forming a large cortical intracerebral hematoma. Since the injury is most frequently the result of a localized blow to the head, there may be a focal neurological deficit without associated loss of consciousness, which develops immediately after the injury. This sudden development of focal neurolgical deficit following a blow to the head may be confused with traumatic thrombosis of the internal carotid or middle cerebral artery. Seizures of either a generalized or focal nature may also be caused by contusion resulting from localized cortical injury or the irritant effect of subarachnoid blood.

The clinical diagnosis of cerebral contusion should be suspected in a patient who develops sudden onset of focal neurological signs immediately following a localized blow to the head without alteration of consciousness. The findings of plain skull radiogram, EEG and isotope scan are nondiagnostic. Angiography may show an avascular mass with stretching and loss of undulation of cortical vessels, usually accompanied by slowing of local blood flow with arteriovenous shunting due to ischemia and vasoparalysis.

This mass effect and associated circulatory abnormalities may rapidly clear. Occasionally in patients with this clinical picture there are no angiographic abnormalities indicative of edema or intracerebral or extracerebral lesions; the diagnosis of cerebral contusion may be inferred by the disparity of significant clinical findings and the normal angiogram.[5] Based on CT findings, the pathological changes of cerebral contusion may be identified. Contusions are visualized as either diffuse or focal low-density areas (4 to 12) located superficially with wedge-shaped deep extension; they may have irregular borders and may be associated with a significant mass effect. The density pattern is nonhomogeneous with a speckled pattern due to punctate hemorrhagic foci. The lesion usually has irregular

borders due to edema and crosses vascular boundaries; this differentiates it from traumatic vascular occlusive findings (Fig. 13–3).

Following contrast infusion enhancement may be seen, related either to the extravascular component of the impaired blood-brain barrier or to the intravascular phase, with circulatory abnormalities visualized by angiography. Maximal diffuse enhancement may be seen in the first week, then diminishing in intensity; it is probably related to extravascular diffusion. From these CT findings contusion may be distinguished from cerebral hematoma but not from traumatic vascular occlusion or laceration, which still requires angiography. Of 10 cases in which contusion was diagnosed clinically, CT confirmed this diagnosis in all; angio-

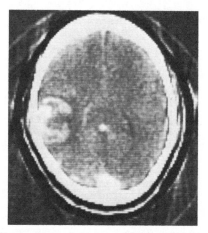

Figure 13–3. A 21-year-old male was hit over the left frontal region and developed an aphasic disturbance several hours after the injury. Neurological findings included a marked receptive aphasic disturbance with no motor, sensory or visual disturbances. EEG showed a focal slow wave focus over the entire left hemisphere but especially in the temporal region; isotope brain scan and angiography were negative. CT showed an irregular nonhomogeneous area of low density with a bandlike enhancement pattern. In addition, there was a small area of high density that did not change after the infusion of contrast and was compatible with hemorrhage. The clinical findings and the negative angiogram were suggestive of cerebral contusion, and the CT pattern was indicative of a cerebral contusion with a slight hemorrhagic component.

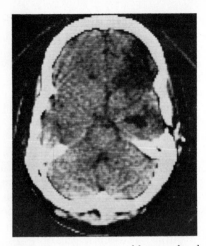

Figure 13–4. A 30-year-old man developed left hemiparesis immediately following a blow to the right side of his head. This condition cleared but he then developed left focal motor seizures four months later. EEG showed mild slow pattern over right hemisphere; isotope scan was negative. CT showed a sharply marginated area in the right frontal parietal area without mass effect or enhancement, a pattern consistent with infarction of the middle cerebral artery that was presumed to be the result of trauma.

graphy was negative in four and isotope scan was negative in eight cases. Traumatic vascular occlusion may show a similar pattern but characteristically reveals a homogeneous low-density wedge-shaped pattern with sharply defined edges (Fig. 13–4).

INTRINSIC BRAIN HEMORRHAGE

Traumatic intracerebral hematoma results from shearing movements with tearing of blood vessels and extravasation of blood into the substance of the brain. The majority of these are found in the frontal and temporal region and less frequently in the parieto-temporal region and cerebellum. If the hemorrhage occurs in the brain stem, pituitary gland or corpus callosum, it is usually fatal. These lesions are superficial in location and frequently may be multiple. Clinically there is usually an immediate onset of symptoms, but in 47 percent there may be a lucid interval with development of symptoms sev-

eral hours later. Impaired consciousness, headache, focal neurological deficit and signs of intracranial hypertension are often present, but clinical diagnosis is not always possible. The hematoma may be causing significant cerebral edema and mass effect, requiring surgical intervention. Based on the clinical symptoms, contusion cannot be differentiated from hemorrhage, and in certain cases CT can define the presence of both lesions, though this is not possible with other studies; with bilateral lesions angiography may not show a midline shift (Fig. 13–5).

The diagnosis of intracerebral hematoma may be suspected by CSF findings, but lumbar puncture is usually contraindicated in head trauma. The most reliable study is angiography, and findings include an avascular mass with evidence of cortical arteries draping around the lesion; the vessels are pushed together, with evidence of extravasation of contrast material from the involved vessel. In

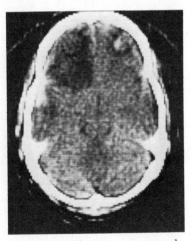

Figure 13–5. Following a motorcycle accident, this patient became dysphasic, with fluctuations in level of consciousness. EEG was diffusely slow, and CSF pressure was markedly elevated, without red cells or xanthochromia. CT findings: a speckled, nonhomogeneous, low-density, wedge-shaped region in the left frontal region, consistent with contusion, and a high-density round lesion surrounded by edema fluid, consistent with an intracerebral hematoma in the right frontal region.

addition, there may be focal circulatory abnormalities and angiographic evidence of herniation, but this is not always specific enough to be differentiated from contusion, and occasionally angiography may be negative.[6, 7]

Since the prognosis and clinical course are better in contusion than in hematoma, with more rapid clearing in the former, this distinction has therapeutic importance. In a patient with a worsening clinical condition in whom it is not possible angiographically to distinguish contusion from hemorrhage, the indication for surgical intervention has relied on identification of the size and location of the lesion and evidence of a possible impending herniation syndrome rather than upon pathological diagnosis.[3]

With CT, the density characteristics of intracerebral hematoma differ from those of contusion, and its location

and shape permit differentiation from extracerebral lesions. These traumatic intracerebral hematomas have attenuation values of 25 to 40 and are surrounded by low-density edema, which may be diffuse or may form a localized circumferential halo. They are usually round in appearance and cause significant mass effect. The lobar location and occasional multiplicity of lesions differentiate them from more usual hypertensive hemorrhages (Fig. 13–6). The shape and location of the hematomas in the temporal region are highly reliable in differentiating them from subtemporal subdural hematomas (Fig. 13–7).[8] The hematoma may be superficial or deeply located; in the latter case there may be intraventricular extension. Extension into the ventricle is established only by CT or necropsy. Although the prognosis is poor, CT studies have shown that its presence may be compatible with survival (Fig. 13–8).

Superficial cortical hematomas represent the confluence of smaller he-

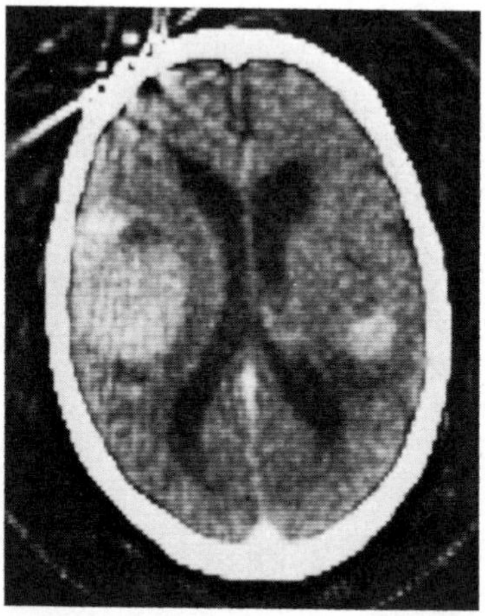

Figure 13–6. An elderly male was struck on the right side of his head and then developed slurred dysarthric speech. EEG showed a bilateral slow wave pattern, more pronounced over the left hemisphere; isotope brain scan and CSF examination were entirely normal. CT showed an area of high density on the surface of the left frontoparietal region. It did not enhance with contrast infusion and was consistent with a diagnosis of traumatic intracerebral hematoma. In addition, there was a second area of high density in the right parietal region, which was also thought to represent a hematoma. Since the patient's clinical condition improved, neither angiography nor surgery was necessary.

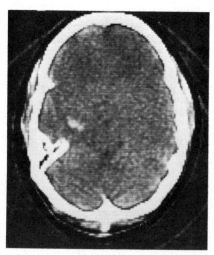

Figure 13–7. This patient struck his head against a steering wheel in an automobile accident. Two weeks later he developed headache and had alternating lethargy–agitated state. CT findings: a small high-density area in the left temporal region that had the configuration of an intracerebral clot. The patient clinically improved and repeat study was normal.

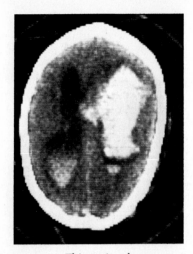

Figure 13–8. This patient became unresponsive after head trauma. Neurological findings included coma, bilateral spasticity and plantar extensor response. CSF was grossly bloody and angiography showed a questionable avascular mass in the right parietal region and ventricular enlargement. CT findings: ventricular enlargement with a high-density lesion, consistent with intraventricular hemorrhage.

matomas and perhaps a more severe stage of cerebral contusion, and this may explain the irregular shape and nonhomogeneous appearance. Contrast infusion may show enhancement of the periphery of the hematoma or a ring pattern. In severe injuries subarachnoid blood may be seen in basal cisterns and over the convexities. Intracerebellar hematoma may be visualized, but brain stem and pituitary hemorrhages are usually too small to be visualized by scan.[1, 4, 9]

In patients with head trauma who develop focal neurological deficit and altered consciousness, the underlying pathological process may be only indirectly related to head injury. Two patients initially suspected of having extra- or intracerebral hematoma were found to have tumor. In one instance there was, hemorrhage into the tumor but in the other no bleeding was found at surgery. In both cases CT showed evidence of an intracerebral lesion that showed more striking enhancement than would have been expected from traumatic hematoma.

Rarely, patients with head injury show definite clinical improvement, with subsequent neurological deterioration up to two weeks later. This is most frequently explained as follows: initial clinical signs are caused by concussional injury, which then clears, but there is a slow increase in intracranial pressure owing to epidural or subdural hematoma. Rarely, this may be caused by late-forming intracerebral hematoma, which occurs because local hypoxia and hypercapnia increase cerebral blood flow and blood pressure. With loss of autoregulation there is hemorrhage into the edematous and necrotic cortex.[6] In one series of delayed intracerebral hematomas angiography was negative in 50 percent of cases, but this lesion is reliably detected by CT, and the evolution of the hematoma may be followed with serial scans.

EXTRADURAL HEMATOMA

This usually results from laceration of the middle meningeal artery but less frequently from tearing of the meningeal emissary veins or venous sinus. The hemorrhage occurs in the temporal region but may also occur in the frontal, parietal or posterior fossa region. A skull fracture that crosses the groove of the middle meningeal artery is almost always seen, as it is the bone fragments that act to shear and tear the vessel. The hematoma consists of a firm clot located external to the dura. Blood extravasates from the meningeal vessels with a force great enough to dissect and strip the dura from the skull, forming an ovoid mass in the epidural space. The lesion is well localized and forms a bulging mass, since the dura at the edge of the hematoma remains adherent to the skull. Because of the acute expansion of this sharply localized mass, there is compression of the adjacent brain, with surrounding edema and atrophy, and there is less likelihood of the formation of surrounding neomembrane, as occurs with subdural hematoma.

Clinically these patients present as acute neurosurgical emergencies, with rapid development of drowsiness, coma, hemiparesis and dilated pupil. A lucid relatively asymptomatic interval may occur, which varies in time from several hours to days but is more prolonged in cases of venous bleeding.[10, 11] The diagnosis may be made by trephination, but with cerebral dehydrating agents there is usually time to perform angiography, which shows an avascular biconvex mass located between the vascularized parenchyma and inner table of the skull, usually directly beneath the fracture line, displacement of the middle meningeal arteries and dural sinus from the skull, extravasation of contrast material from the middle meningeal vessel, and stretching and attenuation of the underlying arteries. Angiographically the biconvex extracerebral space is the most direct sign, but demonstration of this shape may require oblique projections. There is usually a shift of midline structures, as these lesions are often unilateral,

but absence of the shift may be caused by upward rather than medial displacement. The presence of an accompanying intracerebral lesion may diminish the vascular displacement caused by epidural hematoma, and this accompanying lesion may not be detected by angiography.[12, 13]

Utilizing CT, it is possible to visualize the lesion directly because of its characteristic density, pattern and shape and to define more clearly any accompanying intracerebral lesions and mass effect. In uncomplicated epidural hematoma, there is a well-localized, homogeneous, high-density biconvex lesion, which usually shows ventricular distortion and displacement and a thin band of low-density edema or atrophic compressed brain on its medial surface (Fig. 13–9). In addition, the edematous regions may be more widespread, especially in the bifrontal region (Fig. 13–10). If

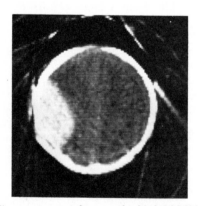

Figure 13–9. A five-month-old child fell from her bed and then was noted to be increasingly irritable, with alternating periods of lethargy. Neurological findings: head and eyes deviated to the left side and she did not move her right side. CT showed a well-localized lesion of uniform high density in the left parietal-occipital region. There were also low-density areas in both frontal regions, a pattern consistent with edema. The diagnosis of an acute epidural hematoma was confirmed at operation.

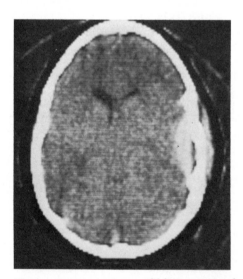

Figure 13–10. A 12-year-old boy was struck in the right temporal region with a baseball bat and then became progressively obtunded. Examination revealed left hemiparesis and a dilated and nonreactive right pupil. CT findings: a high-density lenticular extracerebral lesion in the right subtemporal region, causing mild ventricular distortion and displacement; there were also low-density areas suggesting bifrontal edema. This was consistent with a diagnosis of either a subcortical, subdural or epidural hematoma; an epidural hematoma was found at operation.

the epidural hematoma is bilateral, there may be no shift of midline structures (Fig. 13–11). Venous epidural hematoma less commonly show the characteristic biconvex shape and may be mistaken for a subdural lesion.[14] A well localized lesion in the parietal region is more likely an epidural hematoma but the distinction is not absolute. In suspected posterior fossa epidural lesions, CT is an excellent screening procedure but, even if negative, angiography may be needed. These lesions are always of high density. Since they are contiguous with bone, it is possible to overlook epidural hematoma, which is relatively thin and does not bulge. Svendsen reported CT failure to detect a 4 mm lesion.[15]

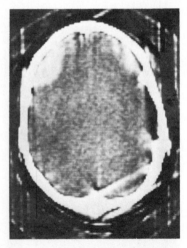

Figure 13–11. A teen-age boy was struck with a blunt object in the right occipital region. Initially he had a brief period of unconsciousness, which was then followed by a lucid interval of 48 hours at which time he wished to be discharged from the hospital. He then began to show signs of progressive lethargy and obtundation but did not have any focal neurological signs. Skull radiogram showed no fracture. EEG was diffusely slow and ECHO was midline. CT showed bilateral high-density lens-shaped lesions in the frontal regions, which were well localized and not associated with any shift of the ventricular system or low-density edema. The initial diagnosis was bilateral acute subdural hematomas. Subsequent angiography and operative findings demonstrated the presence of bilateral venous epidural hematomas.

SUBDURAL HEMATOMA (SDH)

These masses may be unilateral or bilateral; bleeding results from tears in the veins that are located on the brain surface and reach the dural sinuses. These hematomas are clinically and pathologically defined as acute, subacute and chronic. Acute SDH usually results from trauma but occasionally may result from a ruptured intracranial aneurysm or angioma. Clinically patients usually present with altered mentation and subsequent deterioration, and this pattern suggests accompanying parenchymal brain damage, whereas one third have a lucid interval that is then followed by deterioration over several hours. The collection is initially primarily solid and begins to hemolyze over several days. The blood dissects the arachnoid away from the dura and, since there are few thick fibrous adhesions, this produces widespread fluid accumulation, usually located in the fronto-parietal region. This is to be contrasted with the well-limited collection seen in epidural hematoma. Subdural collections that are removed four to 20 days after injury contain some residual solid clot, which is mixed with hemolyzed blood and CSF. Careful analysis of subdural hematomas surgically removed during this period and pathologically examined showed that the hematoma was liquid only in 57 percent, solid in 15 percent, and mixed solid and liquid in 28 percent; in two there was an associated epidural or intracerebral hematoma.[3]

Some episodes of bleeding into the subdural space were caused by trauma not large enough or under great enough pressure to produce symptoms initially; this hematoma may lyse, resulting in a fluid collection. The dural membrane adjacent to the fluid collection then thickens and undergoes fibroblastic proliferation. Capillaries grow into the membrane, which thus becomes vascularized, and this neovascularity is fragile and subject to repeated hemorrhage, which increases the size of the hematoma. It is believed that it requires about three weeks for this membrane formation to occur, although this capsule was found at operation in one third of cases of shorter duration and was not present in 10 percent of cases with a clinical history exceeding four weeks.[16] Diagnosis is established by angiography, in which an avascular extracerebral space, usually widespread and encompassing the fronto-tempo-parietal region, is visualized.

Acute SDH causes a crescentic displacement of the superficial cerebral vessels away from the inner table of the skull. As neomembrane formation occurs, the surface of the lesion becomes less regular in contour, and as the membrane is well established, the hematoma acquires a characteristic biconvex shape.[17] There is midline shift except when the lesion is bilateral (20 percent). In some elderly patients angiography shows a thin crescent-shaped space over the convexity, suggestive of the pattern of SDH, but there is evidence of ipsilateral ventricular dilatation rather than compression, an appearance more compatible with an atrophic than an expanding process. In this case, air study may be required to differentiate focal atrophy from SDH.[18]

In the majority of cases of SDH, the diagnosis may be established by CT and, based upon density values and membrane formation, may also be classified as to pathological characteristics.[4, 5, 15, 19] Acute subdural hematomas have attentuation values higher than normal brain tissue, are located adjacent to the inner table, are widespread in distribution and are crescentic in shape. The presence of a lesion entirely of high density always correlated with a clinical history of less than three days' duration (Fig. 13–12). They are usually located over the convexity region, in the floor of anterior middle or posterior fossa, or against the falx in the interhemis-

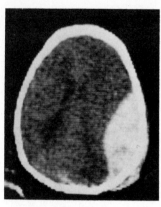

Figure 13–12. This patient fell and struck his right parietal region and became lethargic over 48 hours. CT findings: a large consolidated homogeneous lesion bulging medially to compress the right ventricular system, consistent with acute subdural hematoma.

pheric fissure. Those located over the convexity have a convex-concave lens shape (half-moon). Those located in the middle fossa in the subtemporal region are frequently quite thin in shape and may be difficult to distinguish from adjacent bone. The depth

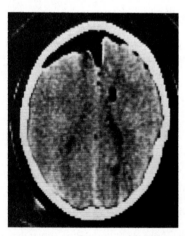

Figure 13–13. A five-year-old fell out of a swing and subsequently developed severe bifrontal headache with nausea; mentation was normal and there were no neurological signs. Skull radiogram showed basilar skull fracture. CT findings: air is present in the epidural and subdural space over the bifrontal convexity region and also within the ventricular and cisternal spaces. The ventricular system appears compressed symmetrically but there is no evidence of an extracerebral hematoma.

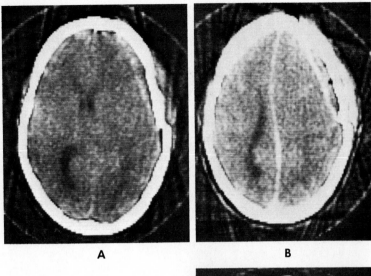

A   B

Figure 13–14. A 24-year-old man suffered a right frontal depressed skull fracture in an automobile accident. Initially, the patient was lethargic but an angiogram showed no evidence of an extracerebral or intracerebral lesion; operation was performed with debridement of the necrotic tissue in the frontal region and elevation of the fracture. Postoperatively, his level of consciousness improved until 17 days later, when he complained of headaches and progressive obtundation without any focal neurological deficit. CT findings: an area of low density beneath the bone flap; this was associated with marked mass effect in the right frontal region, causing bowing of the anterior portion of the falx cerebri with displacement of the anterior portion of the lateral ventricle to the right side (A). Following contrast infusion, there was enhancement of the medial rim of this lesion, a pattern consistent with the presence of neomembrane formation (B); at operation a chronic subdural hematoma with a well-formed membrane was evacuated. One month later repeat CT scan showed ventricular dilatation with prominent temporal horns and a low-density area in the right frontal region (G).

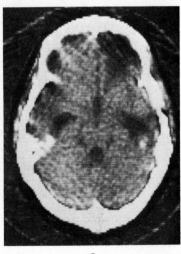

C

of most clinically significant subdural hematomas is 6 to 10 mm and lesions thinner than this may be missed by CT but defined by angiography. In all acute subdural hematomas there is midline shift and frequently underlying low-density edema. In addition, the presence of a concomitant intracerebral hematoma may be reliably detected by CT.

In less acute cases, the lesion shows a mixed-density pattern with high-density material located in the most dependent portion owing to gravitational effect (Fig. 13–19). There is mass effect and no evidence of enhancement along the medial aspect, although there may be extravascular diffusion into the low-density area resulting from an impaired blood-brain

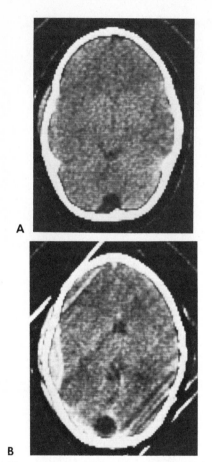

A

B

Figure 13–15.   This patient developed head-ache and mild episodes of confusion one month after trauma. EEG and isotope scan were negative. CT findings: plain scan shows poor visualization of left ventricular system, which appears compressed in comparison with right side, but no hematoma is seen (A). Following infusion, there is enhancement both in the medial capsule and within the subdural hematoma (B).

barrier. These lesions correspond to subacute SDH, but the actual timing of the date of injury is often difficult to correlate based on CT findings.

In chronic SDH the lesion appears of low density, with accompanying ventricular distortion and displacement. The presence of air in the extracerebral space has a shape and density that should be sufficiently characteristic so as not to be confused with chronic SDH (Fig. 13–13). Rarely, in chronic SDH there may be a well-defined linear rim of enhancement along the medial wall of the

hematoma. This enhancement correlates with the pathological finding of well-vascularized membrane (Fig. 13–14).

The role of contrast enhancement in the diagnosis of subdural hematoma is not clearly established other than in defining the presence of a medially located capsule. Infusion may be necessary in all cases. Occasionally plain scan failed to visualize a hematoma, but, following infusion, enhancement occurred in the capsule and within the hematoma. This may be detected only if delayed (3 to 4 hours) scan is performed (Fig. 13–15).

Less commonly it is possible to demonstrate by CT the lack of any extracerebral abnormal density and the presence only of distortion compression and displacement of the ventricle resulting from an isodense SDH (Fig. 13–16). Rarely, bilateral subdural hematomas may be present individually greater than 10 mm in diameter, showing no abnormal den-

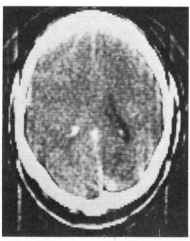

Figure 13–16.   A 36-year-old woman had a two-week history of bitemporal headache not associated with nausea or vomiting and without prior history of head trauma. Findings included early bilateral papilledema and left abducens nerve paresis. Skull radiogram, isotope scan and EEG were negative. CT showed poor visualization of the left lateral ventricle with slight displacement laterally of the contralateral ventricle but no abnormal tissue density or enhancement. Angiogram showed large left hemisphere subdural hematoma. At operation a completely liquefied SDH was found.

sity or shift in midline structures with CT, but clearly demonstrated by angiography.

In patients suspected of having chronic SDH the obliteration of cortical sulcal markings ipsilateral to the lesion, with preservation on the opposite side, is highly suggestive of chronic SDH; conversely, the presence of sulcal and fissure low-density markings with ventricular dilatation usually excludes the presence of a space-occupying lesion. An enlarged extracerebral space caused by cortical atrophy may simulate SDH. In these cases there is no ventricular displacement or distortion and there is interruption of the low-density area by digitation of widened sulci. In some cases the SDH may calcify and this is visualized as a very high-density (50 to 100) peripheral convexity contiguous to bone and surrounding a low-density area (Fig. 13–17).

In some cases an extracerebral lesion is not detected by CT; this was more frequent when an 80 x 80 matrix was utilized or when the scan was degraded by motion artifact. In several series CT infrequently failed to diagnose the SDH; this was more frequent with chronic low or iso-dense lesions. This is consistent with the experimental experience, which demonstrated limited resolution for low-density objects less than 10 mm in thickness. Svendsen reported that of five lesions less than 10 mm in thickness, four were of high density; therefore a thin low-density lesion may be missed by CT, most likely because of the partial volume phenomenon.[15] If there is clinical suspicion, subsequent angiography is necessary. To visualize more adequately thin low-density lesions, oblique positioning of the head may maximize the chance of demonstrating the lesion by lessening the partial volume effect. Utilizing both plain and contrast studies with a high-resolution matrix system and adequate sedation, the detection rate of CT for extracerebral lesions should be in excess of 95 percent.

The pathophysiological mechanism underlying the rapid clinical deterioration that may occur in patients with chronic SDH who have been stable for a period of several months is not known. One possible explanation is that an increase occurs in the size of the collection as fluid shifts; this may result from osmotic differences across the semipermeable arachnoid membrane, in which case CT should show a low-density lesion with well-defined membrane and a shift of midline structures. A second theory relates the increase in size to repeated hemorrhage from the capillaries in the membrane or extravasation of blood from the veins that initially bleed. CT should show a mixed-density pattern with low-density fluid and high-density recent blood (Fig. 13–18).

The conventional management of both acute and chronic SDH is surgical. Following trephination or craniotomy, clinical recovery may be incomplete and further surgery should be contemplated for reaccumulation

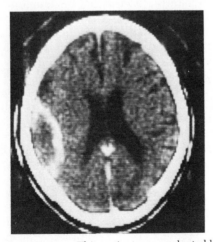

Figure 13–17. This patient was evaluated because of dizziness and isotope scan uptake in the left parietal region. CT findings: a high-density calcified medial capsule with minimal displacement of the lateral ventricle and obliteration of sulci on the ipsilateral side.

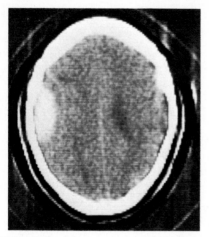

Figure 13–18. A 29-year-old man was struck in the right parietal area. He did not lose consciousness but had right hemiparesis and nonfluent aphasic disturbance. Skull radiogram showed right parietal skull fracture. EEG had delta focus in left parietotemporal region, and isotope scan showed uptake on anterior-posterior but not lateral view. CT showed lenticular mass of high density in left parietotemporal region with medial border of normal density and thin membranous capsule of high density. The mass is compressing the ipsilateral ventricle. This was suggestive of an acute hematoma within a chronic hematoma, with medially located capsule due to neomembrane formation.

or persistence of SDH. Diagnosis of recurrence is difficult because of the persistence of the avascular space, and a shift of the anterior cerebral artery may occur with complete or incomplete clinical recovery.[20] In the absence of reaccumulation of SDH, this is probably due either to cerebral atrophy with failure of the brain to expand or collapse of the arachnoid. Since air study shows normal ventricular size and no filling of the cortical sulcal spaces, this avascular space is most likely caused by collapse of the arachnoid. The most definite angiographic evidence of persistence of SDH postoperatively is failure of the deep midline veins to return to midline position, but this criterion is not of help if SDH is bilateral. In addition, isotope scan may remain positive in patients treated surgically.[21]

CT usually shows a decrease in size of an extracerebral hematoma and a decrease in ventricular dis-placement and compression, but if the lesion is longstanding the underlying brain may fail to expand and a shift of the ventricular system may persist. This CT picture most frequently occurs when clinical recovery is incomplete but may also occur in a scan obtained in asymptomatic postoperative patients. If there is poor clinical response CT should clearly demonstrate a high-density lesion indicative of recent hematoma and may thus obviate the need for angiography. In addition, CT can evaluate the presence of pathological conditions that may be responsible for failure to improve clinically following surgery, including hydrocephalus. In the majority of cases following surgical treatment of SDH, the scan shows no extracerebral abnormal density, and there is no persistent ventricular shift or distortion of the ventricle and no enhancement. If there is a persistent low-density extracerebral space with a displacement of ventricles, this is good evidence for reaccumulation, but the low-density area with *no* ventricular shift or only ipsilateral ventricular dilatation is not evidence of reaccumulation.

Recently, nonsurgical management utilizing corticosteroids and cerebral dehydrating agents has been advocated.[22] If rapid and complete clinical recovery occurs, serial angiography is not necessary, but if recovery is slow or incomplete, this may be necessary to evaluate the size of the avascular space of a midline vascular shift. In patients with slow clinical recovery who had initially showed positive isotope scan and lateralizing EEG, isotope scan took up to 12 months to become negative and EEG was usually normal by eight weeks.[23] In some elderly patients in whom clinical recovery is not complete, the persistence of a positive scan may necessitate prolonged hospitalization and repeat angiography to determine the resolution of the lesions; in certain patients this may be more hazardous than trephination. Serial CT scan is a more reliable and safer technique than EEG, isotope scan or angiography in following patients who are

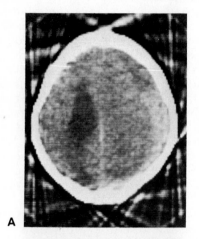

A

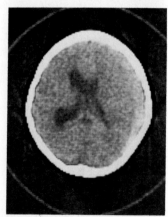

B

Figure 13–19.   An 11-year-old patient with a Fanconi syndrome also had a severe coagulopathy with low platelet count. He became increasingly somnolent and developed right hemiparesis and right pupillary dilatation. EEG showed a diffuse slow wave pattern, and isotope brain scan was negative. CT showed a semilunar area of mixed density in the right hemisphere with high-density material in the most dependent portion of the lesion, consistent with a subacute lesion (A). There is marked distortion and obliteration of the lateral ventricular system. The patient was treated nonsurgically with dexamethasone, and a repeat CT scan one week later showed evidence of distortion of the ventricular system; also, the lesion was less prominent and appeared less dense, as is consistent with liquefaction of the clot and resolution of the underlying edema associated with the hematoma. This improvement in the appearance of the CT scan correlated with the patient's clinical improvement, and surgery was not necessary (B).

not treated surgically. In several instances, management with corticosteroids was associated with a diminution of midline shift and size of mass, a pattern which correlates with clinical improvement (Fig. 13–19).

Subdural hygroma consists of collections of CSF that produce space-occupying masses after head trauma or craniotomy. They result from laceration of the thin arachnoid membrane, which then permits CSF to leak into the dural space. Clinical symptoms and angiographic appearance are identical to those seen with SDH. Isotope cisternography shows an accumulation of isotope in the hygroma, and this permits differentiation from SDH, which does not accumulate isotope. The hygromas are located over the lateral surface of the brain, extend from the frontal to the occipital region and are bilateral in 50 percent of cases. CT shows a semilunar low-density mass (identical to CSF), which causes ventricular compression and displacement if unilateral. In ad-

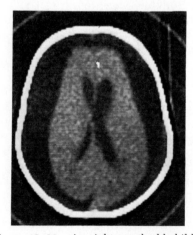

Figure 13–20.   An eight-month-old child underwent craniotomy and postoperatively became lethargic without any focal neurological deficit. EEG showed a diffuse slow wave pattern without any focal abnormalities. CT findings: bilateral homogeneous low-density extracerebral lesions that were compressing the ventricular system and extended from the frontal to the occipital region. These lesions had a density measurement of 4 units, consistent with CSF. The subdural hygromas were then surgically drained.

dition, there is no change with contrast enhancement and no tendency for membrane formation (Fig. 13–20).

DELAYED EFFECT

Localized atrophic regions may result following resolution of intracerebral hematoma, contusion or laceration injury, as the blood and necrotic tissue are replaced by glial proliferation and cavity formation. With CT, a low-density area with widened sulcal and cisternal spaces and ipsilateral ventricular dilatation may be visualized. There may be focal EEG abnormalities localized to the involved hemisphere, and istope scan may be positive, suggesting an expanding mass lesion, but CT may demonstrate its atrophic nature. This is most frequently located in the frontal or temporal region.

In patients who develop a seizure disorder following head injury, there may be localized atrophy or a cyst usually requiring air study for detection. If the patient has clinical evidence of psychomotor seizures and EEG evidence of temporal lobe spike or spike-wave pattern, CT may demonstrate localized dilatation of the temporal horn due to temporal lobe atrophy even when this finding is not documented by air study. In patients with psychomotor seizures, usually accompanied by other focal deficit, or with generalized seizures, CT may show a more widespread loss of brain substance. In one third of cases of head trauma examined by air study, there was evidence of ventricular dilatation, which was due to basilar arachnoiditis with impairment of CSF flow and loss of brain substance. CT may be used serially to follow those patients to demonstrate the extent of ventricular enlargement and to decide if isotope cisternography is indicated.

Following trauma, large cavities may develop within the substance of the brain parenchyma, and communication with ventricular and subarachnoid spaces may exist. Because of CSF pulsation, the mass may enlarge in size, causing development of delayed and progressive neurological symptoms, whereas in other cases the cyst may not increase in size. Angiography may demonstrate an avascular mass without abnormal vascularity but it may not be reliably differentiated from other intracerebral lesions. CT will show a sharply demarcated low-density area that does not enhance. This lesion may be quite large but does not cause significant ventricular compression or displacement and may be associated with ventricular dilatation. This cystic lesion may appear to communicate with the ventricular system, but dynamic communication is best defined by air study or isotope cisternography. Leptomeningeal cysts form when portions of the arachnoid membrane become entrapped within the fracture line. This occurs with dural laceration, allowing loculations of fluid to

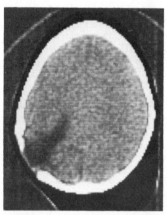

Figure 13–21. A 15-month-old child was injured in an automobile accident and had a left parietal skull fracture. The patient developed increasing head size and the fracture line increased in size. At operation an arachnoid cyst was found with a communication with the left occipital horn. The patient developed a pulsatile mass in the left occipital region. CT showed a defect in the parietal bone with erosion of the bone by an underlying cystic lesion, which was consistent with a leptomeningeal cyst and left porencephaly.

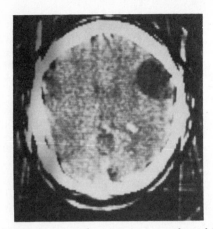

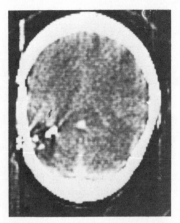

Figure 13–22. This patient was evaluated for persistent postconcussion syndrome; all other neurodiagnostic studies were negative. CT findings: well-circumscribed, round, low-density area in right midfrontal region, extending laterally over convexity. Operative finding: cholesteatoma.

Figure 13–23. High-density metallic fragments are seen in the left hemisphere with associated low-density necrotic tissue four years after this patient was shot in the head.

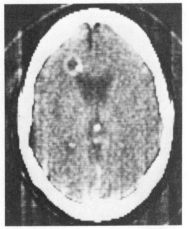

form within subarachnoid spaces. With the pulsation of CSF, there is localized erosion of bone and enlargement of the fracture line, as the dura is not intact over the defect and the arachnoid continues to bulge outward. CT demonstrates the defect in the continuity of the bone with localized erosion and a low-density cyst located underneath the fracture line (Figs. 13–21 and 13–22).

OPEN HEAD INJURY

Shrapnel, bullets and other foreign bodies may be identified and localized by CT. Because of their high-density metallic content, they may produce a sunburst pattern artifact, which makes scan interpretation difficult in delineating other associated lesions (Fig. 13–23). Every foreign body located intracranially is a potential source of intracranial suppuration,

Figure 13–24. This patient had suffered a gunshot wound to the head several years previously, and recently developed headache and nuchal rigidity. CSF examination showed sterile pleocytosis. CT findings: the retained round bullet fragment is contiguous with an enhancing high-density peripheral capsule and low-density core in the left frontal region, consistent with brain abscess.

and both the foreign body and the resultant abscess may be detected by CT (Fig. 13–24).

REFERENCES

1. French BN, Dublin AB: The value of CT in the management of 1000 consecutive head injuries. Surg Neurol 7:171, 1977.

2. Blackwood W, McMenemcy WH, Meyer A, et al: Greenfield's Neuropathology, Williams and Wilkins, Baltimore, 1963. pp 440–456.
3. Brock S: Injuries to the Brain and Spinal Cord. Springer, New York, 1974. pp 136–174.
4. Merino de Villasante J, Taveras JM: CT in acute head trauma. Am J Roentgenol 126:765, 1976.
5. Leeds NE, Reid ND, Rosen LM: Angiographic changes in cerebral contusion and intracerebral hematoma. Acta Radiol (Diagn) 5:320, 1966.
6. Baratham G, Dennyson WG: Delayed traumatic intracerebral hemorrhage. J Neurol Neurosurg Psychiatry 35:698, 1972.
7. Newton TH, Potts DG: Radiology of the Skull and Brain. Vol II, book 4, CV Mosby, St. Louis, 1974. pp 2598–2658.
8. Glickman MG, McNamara TD: Subtemporal subdural hematoma. Radiology 109:607, 1973.
9. Davis KR, Taveras JM: CT in head trauma. Semin Roentgenol 12:53, 1977.
10. McLaurin RL, Ford LE: Extradural hematoma. J Neurosurg 21:364, 1964.
11. Jamieson KG, Yelland JD: Epidural hematoma. J Neurosurg 29:13, 1968.
12. Cronqvist S, Koheler R: Angiography in epidural hematoma. Acta Radiol (Diagn) 1:42, 1963.
13. Ferris EJ, Krich RLA, Shapiro JH: Epidural hematoma. Am J Roentgenol 101:100, 1967.
14. Fager CA: Subacute epidural hematoma. Surg Clin N Am June 1958. pp 877–883.
15. Svendsen P: CT of traumatic extracerebral lesions. Br. J. Radiol 49:1004, 1976.
16. Gilday DL, Eng B, Wortzman G, Reid M: Subdural hematoma: is it or is it not acute? Radiology 110:141, 1974.
17. Radcliffe WB, Guinto FC: Subdural hematoma shape. Am J Roentgenol 115:72, 1972.
18. Ferris EJ, Lehrer H, Shapiro JH: Pseudo-subdural hematoma. Radiology 88:75, 1967.
19. Levander B, Stattin S, Svendsen P: CT of traumatic intra- and extracerebral lesions. Acta Radiol (Supplem) 346:107, 1975.
20. Fogel LM, Capesius P: Postoperative angiographic control of chronic subdural hematomas in adults. Neuroradiology 10:155, 1975.
21. Gildoy DL, Coates G: Subdural hematoma — what is the role of brain scanning in its diagnosis? J Nucl Med 14:283, 1973.
22. Bender MB, Christoff N: Nonsurgical treatment of subdural hematoma. Arch Neurol 31:73, 1974.
23. Lusins J, Jaffe R, Bender MB: Unoperated subdural hematoma. J Neurosurg 44:601, 1976.

Chapter 14 Gait and Movement Disorders

Disturbances of gait and posture are associated with findings of ataxia, unsteadiness, dysequilibrium and incoordination, which may result from pathophysiological disturbances at multiple levels in the CNS, including the cerebellum, brain stem, basal ganglia and frontal and parietal lobes. In some patients who present with gait disorder it is not always possible on a clinical basis to localize the lesion, and in certain cases multiple mechanisms may be involved, making accurate diagnosis more complex. For example, the mechanism of the gait disorder and truncal ataxia that occur with certain posterior fossa tumors is believed to be related to dysfunction of the midline vermal cerebellar structures. If the vestibulo-cerebellum is involved there may be gait and truncal instability without specific limb ataxia, whereas anterior vermal lesions cause predominantly a gait disturbance that is proportional to the limb ataxia. In those patients who initially present with nonspecific dysequilibrium without more definite localizing neurological signs, a medulloblastoma is suspected.[1]

These tumors usually cause early obstruction of the fourth ventricle with resultant hydrocephalus. The mechanism of the gait disturbance is therefore believed to be related to vestibulo-cerebellar disturbance or hydrocephalus. There may be clinical improvement after shunting alone, although it is not clear why the ventricular dilatation causes gait disturbance. In patients whose initial symptom was the characteristic gait dysequilibrium, CT frequently visualized a midline tumor, which was proved to be a medulloblastoma, but in one half of cases the lateral ventricles were not markedly dilated although the temporal horns were prominent (Fig. 14–1). In one third of these patients there was no evidence of papilledema, and all other neuro-diagnostic studies, including skull radiogram, isotope scan and EEG, were negative before the diagnosis was established by CT.

Patients with tentorial meningiomas and acoustic neurinomas initially presented with this type of gait dysequilibrium without other accompanying neurological signs. In 5 percent of patients who were evaluated by CT for gait disturbance alone, CT demonstrated a tentorial meningioma. Because of the lack of accompanying signs and negative diagnostic studies, it is unlikely that contrast radiographic procedures would have been performed. In three patients, the diagnosis of tentorial meningioma was established by CT six to 14 months after the gait disorder had been severe enough for the patient to have sought medical consultation. The diagnosis of multiple sclerosis and hysteria had been initially considered, although there were no accompanying signs or clinical course characteristic of these disorders.

In other patients the gait disturbance was that of stiffness and awkwardness when ambulating. There was difficulty with maintenance of posture and movement of the lower extremities, but the findings were not characteristically that of the apractic gait usually associated with normal pressure hydrocephalus (NPH), festination with stooped posture related to basal ganglia disturbance, or spastic gait consistent with corticopsinal trait involvement. In these patients mentation was normal and there was

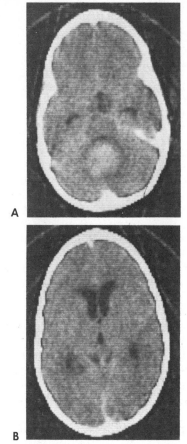

Figure 14–1. A six-year-old boy had a history of several weeks of frequent falls and clumsiness in walking and running. In addition, he had several episodes of nausea and vomiting, which were believed to be caused by "nervous stomach" and responded to sedative medications. The symptoms recurred, and neurological examination showed mild gait ataxia but no other definite cerebellar signs. Skull radiogram and EEG were normal, but CT showed nonvisualization of the fourth ventricle with a midline posterior fossa rim of low density that encompassed an isodense region showing homogeneous enhancement. Immediately anterior to the area of enhancement is a flattened rim of low density which represents the compressed and anteriorly displaced fourth ventricle (A). The lateral ventricles are slightly enlarged and the temporal horns are visualized (B). Operative finding was a medulloblastoma, which compressed the fourth ventricle; it was subtotally removed.

no urinary incontinence. Air study and isotope cisternogram were not performed initially, as other neurodiagnostic studies were negative, and clinically the diagnosis of NPH was considered unlikely. Based upon the CT findings of symmetrical ventricular dilatation including the temporal horns and fourth ventricle, with nonvisualization of the cortical sulci, the diagnosis of NPH was made. A subsequent isotope cisternogram showed reflux of the isotope into the ventricular cavities with persistence at 72 hours and no passage to the parasagittal region.

In most cases, if the CT pattern is consistent with communicating hydrocephalus, contrast infusion CT study is not believed necessary. In one most unusual case there was an enormous fourth ventricle in addition to generalized ventricular dilatation. This was proved surgically to be caused by a fourth ventricular outlet obstruction due to a small ependymoma, which was not visualized even with contrast enhancement or air study (Fig. 14–2).

In patients with characteristic magnetic or apractic gait of NPH, this symptom may overshadow or occur in the absence of dementia and urinary incontinence.[2] This gait disorder is believed to result from transcortical innervatory paresis of the legs due to involvement of the fibers in the anterior portion of the corpus callosum[3] In this disorder the frontal horns are markedly enlarged to a greater extent than the occipital region, but clinical improvement of gait frequently has occurred even if there is no accompanying change in the size of the ventricles. The diagnosis of NPH may be established by CT if there is symmetrical ventricular dilatation and no concomitant increase in size of the cortical sulcal pattern. In addition, there is usually a low-density collar surrounding the anterior frontal horns owing to transependymal resorption of CSF. If the CT pattern is diagnostic of NPH, air study is usually not performed, and the prognostic value of isotope cisternogram has not been established. In all patients in whom CT demonstrated the characteristic pattern, isotope cisternogram was confirmatory. If there were equivocal

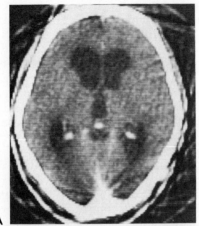

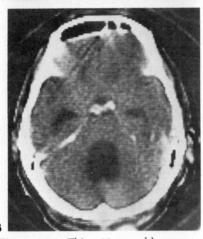

Figure 14–2. This 60-year-old man complained of unsteadiness of gait and dizziness of several months' duration with no history of headache, impaired mentation or incontinence. Neurological findings included slightly broad-based, shuffling and awkward gait but no definite cerebellar abnormalities. All neuroldiagnostic studies were negative. CT showed symmetrical enlargement of the entire ventricular system (A) with an especially large fourth ventricle (B) but no displacement or distortion and no abnormal tissue densities in plain and contrast infusion study. Air study also showed communicating hydrocephalus. At operation, 2 cm ependymoma was found at the outlet foramen of the fourth ventricle that had not been detected by CT or air study. In retrospect, the finding of such an enormous fourth ventricle should raise suspicion of obstruction at the outlet of the fourth ventricle.

CT features, the cisternogram also showed an indeterminant pattern. Neither CT nor cisternographic findings were of value in determining the response to shunt therapy.

In patients with gait disturbance and disorder of mentation CT showed two patterns: (1) ventricular enlargement with no prominence of the sulcal markings; and (2) ventricular enlargement with a prominent sulcal pattern, and in this case the temporal horn and fourth ventricle were not significantly enlarged. In the first instance cisternographic findings were most characteristic of NPH, and following shunt there was good response of gait, whereas in the latter case cisternogram was more typical of an atrophic process and no change was observed after shunt. In several patients CT showed no enlargement of the sulci and cisternogram was typical of NPH: at necropsy two months later there was significant cortical atrophy.

The gait disorder of NPH can usually be distinguished from the characteristic parkinsonian pattern of rigidity, bradykinesia, festination and stooped posture. In certain cases if the resting tremor is absent, differentiation of these two conditions may be quite difficult. Furthermore, it has been reported that certain patients with a clinical pattern of parkinsonism do not respond to drug therapy and reveal on air study and isotope cisternogram a pattern of NPH; these patients respond to shunt procedure.[4] CT was not routinely performed in patients with parkinsonism. If there is a poor response to drugs CT is indicated, as it may suggest the reason for drug failure. Rarely, in drug nonresponders CT scan showed bilateral basal ganglia calcification although there was no laboratory evidence of disorders of calcium metabolism and plain skull radiogram was negative. Other parkinsonian patients showed neither clinical improvement nor evidence of CNS toxicity (mental changes, dyskinesia) on doses well above normal therapeutic dosage, and CT showed evidence of massive ventricular enlargement and cortical sulcal enlargement indicative of severe degenerative change.

Gait ataxia associated with pseudo-cerebellar signs may be the most prominent disturbance in both superficial and deep lesions involving the frontal lobe. Brun divided these patients into those who have gait ataxia involving both legs owing to bifrontal tumor and usually associated with intracranial hypertension and those with unilateral ataxia involving the leg contralateral to the location of the tumor. Although frontal lobe lesions may produce ataxia, dysmetria and dysdiadochokinesia in 50 to 60 percent, nystagmus is present in only 20 to 30 percent.[5] The presence of these pseudocerebellar signs in cases of frontal lesion is believed to be due to functional impairment of the fronto-pontocerebellar pathways. The majority of cases of this syndrome are caused by tumor or trauma and less frequently by vascular occlusion.

Prior to CT, evaluation of these patients with gait impairment alone was quite difficult, as the responsible lesion may be localized to the contralateral frontal or ipsilateral cerebellar hemisphere. If EEG and isotope scan did not give any localizing features or, rarely, falsely suggested, a frontal location, four-vessel angiography was required, but this is no longer necessary with CT. This problem was significant in that in 10 percent of patients who presented with gait disorder without localizing signs were found to have a clinically unsuspected frontal tumor instead of a cerebellar lesion.

Other patients had gait incoordination parallel to the severity of the cerebellar signs; this suggests dysfunction of the rostral part of the anterior lobe of the vermis. If there is no evidence of intracranial hypertension, a degenerative, demyelinating, parainfectious or metabolic etiology is more likely than tumor. In many cases, despite complete investigation, no cause is found, and a degenerative disorder, frequently with a familial basis, is suspected.

The relationship between pneumographic evidence of cerebellar atrophy and clinically apparent cerebellar disease has been investigated by LeMay and Abramowicz.[6, 7] They established that if cerebellar sulci are 2 to 4 mm in width this is consistent with mild to moderate atrophy, and if greater than 4 mm there is marked cerebellar atrophy. When this was correlated with clinical findings, 17 of 28 patients had mild to moderate atrophy and 10 of 11 had severe atrophy. Robertson suggested that the clinicopathological presence of cerebellar atrophy may better correlate with the height of the fourth ventricle, and this measurement is independent of the width of cerebellar sulci.[8]

The most reliable pneumographic assessment of cerebellar atrophy has been obtained by using midline tomography in the sagittal plane; this delineates the folial pattern of the vermis, the height of the fourth ventricle and the dimension of the brain stem and subarachnoid cisterns. Kennedy showed a direct correlation between the severity of clinical dysfunction and the pneumographic pattern, but in 23 of 44 cases of pneumographic atrophy there were no clinical signs present. In two patients with cerebellar signs and pneumographic evidence of atrophy, necropsy examination showed no atrophy, and the explanation for this discrepancy is not known.[9]

Utilizing CT certain correlations between the gait disturbance and cerebellar signs with the pathological site of involvement may also be possible. Several CT patterns in patients with cerebellar atrophic condition have been identified and these include the following: (1) A low-density area in the posterior fossa that does not distort or displace the fourth ventricle; with infusion there is no enhancement. Air study has been performed to exclude nonenhancing neoplasm although lack of mass effect makes this diagnosis unlikely. In other cases CT showed a low-density lesion in the posterior fossa but a poorly visualized fourth ventricle; air study documented cerebellar atrophy (Fig. 14–3). (2) An enlarged fourth ventricle and a cerebellar folial pattern (Fig. 14–4); in this case there may be evidence of brain stem atrophy. (3) A prominent cerebellar folial pattern, fourth ventricle and posterior fossa cisterns; this may represent a more advanced brain stem and cerebellar involvement (Fig. 14–5).

In the olivopontocerebellar disorders, there is a loss of neurons in the cerebellar cortex, basis pontis and inferior olivary nuclei, with latter involvement of the basal ganglia and cerebral cortex. In the cerebellum the major atrophic change occurs in the lobules of the anterior and posterior hemispheres; these areas have important afferent connections to the pontine and olivary nuclei. Air study and CT findings include evidence of widening of brain stem cisterns and enlarged fourth ventricle with minimal widening of the vermal sulcal pattern.

In alcoholic cerebellar degeneration the earliest and most severe pathological change occurs in the anterior superior vermis, and CT scan shows prominence of the superior cerebellar vermian cistern with a normal-sized fourth ventricle and no prominence of a folial pattern.[10] In patients with a history of chronic alcoholism who have other clinical psychiatric and neurological symptoms related to alcohol but no evidence of cerebellar disturbance, CT scan showed no abnormality in the posterior fossa indicative of cerebellar atrophy. Previous pneumographic studies in patients with similar symptoms have occasionally demonstrated gross cerebellar atrophy and this finding was confirmed by necropsy.[9] This may be contrasted with cortical cerebellar atrophy, including that of carcinomatous origin, in which there is prominent widening of the folial pat-

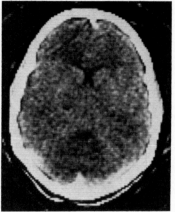

Figure 14–3. A ten-year-old child presented with an 18-month progressive history of limb and truncal ataxia without headache, nausea, vomiting or evidence of papilledema. Skull radiograph and isotope scan were negative. CT findings: a triangular-shaped low-density region crisscrossed by transverse lines, representing folial pattern, no enhancement and normal size and position of the fourth ventricle. The diagnosis of cerebellar atrophy was confirmed by air study.

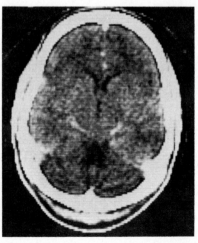

Figure 14–4. In a 21-year-old man with a three-year history of progressive gait disturbance, neurological findings included broad-based ataxic gait, intention tremor of all extremities, truncal titubation, increased tone in all extremities, bilateral Babinski sign, nystagmus on both horizontal and vertical gaze, dysarthria and proximal and distal weakness in both upper and lower extremities. EMG and nerve conduction velocities were negative. CT showed enlargement of fourth ventricle and a midline low-density pattern consistent with cerebellar atrophy.

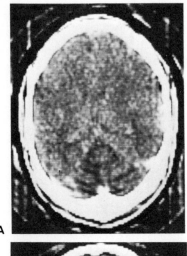

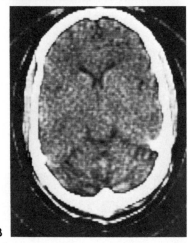

Figure 14–5. In a 50-year-old man with progressive clumsiness in walking, neurological findings included limb and truncal ataxia. CT findings: prominent cerebellar folial pattern, fourth ventricle and basal cisterns consistent with pancerebellar degeneration (A, B). Extensive evaluation for an occult neoplasm demonstrated a lymphoma.

tern extending laterally into the cerebellar hemispheres with a normal-sized fourth ventricle and basal cisterns.

Several patients with systemic carcinoma presented with gait disturbance; CT was performed to exclude a metastatic lesion although there was no clinical evidence of intracranial hypertension and both EEG and isotope scan were normal. Despite the lack of symptoms or signs of intracranial hypertension, one third had CT scan evidence of cerebellar neoplasm. In one half of these cases an-

giography was negative. Conversely, in patients with gait disorder in whom CT scan shows evidence of a widened folial pattern consistent with cortical cerebellar atrophy, this may prompt an investigation for occult malignancy.

In other patients with cerebellar signs due to various causes, including myxedema, Wilson's disease and maple syrup urine disease, no abnormalities have been visualized by CT. In one patient on long-term phenytoin (Dilantin) therapy there was CT scan evidence of cerebellar atrophy. Following surgery, CT scan may show extensive low-density areas with enlarged cisterns and fourth ventricle; lack of mass effect and contrast enhancement exclude tumor recurrence. In patients with dementia without gait disorder, enlargement of folial pattern, cisterns and fourth ventricle may be visualized as part of a generalized atrophic disorder.[11] The CT scan pattern of cerebellar atrophy was not identified in patients without gait disorder or cerebellar signs. In rare instances of patients with gait disorder CT scan was normal but air study showed evidence of an atrophic process, indicating that air study is a more sensitive study. Furthermore, air study also occasionally showed evidence of cerebellar atrophy in asymptomatic patients.

If the gait abnormality is related to multiple sclerosis, the pathological lesion may be in the spinal cord, deep cerebral white matter, cerebellum or brain stem. Pathological studies have shown that 75 percent of plaques were located in white matter and 40 percent were periventricular, usually located around the anterior and posterior horns of the lateral ventricle. These plaques are located in the centrum semiovale and adjacent to the floor of the fourth ventricle but usually not in the cerebellum. Mental changes, including euphoria and denial, are not infrequent in multiple sclerosis, and are believed due to plaques located in the frontal region. Few previous air studies in this con-

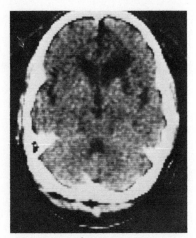

Figure 14–6. Examination of a 50-year-old man with progressive difficulty with gait revealed bilateral spasticity in his legs with Babinski sign, pseudobulbar signs, and dysarthria. CT findings: moderate ventricular dilatation, enlargement of cisterns, and a sulcal pattern with sharply defined frondlike periventricular low-density region adjacent to the posterior area of the right frontal horn, consistent with plaque of demyelination.

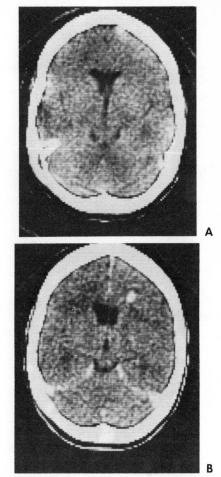

Figure 14–7. A 35-year-old woman had four separate attacks of unsteadiness of gait, vertigo and double vision, which cleared spontaneously. Findings included truncal ataxia, scanning speech, nystagmus and internuclear ophthalmoplegia. CT findings: plain scan was normal (A) but following contrast infusion there were two dense round areas of enhancement (only one shown) in the periventricular region without mass effect, consistent with acute multiple sclerosis (B).

dition have been done but ventricular enlargement is not unusual, and this finding has been confirmed by necropsy studies.

In patients with a clinical diagnosis of probable multiple sclerosis, the incidence of cortical and periventricular involvement has been defined by CT and included a high incidence of evidence of ventricular, central and cortical atrophy with a nonspecific pattern. In addition, in 36 percent there were sharply demarcated low-density areas located in the region of the trigones or the anterior or posterior horn of the lateral ventricle (Fig. 14–6). It is believed that these low-density areas represent areas of demyelination extending into normal parenchyma.[12] In other patients with severe gait disturbance due to demyelinating disease, there was an apparent atrophic process involving the brainstem, with enlarged basilar cisterns and fourth ventricle.

In the acute exacerbations of multiple sclerosis, diffuse enhancement is detected in the periventricular and deep white matter of the cerebral hemispheres without significant edema or mass effect, or other cases show dense enhancement which may represent active demyelination with extravasation through an altered blood-brain barrier. On follow-up scans these may evolve to low-density lesions.[13] The finding of enhancement on CT correlates with the occasional report of positive isotope scan during an acute exacerbation of the condition, which may revert to normal within several months. Another pattern of enhancement that may be seen in an acute exacerbation of multiple sclerosis is a dense, round, multiple, periventricular enhancing lesion, which may resolve following treatment with corticosteroids or may resolve spontaneously (Fig. 14–7). These lesions may be seen in the periventricular region even if the clinical symptoms suggest brain stem and cerebellar involvement (Fig. 14–8). In rare instances, the presence of a positive isotope scan in acute multiple sclerosis may suggest the presence of a neoplasm, and angiography may show an avascular mass; the correct diagnosis may be established only by surgical biopsy.

The diagnosis of multiple sclerosis is usually based on the dissemination of symptoms in time (multiple episodes of clinical worsening) and space (multiple locations of the CNS involved) and, despite the relative specificity of the finding of elevated gamma globulin in the CSF, the diagnosis is established clinically. Huckman reported finding three tentorial meningiomas by CT in which the diagnosis of multiple sclerosis had initially been made. Our experience confirms that the incidence of detecting by CT a structural lesion in patients who were believed to have multiple sclerosis was 5 to 10 percent, and this was highest in those patients presenting with gait disorders. With a recent finding of enhancement in these lesions, clinical judgment is necessary to differentiate them from neoplastic conditions.

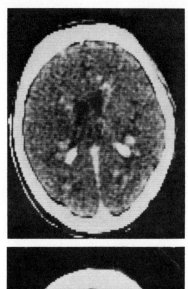

A

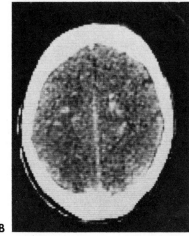

B

Figure 14–8. A 35-year-old man presented with a history of several years of pain in his lower extremities and difficulty ambulating. Findings included spastic paraparesis with patchy sensory loss of vibration and position sensation in his legs. CSF examination showed a count of 65 lymphocytes and protein content of 123 mg per 100 ml. CT findings: plain scan shows no evidence of low-density areas, but following contrast infusion there is periventricular enhancement, especially at the anterior and posterior region (A), as well as in the central white matter (B), a pattern consistent with diagnosis of multiple sclerosis.

REFERENCES

1. Maurice-Williams RS: Mechanism of production of gait unsteadiness by tumors in the posterior fosse. J Neurol Neurosurg Psychiatry 38:143, 1975.
2. Chawla JC, Woodward J: Motor disorder in normal pressure hydrocephalus. Br. Med J 1:485, 1972.
3. Petrovici I: Apraxia of gait and of trunk movements. J Neurol Sci 7:229, 1968.
4. Sypert GW, Leffman H, Diemann GA: Occult normal pressure hydrocephalus manifested by Parkinsonism-dementia complex. Neurology 23:234, 1973.

5. Haymaker W: Bing's Local Diagnosis in Neurological Diseases. CV Mosby, St. Louis, 1969. pp 289–91.

6. LeMay M, Abramowicz A: Encephalography in the diagnosis of cerebellar atrophy. Acta Radiol (Diagn) 5:667, 1966.

7. LeMay M, Abramowicz A: Penumographic findings in various forms of cerebellar degeneration. Radiology 85:284, 1965.

8. Robertson EG: Diagnosis of Cerebellar Atrophy in Pneumoencephalography. CC Thomas, Springfield, Ill., 1967. pp 155–161.

9. Kennedy P, Swash M, Wylie IG: The clinical significance of pneumographic cerebellar atrophy. Br J Radiol 49:903, 1976.

10. Victor M, Adams RD, Mancell EL: A restricted form of cerebellar cortical degeneration in alcoholic patients. Arch Neurol 1:579, 1959.

11. Gawler J, DuBoulay GH, Bull JWD: CT: a comparison with PEG and ventriculography. J Neurol Neurosurg Psychiatry 39:203, 1976.

12. Gyldensted C: Computer tomography of the cerebrum in multiple sclerosis. Neuroradiology. 12:33, 1976.

13. Aita JF, Bennett DR, Anderson RE, et al: Acute multiple sclerosis in CT. Neurology 27:387, 1977.

14. Cohan SL, Fermaglich J, Auth TL: Abnormal brain scans in multiple sclerosis. J Neurol Neurosurg Psychiatry 38:120, 1975.

15. Huckman MS, Fox JH, Ramsey RG: CT in the diagnosis of degenerative disease of the brain. Semin Roentgenol 12:63, 1977.

Chapter 15 Headache

Headache may be the initial symptom of an intracranial lesion. In the majority of cases there are other accompanying neurological abnormalities that may be elicited by careful history and examination, and the diagnosis is confirmed by the results of neurodiagnostic studies. The majority of headache patients evaluated by the neurologist are of the chronic recurring type, and no definite underlying lesion is identified, but in certain instances skull radiograph, EEG and isotope scan have been utilized as screening procedures to exclude an underlying remediable structural lesion. In most cases if the skull radiograph and EEG are negative no further evaluation is performed, with the exception that, if the patient is proved to have or is suspected of having systemic carcinoma, isotope scan is usually included to detect metastatic deposits, although the diagnostic yield is still quite low.

In other patients who present with more acute onset of headache and have not previously had prior headache symptoms, a complete neurodiagnostic evaluation, including EEG, isotope scan, skull radiogram, echoencephalogram and CSF examination, is usually performed, and possible non-neurological systemic causes of the headache are investigated. In these instances the diagnostic yield is somewhat higher and negative results are usually reassuring in excluding a remediable disorder. Contrast procedures are not usually performed unless definite abnormalities are identified by these screening procedures.

With the increasing availability of CT the number of patients referred for evaluation of both "acute" and "chronic recurring" headache has in-

creased. This has afforded the opportunity to compare CT with other diagnostic studies as a screening procedure and to evaluate the incidence and type of abnormalities detected as well as cost versus effectiveness of CT compared to other conventional diagnostic studies.

In patients with chronic recurring headache in whom skull radiogram and EEG were negative, 1.5 percent had lesions subsequently defined by CT, and these included subfrontal meningioma (isotope scan was also negative), chronic subdural hematoma, aqueductal stenosis, subarachnoid and porencephalic cysts. Based upon the chronic nature of the headache, with normal neurological examination and negative studies, contrast studies would not have been performed, and the availability of CT afforded the only opportunity for their diagnosis. It is an important point that several of these patients had recurring headaches that had been present for as long as several years, and with conventional noncontrast studies the possible occurrence of a treatable disorder had not been suggested. In all cases the abnormality was clearly defined by noncontrast CT study, and contrast study was then also performed. Following surgical procedures, the symptoms of the chronic recurring headache persisted in several patients. It is possible that if diagnosis and treatment had been initiated at an earlier stage this outcome may have been more uniformly favorable.

Other conditions that may cause headache only and may not be detected by skull radiogram, isotope scan or EEG include certain intraventricular lesions, especially those causing obstruction of the anterior third ventricle. The most frequent condition to present in this manner is the colloid cyst of the third ventricle. Less frequently, ependymal cyst, choroid plexus papilloma of the fourth ventricle or other midline intraventricular tumors may cause intermittent ventricular obstruction, and these lesions are well defined by CT without the need for performing air study.

In other patients with chronic recurring headache an associated EEG abnormality was the most frequent reason (30 percent) for CT scan, and this is not unexpected since 5 to 8 percent of the normal population may have a mildly abnormal EEG. If the pattern was that of bitemporal or diffuse slowing, CT was uniformly negative, but in rare instances there was a focal delta pattern and subsequent CT study demonstrated a structural lesion. In no instance in which EEG demonstrated a focal delta pattern did CT fail to define the lesion, whereas isotope scan was positive in only one half of such cases. In these cases, CT identified a neoplasm that was believed to be a low-grade astrocytoma or meningioma, but specific pathological diagnosis usually required confirmation by angiography or biopsy. In several instances the lesion defined by CT was a small meningioma and, based on size as defined by CT, the decision not to perform angiography or surgery was made without the necessity for hospitalization.

Ten percent of patients were referred because of an abnormality detected on skull radiogram, including evidence of an old or expanding fracture line, abnormal calcification, sella abnormality, a questionable lucent area and hyperostosis; CT defined the presence of leptomeningeal or subarachnoid cyst, chronic subdural hematoma or hygroma or pituitary adenoma in one fourth of the cases. Air study was required to define the presence of an intrasellar pituitary adenoma and "empty sella syndrome," which were not clearly detected by CT.

In most patients with a negative isotope scan, CT was usually also negative, with the exception of a series of 20 patients with known systemic cancer and recurrent headache, of whom four had metastatic deposits defined by CT. In two patients with headache of 12 to 15 months' duration chronic subdural hematoma was not detected by isotope scan, but the presence of a focal abnormality was detected by EEG and defined by CT; this indicates the lack of sensitivity of isotope scan in this condition. Ten percent of patients with chronic recurring headache had previously been evaluated by physicians and neurological examination had been reported as "negative," but examination by a neurologist demonstrated "soft" neurological signs, including the presence of pronator drift, asymmetrical arm swing, reflex asymmetry, facial asymmetry and focal muscle wasting. Despite normal EEG and isotope scan, one third of these patients had abnormalities identified by CT, usually consisting of focal atrophic lesions, including old infarctions or small cysts that could correlate with the neurological findings, although none of these lesions were evaluated further by contrast studies.

In patients with a more "acute" headache pattern that had been present for less than two months, isotope scan and EEG indicated the presence of a lateralized lesion in 8 percent of cases, and subsequent CT defined the underlying pathological process in all cases. In an additional 2 percent of cases in which these studies were negative, CT demonstrated the presence of an underlying neoplasm or cyst. In this analysis, patients who presented with headache and stiff neck who were suspected of having subarachnoid hemorrhage or meningitis were not included, as CSF was initially performed to establish this diagnosis. In the more acute headache disorders EEG and isotope scan appear to be more sensitive screening procedures for structural lesions, whereas in the more chronic disorders CT is more likely to detect a lesion not detected by EEG, skull radiogram or isotope scan, but the incidence of abnormalities detected by CT is much lower for patients with chronic recurring headache.

MIGRAINE

The majority of patients with chronic recurring headache who had abnormal EEG were classified as having a migraine syndrome. Reports of EEG abnormalities have suggested that up to two thirds of these patients have abnormal EEG findings, which may consist of a generalized slow pattern although there may be a focal spike or slow-wave focus; the latter finding suggests the presence of an underlying structural disorder.[1]

The vascular changes in the migraine syndrome are usually reversible, but it has been postulated that the multiple and frequent attacks cause significant ischemia, which may lead to the development of permanent EEG changes and in rare instances epilepsy.[2] During the migraine attack, EEG changes consist of a spike of slow pattern, usually localized to the occipital region but which may be more widespread; this finding is more frequently seen in complicated migraine and resolves over several days.

Because migraine is almost always a benign disorder, little is known about any resultant cumulative pathological changes other than what has been inferred from EEG findings. Angiography and cerebral blood flow studies obtained during the acute migrainous attack indicate that there is arterial spasm, which results in decreased focal cortical blood flow, and this may lead to cerebral ischemia and cortical atrophy. Dukes and Vieth reported a progressive decrease in filling of the internal carotid artery during the prodromal phase, with normal angiographic findings during the succeeding headache.[3] These findings are in accord with measurements of cerebral blood flow and the belief that angiography is a potential hazard, as confirmed by reports of a high incidence of neurological complications in those studied by angiography during an acute attack. Because of this risk angiography is not a practical or safe modality to study the pathological disturbances of the migraine syndrome.

In studying patients with migraine by CT, several issues may be considered, including the incidence of misdiagnosis with failure to detect tumor or angioma and the presence of any pathological sequelae to the vascular changes. Pearce and Foster evaluated the problem of whether a patient with complicated migraine should be studied by angiography for the possibility of an underlying angioma; of 33 patients only two had angiomas and in these cases the history was not indicative of classical migraine. They concluded that angiography is usually not indicated and that persistent nonprogressive sequelae of an attack, such as hemianopia, are usually caused by secondary cerebral infarction and that only progressive neurological disturbance, papilledema and focal epilepsy should be indications for angiography in patients with migraine. In cerebral angioma located usually in the parieto-occipital region, the symptoms may simulate migraine but the headache is always localized to one side, whereas in migraine the headache may alternate sides or may be bilateral.[4]

Of 100 patients with a diagnosis of migraine syndrome who had CT, only two clinically unsuspected lesions were identified, and in both cases EEG and isotope scan also identified the lesion. Of patients with classical migraine in whom the headache alternated sides, one third had an abnormal EEG. Because of this EEG finding they were referred for CT, and this study was normal in all except two cases in which an angioma and occipital lobe infarction were identified.

During the acute migrainous attack

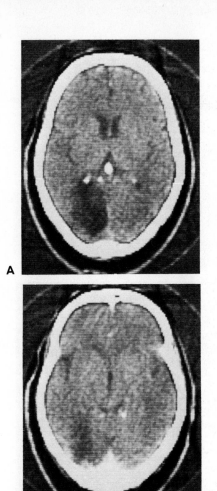

A

B

Figure 15–1. *A* and *B*, This patient presented with left-sided occipital headache and with an aura preceded by flashing lights in the right visual field and then loss of vision in that field. There was a complete right homonymous hemianopia, which cleared over 72 hours, and no bruit was present. EEG showed a slow wave abnormality over the left occipital region; isotope scan was negative. CT findings: vague low-density area in left occipital region without enhancement. Since symptoms rapidly cleared, no follow-up study was obtained.

one third to one half of patients have been reported to have abnormal scans.[5, 6] The abnormal findings include (1) focal low-density areas that do not enhance with contrast, cause no mass effect and resolve completely with serial scans performed four to six weeks later (Fig. 15–1); and (2) diffuse or focal ventricular and corti-

cal atrophic changes. There was little correlation between the CT scan abnormality and the duration and severity of the migraine episode, but there was a correlation between the incidence of finding an abnormal focal low-density area and the presence of focal neurological deficit. In all patients who showed a focal low-density region, usually located in the parieto-temporo-occipital region, there was an accompanying focal EEG abnormality, but the isotope scan was negative. If the isotope scan is positive, this would raise the suspicion of an underlying angioma. The incidence of abnormal CT findings in migraine may be dependent upon when the study is done in relation to the last attack; if it is performed more than one week later, the evidence of low-density ischemia, edema or possibly infarction may be missed. The incidence of abnormal CT scans is highest in complicated migraine.

NEOPLASMS

In the majority of intracranial tumors, headache is often the initial symptom; in one study this was the earliest or principal symptom in 54 percent. There was no difference in the occurrence of this symptom between rapidly and slowly growing tumors, and the incidence of headache in specific tumors is quite similar (meningioma, 46 percent; pituitary adenoma, 51 percent; glioblastoma, 57 percent; metastatic, 65 percent). Although in rare instances the patient may complain only of headache there are usually other neurological findings detected on examination, and screening EEG or isotope scan will be positive.[7]

In meningioma and pituitary adenoma this problem is more complicated because, although the tumor is present this does not necessarily indicate that it is the cause of the headache (Fig. 15–2). Small meningiomas may be found as incidental necropsy

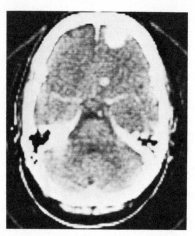

Figure 15–2. A 35-year-old man had a two-year history of classical "cluster" headaches that were pulsatile and located on the left side; they awakened him from sleep and were associated with lacrimation. The headaches responded to treatment with ergot compounds and also to propranolol. Isotope scan, skull radiograph and EEG were negative, but the headache recurred while continuing medication. CT findings: high-density, round, enhancing and homogeneous lesion in the right subfrontal region contiguous with bone, consistent with meningioma.

findings. In one study of 300 asymptomatic tumors found at necropsy, 100 were meningiomas, with a predilection for parasagittal (31 percent), free edge of the convexity (25 percent), sphenoid ridge (16 percent), sella (13 percent), posterior fossa (9 percent), and olfactory groove or basal-frontal region (7 percent). These tumors were sharply circumscribed, well-encapsulated lesions, and 61 percent were less than 1 centimeter in diameter, 22 percent were less than 2 cm, and only 17 percent were greater than 3 cm.[8]

Routine necropsy studies of asymptomatic patients have shown that approximately one third may have pituitary adenoma, and some may have evidence of suprasellar extension. Therefore the finding by CT of pituitary adenoma in patients without visual or endocrine symptoms is not unexpected. Of 300 patients with nonmigrainous headache of the chronic recurring type in which the EEG, isotope scan and skull radio-

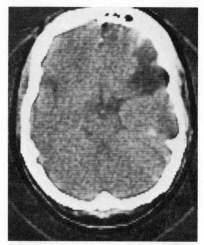

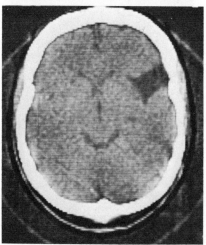

Figure 15–3. A and B, A 20-year-old man who had had no prior history of head trauma developed right-sided headache of 6 months' duration. Skull radiogram, EEG and isotope scan were negative. CT findings: a sharply marginated low-density lesion extending from the sylvian region along the floor of the middle fossa; it was surgically proved to be a subarachnoid cyst.

gram were negative, only two pituitary adenomas and one meningioma were defined. CT has become the most reliable diagnostic study to identify cystic lesions, subdural hematoma and hygroma, even if all preliminary diagnostic studies have been negative. If there has been a history of trauma, CT should be performed, as traumatic lesions may develop and expand, eventually causing neurological deficit (Fig. 15–3).

In the evaluation of the patient with chronic recurring headache, the sensitivity for detection of an occult lesion was greater with CT than with conventional diagnostic studies. At the present time, the cost of performing an EEG and isotope scan is approximately equal to that of a CT scan, and CT is more effective in defining a lesion; EEG and skull radiogram can be performed at one half the cost but with lower sensitivity. If any neurological findings are present, CT is clearly the most sensitive diagnostic study, and in certain patients a negative CT scan may obviate the need for hospitalization or contrast studies. In the evaluation of the more "acute" headache, isotope scan is approximately equal to CT in its ability to detect lesions, but CT provides more specific pathological information. In addition, a skull radiogram may suggest disorders not detected by EEG, isotope scan or even CT. Since CT has detected lesions in only 1.5 percent of patients when EEG and isotope scan have been negative, the cost is quite high for the detection of one lesion by CT.

REFERENCES

1. Hockaday JM, Whitty CWM: Factors determining the EEG in migraine. Brain 92:769, 1969.
2. Hughes JR: EEG in headache. Headache 11:162, 1972.
3. Dukes HT, Vieth RG: Cerebral angiography during migraine prodrome and headache. Neurology 14:636, 1964.
4. Pearce JMS, Foster JB: An investigation of complicated migraine. Neurology 15:333, 1965.
5. Mathew NT, Meyer JS: Abnormal CT scans in migraine. Headache 16:272, 1976.
6. Hungerford GD, duBoulay GH: CT in patients with severe migraine. Neurol Neurosurg Psychiatry 39:990, 1976.
7. Heyck H: Examination and differential diagnosis of headache. In: Handbook of Neurology, PJ Vinken, GW Bruyn (eds). North Holland Publishing Company, Amsterdam, 1968, Vol 5, pp 25–36.
8. Wood MW, White RJ, Kernohan JW: One hundred intracranial meningiomas found incidentally at necropsy. J Neuropath Exp Neurol 16:337, 1957.

Chapter 16 Seizure Disorders and Correlation with Specific EEG Patterns

Since the introduction of CT, we have had the opportunity to investigate over 600 patients in whom the clinical diagnosis of a convulsive disorder was suspected and CT was performed to determine if a structural lesion could be defined. Other patients were referred for CT scan because of an abnormal electroencephalographic (EEG) finding of either diffuse or focal type that was reported as consistent with a convulsive disorder, but the patient had no clinical symptoms and CT was done to exclude a clinically silent lesion.

This chapter presents the results of prospective studies of the incidence of abnormal CT findings in patients with various electroclinical patterns of epilepsy and a comparison of the detection rate compared with isotope scan, skull radiograph, air study and angiography. Since many patients had longstanding and sometimes poorly controlled seizure disorders for which they had taken anticonvulsant medication for many years, an attempt was made to determine if multiple and prolonged convulsions were associated with any CT-definable abnormality. In addition, certain EEG patterns have frequently been associated with pathological processes, including monorhythmic frontal delta activity with increased intracranial pressure and focal delta activity with a vascular or neoplastic lesion. Other EEG patterns have been considered of less pathological significance, including bitemporal slow pattern or slight slowing of the background rhythm, and the sensitivity and specificity of CT in evaluating the significance of these patterns has been assessed.

Sixty patients were evaluated because of "possible convulsive disorder" but the clinical symptoms, lack of associated neurological abnormalities and normal interictal EEG made the diagnosis of primary syncopal disorder more probable. Because of the possibility that these episodes represented convulsive disorders and the possible relationship of syncope to epilepsy, these patients had CT scans, and the complete study, including contrast infusion, was normal; in no case did other neurodiagnostic studies demonstrate any abnormality.

In 25 other patients the episodes of loss of consciousness were of recent onset and were not associated with tonic-clonic activity, incontinence, tongue biting or postictal confusion or paralysis, but the interictal EEG was abnormal, showing either a diffuse slow pattern, bitemporal slow wave or spikes in either focal or generalized distribution. Seven of these patients had abnormal scans, of which five were consistent with cerebrovascular disorder and two showed tumor. In five cases the CT scan showed a focal wedge-shaped low-density area without mass effect in the distribution of the middle cerebral artery, with a slight enhancement pattern, consistent with recent infarction. Despite the CT evidence of cerebral infarction, there was no evidence of a focal neurological deficit; isotope scan was negative and EEG showed either a unilateral or bilateral temporal slow pattern.

Focal cerebral ischemia caused by carotid insufficiency has been reported to produce syncope, but this etiology would appear to be an unlikely explanation in the absence of associated neurological signs. It is not probable that the CT patterns of infarction in these cases were incidental findings. In three cases syncopal attacks ceased in two months and the CT scan abnormality disappeared, whereas in two the attacks persisted as did the CT scan abnormality. Vertebral-basilar insufficiency may cause "drop attacks" and, rarely, syncope, but brain stem ischemia or infarction is not usually detected by CT.

Rarely, syncope may occur with intracranial tumors, and it has usually been presumed to be due to brain stem compression, but neurological findings and intracranial hypertension are invariably present. One patient with postural syncope was found by CT to have a pituitary tumor and the episodes were caused by secondary adrenal insufficiency; CT had preceded a skull radiograph, which clearly showed an enlarged eroded sella turcica. In another case the syncopal episode was preceded by severe unilateral headache without any visual prodromata. EEG showed a focal spike pattern in the parieto-occipital region, whereas isotope scan and skull radiogram were negative. CT showed a low-density region in the occipital region without mass effect or enhancement, a pattern consistent with ischemia as seen in migraine syndrome. This CT scan pattern was sufficient to exclude a possible an-

giogma without the need for angiography in this clinical setting. One patient with syncope had a parietal convexity tumor, but after removal of the meningioma the attacks persisted (Fig. 16–1). The results of CT findings in patients with syncope suggest that occasionally cerebral ischemia and infarction or an underlying structural lesion may be defined by CT, but the potential yield is quite low in these cases.[1]

In patients with more definite electroclinical evidence of a convulsive disorder, an attempt was made to classify these disorders, utilizing the International League Against Epilepsy so as to compare our CT scan results with other studies that have recently been reported.[2] Primary generalized epilepsy (PGE) refers to attacks characterized by sudden loss of consciousness with symmetrical generalized tonic-clonic activity or brief episodes of unawareness without accompanying motor activity (absence attack). These episodes begin before age 20 and frequently have a familial and genetic basis; they are

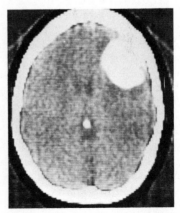

Figure 16–1. A 45-year-old woman was evaluated because of episodes of unconsciousness that were not associated with abnormal motor activity, tongue biting or incontinence. Skull radiograph was negative but EEG showed bitemporal slow pattern, more pronounced on the right side. CT scan showed a high-density (25 to 40) consolidated round mass which did not enhance and was consistent with convexity meningioma. This was removed surgically but there was no change in the pattern or frequency of syncopal attacks.

believed to be caused by some un-identified factor. A generalized cere-bral electrophysiological disturbance is present but no structural pathologi-cal abnormality is identified. The neurological examination is normal in these patients.

The interictal EEG in patients with the major motor disorder may show spike discharges or be entirely nor-mal, whereas in petit mal there is the characteristic 3 cps spike-and-wave discharge. There have been rare re-ports of absence attacks associated with a structural lesion in children, but it seems more likely that these were psychomotor attacks or tumors not directly related to the clinical at-tack.[3] Conversely, it is not unusual for patients with "absence attacks" to have certain asymmetrical or atypical EEG variants of the classic spike-wave pattern, and these minor variants do not suggest an underlying structural lesion unless the EEG pat-tern is less thant 2.5 cps.[4]

Despite the previously reported very low incidence of pathological le-sions associated with PGE, Gastaut reported 10 percent abnormal CT scans, whereas other studies of CT in this condition showed only 0 to 2 percent abnormalities.[2] In patients with "absence attacks" CT has been normal in all cases, even in those performed because the spike-wave pattern was slightly less than 3 cps or showed an asymmetry, although we did not include cases in which EEG was as slow as 2 cps, in which the incidence of CT abnormalities was significantly higher. (See Infantile Spasms, discussed later.) Of those pa-tients less than 25 years old with a major motor pattern of PGE in whom the neurological examination was normal and EEG was normal or showed only a focal spike pattern, CT was invariably normal. In four of six patients studied who had a focal delta pattern, CT identified a strucutral le-sion (vascular angioma, dermoid or subarachnoid cysts). In these cases the presence of the lesion was detect-ed by preinfusion study, and the le-sion was more precisely classified pathologically by infusion study. In three of these cases the isotope scan had been negative.

If a focal slow-wave abnormality is detected by EEG and CT is negative, isotope scan should also be done be-cause it may be a more sensitive technique to detect angioma, but air study is probably not necessary. In patients with PGE who showed focal delta activity with negative CT and isotope scan, subsequent angiography was also negative. In one most unu-sual patient who presented with PGE, all studies were negative and CT was performed because of poor seizure control despite adequate anti-convulsant levels; the scan demon-strated epidermoid cyst (Fig. 16–2).

In these patients with PGE, CT makes it possible to determine if the length of the seizure disorder, ade-quacy of control or type of medica-tion produces any change in the size

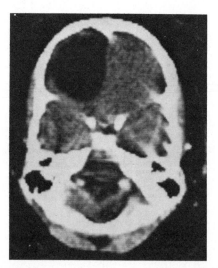

Figure 16–2. A 13-year-old with a general-ized seizure disorder had a normal neurological examination, EEG, skull radiograph and isotope scan. CT was performed because of poor control with medication and showed a well-circumscribed round low-density lesion in the left inferior frontal region which showed no evi-dence of enhancement. This was consistent with epidermoid cyst; this diagnosis was confirmed at surgery without other contrast studies.

of the ventricles and subarachnoid space or causes any abnormal focal density pattern. In comparing those patients who had more than two seizures per month with those who had only infrequent attacks (one to two per year) and matching those patients with normal controls of the same age and sex, no differences were detected in the incidence of focal lesions or evidence of cerebral atrophy. The only exception was that several patients who had previous episodes of status epilepticus had generalized cerebral atrophy. In addition, two patients with PGE who had been treated with phenytoin (Dilantin) for more than five years had some CT evidence of a cerebellar folial pattern prominence, consistent with mild cerebellar atrophy, but no clinical cerebellar findings. With further refinements in CT, including thinner tissue sections, it may be possible to detect the cumulative effect of multiple seizures, including temporal lobe gliosis and ischemic changes in the thalamus, hippocampus and cerebellum, which have been found by necropsy in patients with "idiopathic" epilepsy.[6]

The partial (focal) epilepsies are acquired disorders, and the results of CT in these patients were expected to show a higher incidence of abnormalities. Gastaut reported that 63 percent had abnormal studies of which 78 percent had focal and 22 percent diffuse abnormalities. The incidence of abnormal CT scans in patients with partial epilepsy is dependent upon the specific electroclinical pattern; these cases include attacks that appear to be generalized from the onset, those that begin with focal elementary motor or sensory symptoms, and those characterized by complex behavioral and automatic-stereotyped motor activity.

If primary generalized seizures occur after age 20, neurodiagnostic studies are necessary to exclude the presence of a structural cause but the extent of the work-up has not been definitely established. Penfield stated that the most common cause between ages 20 and 35 was related to head injury or tumor; between 35 and 55, vascular disorders; and after age 55, degenerative disorders.[6] Therefore, air study and angiography are frequently indicated in the initial diagnostic work-up, but others have suggested that, if there are no neurological findings and EEG and isotope scan are negative, then contrast studies are not indicated. Previous clinical studies have shown that many lesions will be initially missed by this approach, and it is expected that CT would further limit the necessity for contrast procedures. In one study of 66 patients with late onset generalized seizures in whom the neurological examination was normal, 26 had an abnormal isotope scan; 18 had cerebral neoplasm, four had cerebral infarction, three had lesions related to trauma and one had a brain abscess. In two patients astrocytomas were not detected by isotope scan, and subsequent contrast studies and surgery were necessary to determine the exact pathological etiology.[7]

Gilday found that 22 percent of patients with generalized seizures evaluated by isotope scan were found to have a cerebral neoplasm, but that the incidence was extremely low in those under 30 years old.[8] In these studies the lesions detected were greater than 2 cm in diameter, and despite the nonfocal nature and absence of neurological findings, some lesions were in excess of 5 cm. Rarely, the initial scan was negative and repeat study several months later was positive; the presence of a negative scan one year after the onset of seizure is strong evidence against a neoplasm, but there have been reports of seizures of up to 15 years' duration before the diagnosis of neoplasm is established.

Raynor reported an 18 percent incidence of neoplasm in adult onset generalized seizure disorders. If the EEG showed a focal abnormality and neurological findings were present, the incidence was higher. Others have indicated that the accuracy of combined EEG and isotope scan in detecting neoplasm should be greater than 90 percent.[8, 9] Mosely and Bull reported that if neurological examination was abnormal, CT demonstrated tumor in 40 percent, but if examination was normal, CT demonstrated tumor in only 7 percent. In 20 percent of patients with normal EEG, CT demonstrated an underlying neoplasm.[10] Gastaut reported the diagnostic accuracy of CT in 47 patients with cerebral neoplasms; CT was positive in all cases, but only 21 percent had a progressive neurological deficit or intracranial hypertension, 30 percent had a continuous focal or projected delta slow-wave pattern, and in only 59 percent was angiography or air study positive.

From our experience in patients with adult onset primary generalized seizure, CT demonstrated neoplasm in 20 percent with nonfocal EEG, 40 percent had negative isotope scan, and 20 percent had a normal neurological examination. The presence of focal postictal neurological deficit, focal spike focus on EEG, and difficulty in control of the seizure disorder did not correlate with the likelihood of underlying neoplasm by CT. In our experience to date no patient who had generalized seizure and normal CT has later been found to have neoplasm detected by subsequent scan or other neurodiagnostic studies. The neoplasms most frequently causing seizure without localizing neurological signs included low-grade astrocytomas, and CT demonstrated a high incidence of cystic lesions (Fig. 16–3). CT studies confirm that the neoplasm usually originates from the frontal or nondominant temporal region, although in 10 percent of cases the neoplasm was located in the centro-parietal region, in which case it is believed that the focal origin has not been detected.

Non-neoplastic etiologies that may

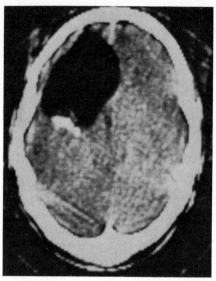

Figure 16–3. A 33-year-old man was examined following an episode of generalized seizure. Neurological examination was negative; skull radiograph showed a curvilinear calcification in the left frontal region, but EEG and isotope scan were negative. Plain scan showed a large low-density region in the left inferior frontal and temporal region, which extended to the falx and suprasellar region. The density values were negative (+4 to −10) and there were peripheral high-density calcified nodules. Angiography showed an avascular mass. A dermoid tumor was found at operation.

be delineated by CT more accurately than by other diagnostic studies include vascular, traumatic, infectious and degenerative disorders. In nonembolic cerebral infarction, 6.7 percent had nonfocal seizures; in 1.6 percent this was the initial clinical manifestation and in several instances the *only* manifestation of the seizure disorder.[11] Ten percent of patients with cerebral emboli and 15 percent with intracerebral hemorrhage present with generalized seizures, and the diagnosis is established by the apoplectic onset of a focal deficit and EEG, isotope and CSF findings.[12] In 20 percent of patients with generalized seizure, CT established the diagnosis of nonhemorrhagic infarction despite negative EEG and isotope scan. In Alzheimer's disease the incidence of seizure may be 25 to 33 percent and may occur before there is any clinically detectable deterioration in memory, intellect or personality, whereas in Pick's disease seizures are less common.[13] Results of CT have shown definite cortical atrophy and ventricular enlargement in 26 to 40 percent of patients with adult onset nonfocal seizures. In many of these patients initially there was no evidence of dementia but this developed 6 to 11 months later.

In patients with a previous history of head trauma, seizure may be a result of gliotic scar, atrophy, cyst formation or residual hematoma of either intracerebral or extracerebral origin. Subdural hematomas are not usually associated with seizure unless there is an underlying intracerebral lesion, and results of CT findings confirm this belief. In several cases of patients with extradural hematoma, CT accurately demonstrated an intracerebral hematoma or contusion not shown by angiography.

In evaluating patients with partial seizures of the nonfocal type by CT, 35 percent were found to have abnormalities, of which 40 percent were focal and 60 percent were diffuse. In all except certain vascular lesions the CT abnormality was detected by plain scan, but pathological characterization frequently required postinfusion study. The importance of an initial plain scan cannot be overemphasized, as certain lesions, including infarction, angioma, and glioma, may initially appear as low-density regions that cause minimal or no mass effect; they may then appear isodense after contrast infusion and not be detected unless both studies are performed. In only two of 400 instances (infarction, neoplasm) was the lesion detected only after contrast infusion (Fig. 16–4). If metastases, angioma or infarction are suspected, contrast infusion is still indicated if plain scan is normal. Isotope scan was not a sensitive screening procedure, since only 33 percent of CT-positive cases were positive by isotope scan; one half showed a focal slow-wave pattern; neurological ex-

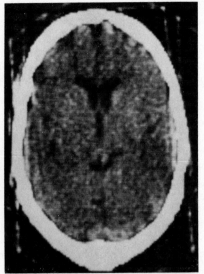

A

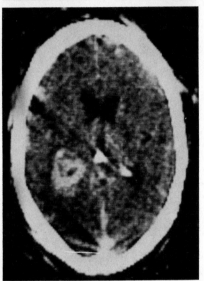

B

Figure 16–4.   A 40-year-old man experienced a sudden onset of generalized motor seizures. Neurological examination and isotope scan were negative but EEG showed a delta slow wave pattern most pronounced in the left temporal parietal region. Preinfusion CT scan was negative, with no evidence of mass effect or abnormal tissue density (A), but contrast study showed a complex circular pattern of enhancement (B). Angiography revealed a diffuse stain and early draining vein pattern consistent with malignant neoplasm.

amination showed an abnormality in only 40 percent.

In patients with no neurological deficit the results were most remarkable in defining the presence of lesions that usually required angiography or air study. Two patients had aqueductal stenosis, which was confirmed by subsequent air study although there was no clinical or radiographic evidence of intracranial hypertension; because of the lack of neurological findings, it is not likely that air study would have been performed. In addition, multiple nontumorous cystic lesions that were quite large were easily detected by CT although no focal signs were present.

It has been suggested that all patients who present with partial epilepsy having attacks characterized by focal motor or sensory or behavioral psychomotor symptoms should undergo angiography or air study because the statistical probability of detecting a structural lesion is very high even if neurological examination is normal. Despite complete studies 25 to 35 percent of adult patients with these partial motor or sensory studies are classified as idiopathic, and this incidence of negative studies is higher in children.

In determining the extent of studies to be performed in an individual case, certain findings have suggested the need for angiography. These include focal attacks limited to one side of the body, the presence of interictal neurological deficit, positive isotope scan, focal EEG abnormality and abnormal skull radiogram. In one study isotope scan detected 90 percent of neoplasms but was less sensitive in detecting other conditions. The EEG finding of a focal slow-wave pattern is more frequently associated with an identifiable structural lesion than is sharp or spike activity.[7] The presence of an interictal neurological deficit in a patient with a focal seizure was associated with neoplasm in approximately 60 percent of cases.[14] Neoplasms are considered the most common etiology for focal seizures, but this may reflect a bias, in that our diagnostic studies are most reliable in detecting these tumors and less sensitive in detecting non-neoplastic disorders. Necropsy and angiographic studies have shown that vascular disorders are the most frequent cause but in these cases EEG and isotope scan are usually negative and angiography is necessary. In one study of 23 patients with "idiopathic" focal motor seizures angiographic analysis showed occlusion of the small vessels supplying the pre-Rolandic region in 16 and in seven others the arterial supply to the motor cortex was vestigial. This vascular disturbance was not large enough to cause a neurological deficit or positive isotope scan but produced an epileptogenic focus.[12]

The utilization of CT provides a new approach to focal seizures, with decreasing reliance on angiography or air study. Bogdanoff performed CT in 50 patients whose seizures had focal features based on a clinical pattern or EEG pattern and he found 30 percent abnormal. Two were neoplasms but the others included conditions which previously required air study (focal or diffuse atrophy, hydrocephalus, cerebral or cerebellar hypoplasia). Of eight patients with interictal neurological deficit six had abnormal CT study. If the EEG showed only paroxysmal sharp or spike activity, 15 percent had abnormal CT compared to 66 percent with a focal slow-wave pattern. According to the belief in the pre-CT scan era that all adult focal seizures require contrast study, 37 patients would have required hospitalization and contrast study, but this was necessary in only three cases, whereas in three children CT defined an abnormality.[16]

Confining our definition of focal seizures to only those patients who have clinical evidence of focal disorder, CT was positive in 90 percent. Of those with abnormality defined by CT, at least 40 percent of patients had a normal interictal examination; isotope scan was negative and EEG showed only a spike focus. In all cases CT was sensitive and reliable in differentiating specific pathological etiologies, and in no case was CT negative and a lesion defined by other contrast studies. In one patient initial CT was negative, as were isotope scan and angiography, but repeat CT scan demonstrated a metastatic neoplasm three weeks later. Of 10 children with focal seizures only, one had evidence of subarachnoid cyst and there were focal neurological ab-

normalities; follow-up for 18 months has been negative in the others, as is consistent with the benign nature of focal seizures in children.[17]

In five patients who presented with focal motor seizure only and had an extensive delta focus on EEG, the suspicion of neoplasm was quite high, but CT showed evidence of recent cerebral infarction and angiography showed branch occlusion of the middle cerebral artery (Fig. 16–5). On the basis of a single EEG rec-

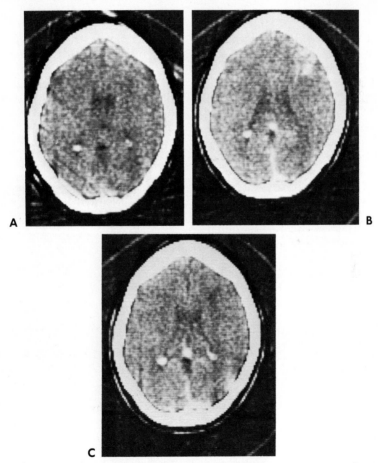

Figure 16–5.   A 36-year-old woman experienced left-sided focal motor seizures and two episodes of generalized motor seizures without focality. Interictal neurological examination was entirely normal. EEG showed right frontoparietal slow wave focus with spike discharges; isotope scan was positive. CT findings: plain scan was negative (A), but contrast enhancement study showed an area of high density in the mid- and posterior frontal region with an intervening low-density area and no mass effect (B). The CT findings were most consistent with enhancing cerebral infarction, but clinical presentation and isotope scan were suggestive of neoplasm. Angiography showed branch occlusion of the middle cerebral artery, and no mass effect. Follow-up CT three months later showed a focal nonenhancing low-density area consistent with an infarction (C).

ord, it is not always possible to differentiate infarction and hemorrhage from neoplasm. The degree and extent of focal delta activity correlates directly with the size of the lesion. In most cases the smaller the lesion, the fewer the number of involved electrodes, and if the lesion is deeply placed there may be a bilateral slow pattern without focal abnormality. In addition, serial tracings may be confusing, as tumors may not always show an increasing focal or diffuse abnormality, and EEG abnormality may disappear, whereas in infarction the slow-wave pattern may increase in size.

A useful clinical rule is that a large delta focus associated with only mild clinical deficit is most usually associated with neoplasm, whereas if a severe clinical deficit is present differentiation from non-neoplastic etiologies is not possible. In addition, immediately following a seizure isotope scan may yield positive results in the absence of neoplasm or infarction and then revert to normal several weeks after the seizure activity ceases. The initial positive isotope scan may be related to hyperperfusion secondary to the seizure and not to infarction.[18, 19] In this post-seizure state CT may rarely show an area of enhancement, which then rapidly and completely clears without leaving a residual focal low-density region, as contrasted to the CT pattern seen in nonhemorrhagic infarction. In patients with focal seizure without neurological deficit who had extensive delta focus on EEG, CT reliably distinguished neoplasm from infarction and this diagnosis was confirmed by angiography.

The results of isotope scan and CT scan in rare instances may not permit differentiation between cerebral infarction and the immediate postictal seizure state, although the following favor the latter diagnosis: (1) isotope scan showing normal flow with uptake immediately following seizure, which clears in 72 hours; (2) normal plain CT scan with enhancement in the gyral pattern without mass effect immediately after the seizure, which clears in 96 hours. Other pathologic conditions, including cystic and focal atrophic lesions, were demonstrated by CT, which obviated the need for angiography or air study (Fig. 16–6).

Partial seizures with complex symptomatology have been found to have an underlying pathological process in 25 percent of cases, and this may be as high as 75 percent if necropsy and surgical specimens showing Ammon's horn sclerosis are included. The majority of the tumors are slow-growing gliomas but meningiomas, cysts, hematomas, angiomas and inflammatory disorders have also been found.[20] In addition, Currie described abnormal angiographic findings and pneumographic abnormalities of the temporal horn due to nontumorous conditions in 33 percent.[21] It has been postulated that dis-

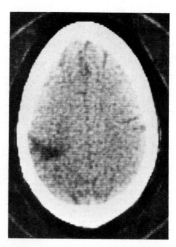

Figure 16–6. A 25-year-old man was initially evaluated because of episodes during which he felt that his right arm was being drawn up; this was followed by paresthesias beginning in his thumb and spreading up to his shoulder. These episodes began six months after he was hit with a heavy blunt metallic object over the left temporal region. There were no abnormal neurological findings and EEG showed random spikes in the left parietal area. CT scan showed a focal wedge-shaped, low-density region in the left parietal area that did not enhance or cause mass effect, a pattern consistent with focal atrophy.

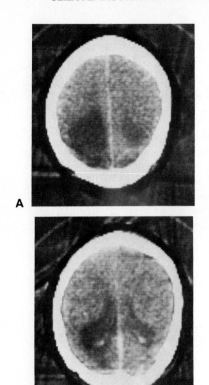

A

B

Figure 16–7. Examination of a 19-year-old woman who had psychomotor seizures showed right hemiparesis and homonymous hemianopia. EEG showed a delta pattern in the left parieto-occipital frontal region. CT findings: a large low-density, round, sharply marginated lesion in the left parieto-occipital region *(A)*, associated with dilatation of the atrial and occipital horn *(B)*. In addition, there is a similar but small region in the right hemisphere.

who, in addition to their psychomotor attacks, were also mentally retarded and had hemiplegia and visual field deficit. CT scan showed a focal well-marginated lesion located in the temporo-parietal-occipital region, which derived its arterial supply from the posterior cerebral artery.[22] These lesions were porencephalic cysts, which probably resulted from old cerebral infarctions, and this conclusion was consistent with the angiographic and pneumographic findings in such patients (Fig. 16–7). In addition, several patients with psychomotor epilepsy who showed a significant atrophic process by CT were found to have a characteristic isotope scan finding of decreased perfusion to the atrophic hemisphere with more prominent isotope uptake on the noninvolved side (Fig. 16–8). In the majority of patients with psychomotor epilepsy with abnormal CT findings, neurological examination was entirely normal, and the scan showed focal at-

turbances of the posterior cerebral artery cause infarction in the occipital, inferior and medial temporal cortex, and parahippocampal gyrus. Air studies have shown localized expansion of the temporal region adjacent to the uncus and hippocampus in two thirds of cases, and if the seizure disorder is poorly responsive to drug therapy, temporal lobectomy may be indicated.

Of 50 patients who were investigated because of psychomotor seizures, 40 percent had abnormal findings as compared with the results obtained by Gastaut of 30 focal and 20 diffuse lesions in 84 patients studied. The latter study included nine patients

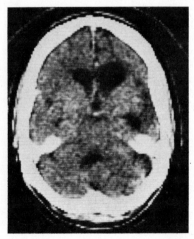

Figure 16–8. A 26-year-old man developed both primary generalized and psychomotor seizures four years following a blow to the right temporal region. EEG showed right temporal polymorphic delta activity intermixed with frequent spike discharges. Isotope scan revealed decreased perfusion in distribution of the right middle cerebral artery. CT findings: enlargement of right lateral ventricular system including temporal horn and sylvian cistern, consistent with focal atrophic process.

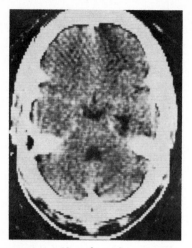

Figure 16–9. Neurological examination was normal in a 30-year-old man with psychomotor seizures. EEG showed a focal delta pattern with frequent spikes in the right temporal region; isotope scan, skull radiogram and echoencephalogram were negative. CT findings: the ventricular system was normal except for dilatation of the right temporal horn.

INFANTILE SPASMS (WEST SYNDROME)

This is associated with a characteristic hypsarrhythmia EEG pattern, and may occur in children who have a prior history of birth injury or pre- or postnatal infection and have had poor development prior to the onset of seizures, but may also occur in those who were entirely normal prior to the development of seizures. In those infants who were previously normal, evaluation should include metabolic studies and a careful search for any stigmata of neurocutaneous disorders. The most frequent as-

rophy, cystic lesions, or infarction. In rare cases patients who had had long-standing seizure disorders and had been well controlled on medication were proved by CT to have temporal gliomas.

Previous studies of patients with psychomotor epilepsy have indicated that the tumor may be located outside the temporal region. Analysis of CT findings revealed that one fourth of patients with psychomotor seizures and temporal lobe localization by EEG had lesions not involving the temporal lobe. If the epileptogenic foci are due to ischemic and gliotic pathological changes in the medial temporal region, air study is more sensitive in visualizing the temporal horns than CT utilizing the 13 mm tissue section. Because of the partial volume effect, these are poorly visualized unless enlarged by cortical atrophy or atrophic process (Fig. 16–9). In several cases in which unilateral temporal horn dilatation was detected by air study, this finding was not confirmed by CT.

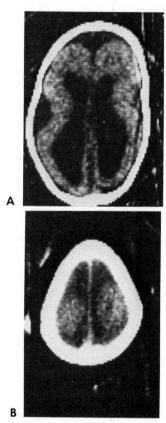

Figure 16–10. A and B, A nine-month-old child had poor neurological development and frequent seizures, poorly responsive to medication. EEG showed a hyporhythmic pattern without any focality. CT findings: dilated ventricular system and subarachnoid spaces with no evidence of sulcal markings over the convexities. Necropsy findings confirmed the diagnosis of lissencephaly. (Courtesy of Dr. David Dunn.)

sociated syndrome is tuberous sclerosis, and a skull radiogram may not show evidence of intracranial calcification; hypopigmented skin lesions or adenoma sebaceum also may not be clinically detectable at the early stage. With CT, it is frequently possible to identify the subependymal calcifications characteristic of this disorder. In addition, with CT it may be possible to define other developmental anomalies, including agenesis of the corpus callosum and focal or diffuse cortical atrophy, which have been associated with infantile spasm (Fig. 16–10).

LENNOX-GASTAUT SYNDROME

These children with petit mal variant (mixed minor motor seizures) characteristically are found to have symmetrical or asymmetrical slow spike and wave variant and are usually mentally retarded. As the child with infantile spasms matures, he may develop this seizure pattern and EEG may show this slow spike-and-wave pattern. Of 42 patients studied with CT by Gastaut, 60 percent showed abnormalities, which most frequently consisted of global or focal atrophy but also included several focal lesions, one a tumor localized to the parieto-occipital region. This is quite unexpected since it is believed that a diffuse process underlies this disorder.

EEG ABNORMALITIES

FOCAL SLOW PATTERN

In certain cases CT was performed because preliminary EEG studies were consistent with the presence of a focal structural lesion, despite the absence of neurological findings or a history of seizures. This EEG pattern usually consisted of unilateral theta or delta focus. In previous studies, Joynt investigated the predictive diagnostic value of focal delta activi-

ty; 70 percent of these patients had abnormal neurological findings and two thirds were proved to have vascular disease or neoplasm.[23] In one fifth of patients the delta pattern was not associated with any abnormal neurological findings on examination, and in these cases it was presumed to be related to epileptic disorder. In 10 percent the EEG abnormality was not associated with any definable neurological conditions. In these latter cases adequate follow-up was not available, but it was suggested that this electrophysiological pattern was an earlier sign of a focal structural lesion than epilepsy or clinical neurological findings.

The delta pattern was most usually located in the temporal region, and this localization is frequently a source of false EEG localization, as lesions in other areas may cause a delta pattern in the temporal region. Kooi has reported that after the age of 40 there is an increase in the incidence of this abnormality and this is postulated to be related to ischemia in this region. EEG focal or bilateral abnormalities are most prominent in the temporal region in cerebral infarction, regardless of the actual pathological site of the infarction.[24]

In addition, it is possible that localized degenerative pathological processes and normal aging changes first occur in the temporal region, and there is histological evidence that initial neuronal depopulation is most prominent in the temporal and frontal areas. Of 50 consecutive patients who were found to have a unilateral temporal delta pattern associated with either focal or diffuse neurological findings (not including clinical seizures), CT scan showed evidence of focal abnormality in 30, diffuse cerebral atrophic process in eight, hydrocephalus in two, and was normal in the remaining 10 patients. Of the 30 focal lesions, 20 were neoplasms, and in seven of these CT showed that the tumor predominantly involved areas other than the temporal region (including two cases in which the lesion was located in the posterior fossa), although necropsy and surgical confirmation was not always obtained. In 10 cases both plain and contrast CT scans were normal although three of these patients had mild focal neurological disturbances. Subsequent isotope scan and angiography were negative in these cases, and serial CT scans six to 12 months later were also normal.

In 20 other cases, a unilateral delta pattern was reported but was not associated with *any* abnormal neurological findings. Of these patients, three had CT evidence of a cerebral atrophic process, and within six months one patient showed clinical evidence of dementia. In two other patients, CT showed a pattern consistent with old middle cerebral artery syndrome. In 20 patients with bitemporal slow-wave pattern and no clinical symptoms. CT was entirely normal in all, and no further diagnostic studies were performed.

DIFFUSE SLOW PATTERN

There is general agreement that in senescence the frequency of the alpha rhythm is decreased, and that the amount of theta and delta activity increase. It is believed that the presence of diffuse slow-wave pattern is correlated with evidence of intellectual deterioration, and that the reduction in frequency of normal background pattern is an unusual finding in normal elderly patients.[25]

Also, the presence of a diffuse slow-wave pattern has been used to differentiate functional from organic brain disorders in some elderly patients.[26] Stefoski (1976) studied 35 patients with clinical evidence of dementia who were older than 59 years and then attempted to correlate CT estimation of ventricular size with the alteration of background pattern demonstrated on EEG.[27] Twenty-three percent of these patients with clinical evidence of dementia had normal EEG, 40 percent had mild generalized abnormality and 37 percent had severe generalized slowing of background pattern, but there was no significant correlation between mean ventricular size and diffuse EEG abnormality. Despite this general lack of correlation between EEG abnormality and CT scan evidence of a diffuse atrophic process, we have found that in those patients with dementia who also show evidence of generalized neurological disturbance (gait impairment, presence of primitive reflexes) almost all showed a bilateral slow-wave pattern with moderate to severe ventricular enlargement. In several cases, because of the gait impairment isotope cisternography was performed and was characteristic of hydrocephalus ex vacuo rather than communicating hydrocephalus.

Twenty patients were found to have a diffuse slow-wave pattern but had no clinical evidence of dementia, although complete psychometric evaluation was not performed. Of these, 10 had CT evidence of ventricular and sulcal enlargement as compared to controls matched for sex and age, and follow-up studies of these patients are presently being performed. It is suggested that the EEG is an earlier indicator of the presence of underlying pathological disorder than is clinical evaluation, and the CT scan is a still later indicator, which becomes abnormal only when there is significant loss of cerebral tissue.

MONORHYTHMIC FRONTAL DELTA PATTERN

The presence of the EEG pattern of monorhythmic frontal delta (MRFD) activity is usually believed to be an indicator of increased intracranial pressure, which on a statistical basis is most likely to be associated with a deep medio-frontal tumor. This is not a specific finding for either ventricular obstruction with resultant intracranial hypertension or tumor, as this pattern has been reported in multiple conditions, including idiopathic convulsive disorders, degenerative conditions, head injury and toxic-metabolic disturbances. The rhythmicity of the discharge may indicate that the region under suspicion is located at a distance and may only indirectly affect the frontal region. Of 100 cases of MRFD, 12 had lesions directly involving the brain stem, the deep midline structures or the posterior fossa, and of 37 lesions of these areas, 11 percent showed MRFD. Cordeau has suggested that supratentorial lesions may cause indirect brain stem compression to produce this discharge pattern.[28]

Ten patients were found to have this EEG pattern, and in all cases the patients presented with signs of intracranial hypertension and were found by CT to have obstructive hydrocephalus caused by neoplasm. In five cases the tumor was located in the medial temporal or deep frontal region, and in five the tumor was located in the posterior fossa. Eight other patients were found to have MRFD and clinically this was always associated with confused or delirious mentation but no funduscopic evidence of papilledema. CT was entirely normal in all cases and the etiology was toxic-metabolic abnormality. In these cases normal scan was reassuring to exclude mass lesion or ventricular obstruction and obviate the need for angiography.

REFERENCES

1. Wayne HH: Syncope. Am J Med 30:419, 1961.
2. Gastaut H, Gastaut JL: Computerized transverse axial tomography in epilepsy. Epilepsia 17:325, 1976.
3. Stevens JR: Focal abnormality in petit mal: intracranial recordings and pathological findings. Neurology 20: 1069, 1970.
4. O'Brien JL: EEG abnormalities in addition to bilaterally synchronous 3 per second spike and wave in petit mal. Electroencephalog Clin Neurophysiol 11:747, 1959.
5. Blackwood W, McMenenemy MA: Greenfield's Neuropathology. Arnold Co., London, 1963. pp 602–615.
6. Penfield W, Jasper HH: Epilepsy and the Functional Anatomy of the Brain. Little, Brown and Co, Boston, 1954. pp 50–65.
7. Wallace JC: Radionuclide brain scanning in investigation of late onset seizures. Lancet 2:1467, 1974.
8. Gilday DL, Reba HC: The role of brain scanning in the differential diagnosis of seizures. Canad Med Assoc J 106:1091, 1972.
9. Raynor RB, Paine RS, Carmichael EA: Epilepsy of late onset. Neurology 9:111, 1959.
10. Mosely IF, Bull IWD: CT in epilepsy. Epilepsia 17:339, 1976.
11. Richardson EP, Dodge PR: Epilepsy in cerebrovascular disease. Epilepsia 3:49, 1954.
12. Louis S, McDowell F: Epileptic seizures in non-embolic cerebral infarction. Arch Neurol 17:414, 1967.
13. Radermecker J: Epilespy in the degenerative diseases. In: Handbook of Clinical Neurology, PJ Vinken, GW Bruyn (eds), North Holland Publishing Co., Amsterdam, 1974. Vol 13, pp 342–346.
14. Sumi SM, Teasdall RD: Focal seizures. Neurology 13:582, 1963.
15. Vermess M, Stein SC: Angiography in idiopathic focal epilepsy, Radiology 111:120, 1972.
16. Bogdanoff BC, Stafford CR: Computerized transaxial tomography in evaluation of patients with focal epilepsy. Neurology 25:1013, 1975.
17. Golden GS: Radionuclide brain scan in convulsive disorders. Pediatrics 49: 787, 1972.
18. Prensky AL, Swisher CN, DeVivo DC: Positive brain scans in children with idiopathic focal epileptic seizures. Neurology 23:798, 1973.
19. Yarnell PR, Burdick D, Snaders B: Focal seizures, early veins, and increased flow. Neurology 24:512, 1974.
20. Falconer MA, Serafetinides EA, Corsellis JA. Etiology and pathogenesis of temporal lobe epilepsy. Arch Neurol 10:233, 1964.

21. Currie S, Heathfield WG, Henson RA, et al: Clinical course and prognosis of temporal lobe epilepsy. Brain 94:173, 1971.
22. Remillard GM, Ethier R, Andermann F: Temporal lobe epilepsy and perinatal occlusion of the posterior cerebral artery. Neurology 24:1001, 1974.
23. Joynt RJ, Cape CA, Knott JR: Focal delta activity in adult EEG. Arch Neurol 12:631, 1965.
24. Kooi KA, Guvener AM: Electroencephalographic patterns of the temporal region in normal adults. Neurology 14:1029, 1964.
25. Obrist WD: EEG of normal aged adults. Electroencephalog Clin Neurophysiol 6:235, 1954.
26. Tomlinson BE, Blessed G, Roth M: Observations on brains of demented old people. J Neurol Sci 11:205, 1970.
27. Stefoski D, Bergen D: Correlation between diffuse EEG abnormalities and cerebral atrophy in senile dementia. J Neurol Neurosurg Psychiatry 39:751, 1976.
28. Cordeau JP: Monorhythmic frontal delta activity in the human EEG. Electroencephalog Clin Neurophysiol 11:733, 1956.

Chapter 17 Visual Symptoms

CT examination of the orbital region is possible by means of the head scanner, but complete examination with detailed anatomical resolution requires special x-ray beam collimation to reduce tissue section thickness to 3 to 4 mm. The orbital scan is usually performed with zero degree angulation but 10° angulation may be necessary to visualize completely the course of the optic nerve. Utilizing standard 8 mm collimators, a single scan sequence will examine a pair of 8 mm transverse sections above and below midplane of the orbit, whereas with 3 to 4 mm collimation, six to ten consecutive sections provide detailed orbital anatomy with no significant increase in total radiation dose.[12] A window width of 200 provides optimal contrast resolution to outline low-density retrobulbar fat space and to contrast this with high-density thin orbital bone, optic nerve and extraocular muscles, with minimal computer artifact.

The normal anatomical structures visualized by CT include the following:

1. Medial and lateral walls of the orbit, which meet at the posterior limit of the orbit (apex) to form a triangular space, with the globe forming the anterior junction.

2. The confluence of recti muscles (muscle cone) is seen as a high-density region at the posterior apex and may stimulate a pathological lesion, especially if the insertion of the individual muscles is not seen, as may occur with an 8 mm tissue section.

3. Extraocular muscles are best individually visualized with thin sections and are inconsistently seen with 8 mm sections. The medial and lateral recti are most frequently visualized at the midorbital level; they parallel the orbital walls and, if contiguous, may not be seen. The superior and inferior recti are seen only if they are pathologically enlarged, and the oblique muscles are not visualized because of their position relative to the scanner angulation.

4. The optic nerve has a thickness of 5 to 6 mm and with 8 mm sections it may be subject to a partial volume effect, but its entire course may be outlined by thin sections. The nerve has a uniform density and thickness and its course is fairly straight but may be slightly curved; an increase in density, nodularity or distortion of its course should raise suspicion of a retro-orbital lesion.[1]

5. Retro-orbital fat has a density of −10 to +10 and this provides good contrast to accentuate the relatively higher density of muscle cone, optic nerve and most orbital pathological lesions, which are almost always of high density.

6. The globe appears as a round structure that has a high-density peripheral rim due to the sclera and attached musculature. The lens has horizontal orientation and appears as an oval high-density structure; the central portion of the globe is of low density, consistent with the fluid content of vitreous and aqueous.

7. The lateral wall of the orbit is made up of the greater wing of the sphenoid and this separates the orbit from the middle cranial fossa. The medial wall of the orbit separates the orbit from the ethmoid and sphenoid

sinuses, and since it is thin in several regions it may appear discontinuous, simulating erosive change. If the section includes the roof or floor of the orbit, this may simulate a high-density lesion.

8. The optic canal and superior orbital fissure are usually visualized at the orbital apex, and may be distinguished only with thin section.

CLINICAL APPLICATIONS

Evaluation of the patient with exophthalmos is the most frequent reason for referral for orbital CT scan. It may be defined as the abnormal prominence of one or both globes, resulting from a neoplastic, vascular, inflammatory or endocrine process.[3, 4] In addition, there are cases in which there is globe prominence due to an asymmetry of the orbit or face but no definite anterior displacement of the globe. The actual degree of displacement may be measured with the Hertel exophthalmometer, and may also be accurately confirmed by midorbital CT section by measuring a line drawn from the anterior portion of the globe directly through the lens to a point drawn between the zygomatic processes, with correction for scan size factor; this measurement is normally less than 21 mm.[1]

Thyroid Ophthalmopathy

This is the most frequent cause of bilateral or unilateral exophthalmos, and if unilateral the suspicion of an orbital neoplasm is raised. Most patients have clinical and laboratory evidence of thyroid disease when visual symptoms occur, including exophthalmos, limitation of extraocular muscle motility and visual loss, but rarely ophthalmopathy may precede clinical hyperthyroidism. The patient may be euthyroid by measurement of thyroxine or triiodothyroxine, although antithyroid antibodies and an elevated titer for long-acting thyroid stimulator may be present or an abnormal eight-day tri-iodothyroxine suppression test may be recorded.[5]

If the eye findings are unilateral, orbital venography may need to be performed but this may be unsuccessful because of high intraocular pressure. This is the most sensitive invasive diagnostic study to differentiate endocrine ophthalmopathy from neoplasm. With ophthalmopathy there may be swelling of the muscle cone at the orbital apex with minimal displacement of veins, although this finding is quite rare in the absence of neoplasm.[6] Orbital neoplasms show early compression or displacement of the superior ophthalmic vein. A normal venogram usually excludes orbital apical tumor, whereas negative angiography is of little diagnostic help.

Orbital (B-mode) ultrasonography is a most sensitive study to detect the swollen muscles in ophthalmopathy and may show abnormalities even if patients have no clinical symptoms. Other findings include erosion of retrobulbar fat and reduplication echoes of the optic nerve, consistent with perineural inflammation. If clinical findings are unilateral, ultrasonography is sensitive enough to detect subclinical change in the opposite eye, and this may obviate the need for contrast procedures.[7, 8] Initial studies indicated that CT was less sensitive than ultrasound, and CT abnormalities were visualized only if the patient had limitation of eye movement, visual loss or proptosis, but if the symptoms were present in one eye, CT detected abnormalities in the opposite clinically uninvolved eye.[9]

Midorbital CT sections most frequently demonstrate enlargement of the extraocular muscle in the lateral and medial recti; superior and inferior recti enlargement may be seen with additional sections but oblique muscles are not usually seen. In the majority of cases the apex of the mus-

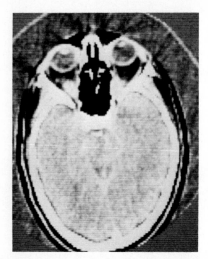

Figure 17–1. This patient underwent thyroidectomy three months previously and has developed bilateral proptosis. CT findings: bilateral proptosis, greater on right side, with enlargement of apical muscle cone with both lateral and medial recti enlargement. Ultrasound demonstrated enlarged muscles, consistent with endocrine ophthalmopathy.

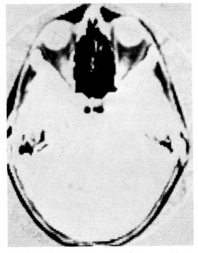

Figure 17–2. A patient with a previous history of medically treated hyperthyroidism, which was in remission, with normal thyroid function studies (including LATS, titer and antithyroid antibodies) has now developed proptosis, diplopia and impaired ocular motility but no visual impairment. CT findings: enlargement of lateral and medial recti with marked prominence of apical muscle cone. In addition, it appears that the optic nerve is thickened and is of homogeneous density, extending to the posterior portion of the globe.

cle cone is enlarged, and this is usually associated with medial and lateral recti thickening (Fig. 17–1). Utilization of thin section has made possible resolution of certain apical lesions — for example, an enlarged inferior rectus muscle which may be confused with tumor — and Hilal has emphasized the well-marginated lateral boundary of the muscle with a feathering effect anteriorly.[1, 6]

The following CT findings have been detected in endocrine ophthalmopathy: proptosis alone, muscle enlargement. thickening of the optic nerve, and anterior prolapse of the orbital septum due to excessive orbital fat; however, the density of the retro-orbital fat does not differ from that in normal patients, as fat erosion and polysaccharide deposits have not been detected by CT (Fig. 17–2). The CT scan finding of thickening of the optic nerve with no change in density did not correlate with clinical evidence of visual loss or optic atrophy, but others have reported optic nerve thickening only in the most severe cases of ophthalmopathy.[6]

PROPTOSIS WITHOUT ANY DEFINABLE ETIOLOGY

If the head is positioned slightly oblique to the x-ray source, the beam cuts through the globe and lens at different levels on the two sides; this has the effect of making one eye appear larger and seem to extend further forward, creating the illusion of proptosis. In other cases marked proptosis may be present, but CT may show no abnormal density or muscle enlargement and no abnormality is subsequently defined by ultrasound or venography. In the absence of thickened extraocular muscles it is unlikely that this represents endocrine ophthalmopathy, but it may be due to orbital pseudotumor (Fig. 17–3); however, Jacobs reported one patient with breast carcinoma whose scan showed only proptosis

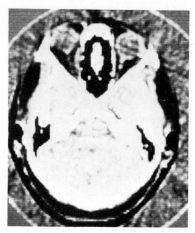

Figure 17–3. A 30-year-old woman with un-ilateral exophthalmos and limitation of move-ment in the left eye only had negative thyroid studies. CT findings: proptosis of left eye with enlarged left medial rectus, consistent with orbital inflammatory disease. Tomogram of orbits and sinus showed no bony abnormality; ultrasound demonstrated left medial rectus enlargement.

but orbital exploration subsequently revealed orbital metastases.[2]

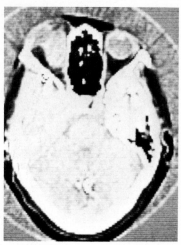

Figure 17–4. An elderly patient who had painless proptosis in the left eye for 12 years recently developed visual impairment in that eye. CT findings: a dense nonenhancing, nonhomo-geneous mass displacing the globe laterally and causing proptosis; this extends anteriorly without displacement of the left optic nerve. Angiography was negative and venography showed vascular displacement; surgical exploration showed lym-phocytic infiltration and diffuse edema, consis-tent with diagnosis of orbital pseudotumor.

ORBITAL INFLAMMATORY DISEASE

Pseudotumor of the orbit is a dis-order characterized clinically by proptosis, impaired ocular motility, visual loss and orbital pain. If the findings are unilateral it may simulate orbital neoplasm or endocrine ophth-almopathy, and if bilateral this dis-order must be differentiated from en-docrine disease by exclusion of clinical or laboratory evidence of thy-roid disease.[10] Ultrasound may detect generalized or focal areas of widely spaced echoes due to edema, gran-uloma formation and lymphocytic in-filtration of normal retrobulbar fat. Bi-opsy shows evidence of lymphocytic infiltration with fibrosis and nonspe-cific granuloma and there is clinical response to corticosteroid therapy, al-though differentiation from euthyroid ophthalmopathy is not always possi-ble. The clinical course is frequently nonprogressive, which permits dif-ferentiation from neoplastic condi-tions (Fig. 17–4). Enzmann reported

CT findings in this disorder included the following: (1) high-density lesions in the retro-orbital space that were asymmetrical; they encircled and at-tached to the globe posteriorly; (2) vague poorly marginated thickening of recti muscles; (3) an enlarged optic nerve most prominent at the posterior edge of the globe, obliteration of low-density retro-orbital fat space, and oc-casionally a diffuse enhancement pat-tern.[11]

Since the clinical findings in orbital pseudotumor are usually unilateral, the finding of bilateral abnormalities vis-ualized by CT scan would exclude mass lesion, but differentiation from endocrine ophthalmopathy is more un-certain. Hilal has reported the follow-ing patterns in this disorder: proptosis alone; enlargement of muscles and high-density lesion in retrobulbar fat. In the latter group, orbital venography may still be required to exclude neo-plasm, but an alternate approach would be a therapeutic trial of corticosteroids and repeat CT scan one month later. In addition, CT distinguishes orbital myositis (myositic pseudotumor) from nonmyositic pseudotumor, and following treatment the abnormal densities revert to normal. CT may demonstrate extension of certain inflammatory conditions to retrobulbar fat space, and define the presence and location of the involvement. Systemic granulomatous disease, including sarcoidosis, histiocytosis, and Wegener's and midline granulomatosis, may also involve the retro-orbital space, and CT shows a diffuse speckled high-density appearance, which may completely fill the retro-orbital space, with loss of detail of the optic nerve and muscles.[1]

ORBITAL TUMORS

The incidence of orbital tumors includes metastatic tumors and those arising from direct spread from carcinoma of the sinus (10 percent), vascular malformation (15 percent), orbital pseudotumor (13 percent), lymphoma (9 percent), glioma (7 percent), meningioma (5 percent), rhabdomyosarcoma (5 percent), lacrimal gland tumor (5 percent), melanoma (4 percent) and dermoid (4 percent), although the most frequent cause of unilateral exophthalmos is still endocrine ophthalmopathy.[3]

Initial evaluation of patients with unilateral exophthalmos and visual loss should include plain skull radiograph with views of the superior orbital fissure and optic foramina; a diameter of greater than 6.5 mm or an asymmetry of more than one millimeter of the optic foramina is suggestive of an optic glioma. If the lesion extends intracranially, abnormalities of the sphenoid bone and sella region may be detected most sensitively with polytomography. In addition, the paranasal sinus and nasopharynx region must be completely evaluated radiographically for evidence of bony change by tumor arising in this region.

Ultrasound is a highly sensitive procedure to detect the presence of a retro-orbital mass, especially those located anteriorly toward the globe, but it is less sensitive if the lesion is located adjacent to the orbital walls or near the apex. This technique utilizes ultrasound to produce echoes at physical interphases between structures having differing acoustical transmission qualities. In B-scan display a transverse axial section is visualized with the amplitude of the echo modulating its brightness; the display orientation is similar to that of CT.

Orbital tumors distort the retro-orbital fat pattern and may be classified as solid if they transmit sound poorly, whereas cystic and vascular tumors, which are fluid-filled, have good acoustical transmission properties. Of those with good sound transmission, cystic tumors have a rounder anterior border because of tissue homogeneity, whereas angiomas have irregular borders. Of the solid tumors with poor acoustical properties, malignant infiltrative tumors have irregular borders, whereas neurogenic tumors have a regular rounded anterior border.[12]

Carotid angiography is most helpful to define intracranial extension of orbital tumors and to detect carotid-cavernous fistula. It is frequently negative in orbital tumors, including vascular tumors such as hemangioma, even if magnification and subtraction techniques are used, because of vascular anatomical variability and lack of vascular displacement. In certain vascular malformations (hemangioma, orbital varix), the major arterial supply is less prominent than the venous circulation, and orbital venography is more sensitive in detecting venous displacement and pooling of dye.[13, 14]

In one study assessing sensitivity of CT in the diagnosis of the orbital tumors, CT had 93 percent accuracy with 8 mm section and fine matrix system compared with 71 percent for axial hypocycloidal tomography, 76 percent for ultrasound, 84 percent for venography and 25 percent for carotid angiography. CT was inaccurate in three cases. One tumor of the anterior portion of the optic nerve was detected by ultrasound and not by CT. One recurrent tumor was obscured by scar tissue and not detected by ultrasound or CT. One lesion was defined as tumor by CT and ultrasound, but biopsy showed granuloma.[13]

In the evaluation of suspected orbital lesions, CT is complementary to hypocycloidal tomography and ultrasound and may decrease the need for venography and angiography unless an intracranial component or carotid cavernous fistula is suspected. CT is superior to ultrasound in the posterior orbital region but may be less sensitive for small tumors of the optic nerve sheath; combined CT and ultrasound accuracy was reported as 97 percent for orbital tumor diagnosis. Conventional tomography may be superior for small lesions along the ridge of the sphenoid bone or tumors arising from the roof or floor of the orbit before they extend into retrobulbar fat space, but may be negative for many intraorbital tumors if clinical symptoms develop before invasion of bone has occurred.

Optic Glioma. Plain skull radiogram shows abnormalities of the optic foramina, chiasmatic sulcus, or shape of sella in 90 percent of cases. Ultrasound is highly reliable in showing localized widening of nerve, with sharply defined round anterior borders having poor acoustic transmission, thus differentiating this from malignant, cystic and vascular tumors. These findings may be identical to those in meningioma except that meningiomas show more widespread thickening of nerve. CT shows fusiform expansion of the optic nerve with nonhomogeneous increased density and only slight enhancement (Fig. 17–5). Because of the high contrast provided by the retro-orbital fat space, it has been possible to detect gliomas less than 13 mm in diameter.[1, 2]

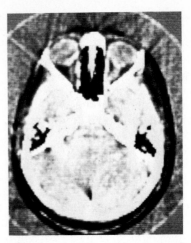

Figure 17–5. A patient with a previously documented optic glioma in the right eye; scan shows irregularly shaped fusiform dilatation of the right optic nerve. No enhancement was detected.

Because of the possibility of intracranial extension to the anterior suprasellar region, visualization of the suprasellar cistern following contrast enhancement should always be performed.

Meningioma. In patients who present with proptosis, meningioma arising from four sites should be considered, including the sphenoid ridge, olfactory groove, tuberculum sellae, and intra-orbitally from the sheath of the optic nerve. Conventional radiography and ultrasound may fail to detect small tumors of the nerve sheath or posterior apex region. CT may show evidence of diffuse and smooth thickening of the optic nerve, with a denser enhancement pattern than that of glioma, and both tumors may cause intracranial extension.[8] The tumors may show round calcific areas and are characteristically round and lobular, whereas gliomas are fusiform and elongated (Fig. 17–6).

Hemangioma. These have been found to be the most common primary intraorbital tumor. Patients may present with proptosis, which may be pulsatile, and there may be other associated vascular lesions in the eyelid and subconjunctival space. Radio-

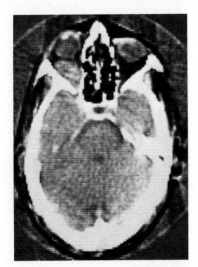

Figure 17–6. A patient with proptosis and decreased acuity in the left eye. Skull radiograms including optic foramina views, were negative. CT findings: plain scan shows speckled, calcific oval mass which enhances in left retrobulbar space. Operativé diagnosis: intraorbital meningioma.

gram may show erosion and enlargement of the optic foramina, soft-tissue density or calcification in the orbit. Ultrasound shows an irregularly shaped mass with excellent acoustical qualities due to blood-filled spaces,

whereas circulation is most reliably detected by venography. CT shows an encapsulated lesion that displaces the optic nerve and extraocular muscles medially and is completely separated from these structures. Diverse results have been reported with contrast infusion. Although angiography shows these tumors to be avascular there may be dense enhancement; others have reported no density change following infusion (Fig. 17–7).

Metastatic Tumors. In children neuroblastoma and leukemia are the

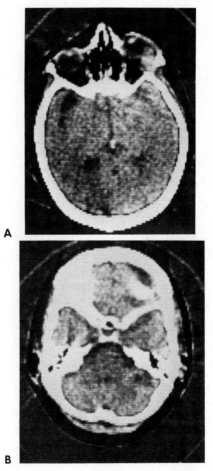

A

B

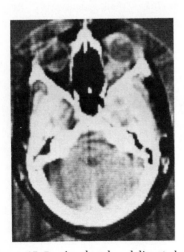

Figure 17–7. A sharply delineated high-density retro-orbital mass extends medially to involve the sinus; it did not enhance following infusion. The optic nerve was normal and well visualized on a lower section. Operative findings: orbital hemangioma. (Courtesy of Dr. Roger Tutton, Ochsner Foundation Hospital.)

Figure 17–8. A 70-year-old woman with proptosis, which developed two years after surgical treatment for right lacrimal gland adenocarcinoma. CT findings: proptosis, with medial and forward displacement of the right globe by tumor in right superior lateral aspect of the globe (A); tumor extends posteriorly (B).

most frequent causes of orbital involvement, whereas in adults lymphoma and myeloma are most frequent.[4] Radiogram shows bony change and ultrasound shows an irregular poorly marginated lesion with poor sound transmission. CT may show an irregularly shaped mass that extends to bone, but these do not have distinctive enough CT features to differentiate from other orbital tumors.

Lacrimal Tumors. They arise in the upper outer quadrant of the orbit and may extend into retrobulbar space and medially displace the lateral rectus muscle. These tumors may be benign (dermoid or epidermoid). CT scan shows a sharply marginated high-density lesion, whereas lacrimal gland carcinomas have poorly defined margins (Fig. 17–8).

Paranasal Sinus Tumors. Tumors of the ethmoid and sphenoid sinuses may be visualized by CT, showing bony change in the sinus, displacement of orbit and muscle but usually no involvement of the optic nerve.

Cysts. Dermoids, epidermoids and mucoceles are cystic tumors that are well defined by ultrasound. Because of their fat content and low-density appearance with CT, it may be possible that they are not visualized owing to lack of effective contrast, but dermoids have also been found to be round, smoothly contoured high-density lesions. Because of the variable CT appearance, ultrasound is a more reliable diagnostic study.

TRAUMA

Proptosis may develop following direct injury to the eye, which may involve a retrobulbar hematoma, inflammation or a foreign body. Metallic objects are well detected as very high-density lesions, but they cause

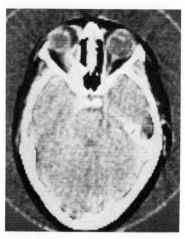

Figure 17–9. This patient lost vision in his left eye following an automobile accident and 14 months later began developing proptosis in the left eye. CT findings: a high-density mass in the medial region of the left orbit; it does not involve the optic nerve and does not enhance. Orbital exploration showed this to be a foreign body — a fragment of wood — without surrounding granuloma formation.

significant artifact; and glass is poorly detected. Occasionally wood may be detected as a high-density mass even if significant granuloma formation has not occurred (Fig. 17–9). Following surgery, CT may reliably detect hematoma as well as ultrasound can, and serial studies may obviate the need for surgery.

NONTUMOROUS OPTIC NERVE ABNORMALITIES

In rare instances of optic atrophy that has resulted from prolonged intracranial hypertension, there may be thickening of the optic nerve. In other patients with bilateral optic atrophy of unknown etiology, a similar change may be detected. Following operations, a high-density linear pattern may suggest the presence of "phantom" optic nerve, and this may be due to fibrosis.[1]

REFERENCES

1. Hilal SK, Trokel SL: CT of the orbit using thin sections. Semin Roentgenol 12:137, 1977.
2. Jacobs L, Kinkel W: CT in the diagnosis of orbital tumors. Trans Am Acad Ophthalmol Otolaryngol 81:305, 1976.
3. Grove AS: Evaluation of exophthalmos. N Engl J Med 292:1005, 1975.
4. Smigiel MR, MacCarty CS: Exophthalmos. Mayo Clin Proc 50:345, 1975.
5. Werner SC, Coleman DJ, Franzen LA: Ultrasound evidence of a consistent orbital involvement in Graves disease. N Engl J Med 290:1447, 1974.
6. Brismar J, Davis KR, Dallow RL, Brismar G: Unilateral endrocrine exophthalmos — diagnostic problems in association with computed tomography. Neuroradiology 12:21, 1976.
7. Coleman DJ, Jack RL, Franzen LA: Eye changes in thyroid disease. Arch Ophthalmol 88:465, 1972.
8. Dallow RL, Momose KJ, Weber AL, Wray SH: Comparison of ultrasonography, computed tomography, and radiographic techniques in evaluation of exophthalmos. Trans Am Acad Ophthalmol Otolaryngol 81:305, 1976.
9. Enzmann D, Marshall WH: CT in Graves ophthalmopathy. Radiology 118:615, 1976.
10. Jellinek EH: The orbital pseudotumor syndrome and its differentiation from endocrine exophthalmos. Brain 92:35, 1969.
11. Enzmann D, Donaldson SS: CT in orbital pseudotumor. Radiology 120:597, 1976.
12. Coleman DJ: Reliability of ocular and orbital diagnosis with B-scan ultrasound. 2. Orbital diagnosis. Am J Ophthalmol 74:704, 1972.
13. Gawler J, Saunders MD: CAT in orbital disease. Br J Ophthalmol 58:571, 1974.
14. Hobbs HE, duBouloy G, Davis RE: Orbital angioma diagnosed by phlebography. Br J Ophthalmol 44:551, 1960.

Chapter 18 Calcification

Deposition of calcium is frequently found at routine necropsy examination in the brain parenchyma, blood vessels, and surrounding structures, although this is less frequently detected by plain skull radiograph. Histochemical studies may show basophilic vascular granular deposits containing iron and copper that are not detected radiographically because they are not sufficiently dense or radiopaque; therefore, the presence of radiopacity usually correlates with the histochemical demonstration of calcium.[1]

These deposits in brain parenchyma or blood vessels may be caused by pathological processes or may occur in the absence of any known pathological disorder. Since calcification is exceedingly rare in children and increases in frequency with age, it has been suggested that this represents a degenerative or "aging" process. These siderocalcific deposits may be detected most frequently in the globus pallidus, striatum, hippocampus and cerebellar white matter. Iron deposits have been reported in the basal ganglia in both Hallervorden-Spatz disease and infantile neuroaxonal dystrophy, and copper is deposited in the basal ganglia in Wilson's disease but is not detected by radiographic analysis. In patients who are at risk for having Wilson's disease but are neurologically asymptomatic, CT may detect high-density areas due to copper deposition or low-density areas due to degenerative change in the basal ganglia and thus afford another indicator of CNS involvement. With CT, the sensitivity for detecting intracranial calcification is greater than with conventional radiography and tomography but the *spatial* resolution is less accurate in defining the specific pattern.

Pineal body calcification may be detected in 60 to 80 percent of radiographs of patients 20 years or older. It is most readily appreciated on lateral skull radiograph but determination of a shift from its usual midline position is most readily evaluated from the anteroposterior projection, since this requires a simple measurement rather than complex formulae. Occasionally, the pineal may be obscured by the thick midline occiput in Towne views or the frontal sinus in frontal projection. If frontal tomography is also utilized, it is possible to visualize the pineal in 40 percent of cases in which it is not clearly detected by routine view.

In routine CT scan, the pineal was visualized in 75 percent of patients older than 20 and 94 percent over age 40. Because the pineal is surrounded by low-density CSF, it may be visualized with CT even if it is not calcified; this accounts for more frequent detection with CT. It is significant that in patients who had funduscopic evidence of papilledema and increased intracranial pressure determined by CSF examination, this structure was visualized in a significantly lower incidence (40 to 50 percent), suggesting that there was demineralization analogous to sella turcica changes in long-standing intracranial hypertension. In addition, if there were plain skull radiographic changes of intracranial hypertension in the absence of papilledema, the pineal was also usually poorly visualized by CT.

Because of the small size of the Polaroid picture, it may be difficult to make an accurate assessment of pineal displacement. In most cases a significant shift may be appreciated without difficulty but occasionally the shift is small or equivocal. Hahn has devised a technique that magnifies the scan picture and then measures the calvarial diameter and pineal distance from the inner table and expresses the percentage of pineal shift normalized to the calvarial diameter. The diameter ranges from 31 to 37 mm so that a shift of 0.9 mm represents a 2.6 percent shift; 99 percent of normal cases show less shift.[3]

In 5 percent of cases, CT was performed because the skull radiograph visualized a pineal shift. CT scan demonstrated that multiple calcifications were present, especially in the ambient or quadrigeminal cisternal region and the tentorium, which perhaps had been incorrectly identified as the pineal by skull radiograph. CT reliably identified the midline pineal position.

Other intracranial structures that are infrequently seen on plain skull radiograph include the glomera of the choroid plexus (10 percent), the habenular complex (30 percent), the basal ganglia and dentate of the cerebellum (2 percent) and the falx cerebri (7 to 9 percent), but these are more frequently detected by CT.[4] In addition, the finding of intraparenchymal calcification by CT has led to subsequent angiography for suspected angioma or neoplasm, but in many cases no etiology was detected. Dense calcification in the atrial portion of the lateral ventricle is common and asymmetrical displacement may indicate the location of the tumor. Unfortunately, asymmetrical location of this calcification in different portions of the glomera may falsely suggest the presence of the tumor. The choroid plexus is visualized on 77 percent of CT scans in patients older than 45 and in 40 percent in patients 20 to 44 years old; in one third of cases they are asymmetrical in location.

The falx may show calcification, especially in its anterior aspect; this may be a linear band or a thick plaque and may be visualized by CT even when it consists of thick fibrous sheets without calcification.[5] The finding of dense plaque in the falx with CT was suggestive of meningioma, but failure to enhance following infusion and negative isotope scan made this diagnosis unlikely, and in several cases angiography was subsequently negative.

Calcification in the petroclinoid ligament, arachnoid granulation, and diaphragma sella are better visualized with conventional radiography. The presence of intrasellar calcification occurring in association with an otherwise normal sella turcica may occur with tumor or aneurysm but may also occur with pituitary calculi. In these cases, the patient has no endocrine or visual symptoms and the contrast CT study shows no enhancement.[6]

In pathological conditions, calcification occurs in tissue undergoing necrosis and hyaline degeneration. If it is of sufficient size and density, it may be seen on radiogram but more frequently it is visualized by CT. In certain cases, the CT findings are so diagnostic that they may obviate the necessity for angiography.

Tuberous Sclerosis. In 40 to 50 percent of cases, calcification is demonstrated by radiography as multiple round radiopaque areas located along the walls of the lateral ventricles as well as in the superficial cortex. These are believed to represent foci of cortical gliosis containing abnormal neuronal and glial elements. If the periventricular tubers are not sufficiently calcified, air study is necessary to outline the nodular masses projecting into the surface of the ventricles. Some children may initially present with mental retardation and seizures but lack the cutaneous manifestations of the disorder, and CT may suggest the diagnosis without an air study (Fig. 18–1). In addition, subependymal and intraventricular giant cell astrocytomas may occur in this disorder, and these round high-

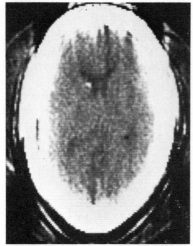

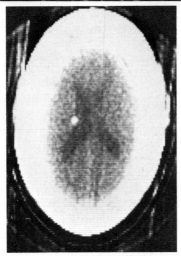

Figure 18–1. A and B, A two-year-old child with delayed development was evaluated for seizures; there were no abnormalities of skin, bone or viscera. CT shows multiple round, high-density, periventricular areas, with normal ventricular system, a pattern characteristic of tuberous sclerosis.

in the walls of the capillary-venous malformation. The complete syndrome includes trigeminal port-wine stain due to the angioma, seizures, mental retardation and intracranial calcification but may be incomplete; CT may demonstrate calcification before radiogram. Although the high-density region is believed to represent calcification in the cortical gyri, it may partly be related to the malformation itself, since enhancement may occur.

Disorders of Calcium Metabolism.
In idiopathic hypoparathyroidism, pseudohypoparathyroidism and hyperparathyroidism there may be metastatic calcification with deposition of calcium intracranially, especially in the basal ganglia, dentate nucleus, and rarely in the cortex. It is believed related to deposition of colloid material in and around walls of blood vessels; the material then calcifies. The specific predilection for these anatomic sites is not known.[7] Despite the frequency (45 to 55 percent) of these calcifications, clinical symptoms are

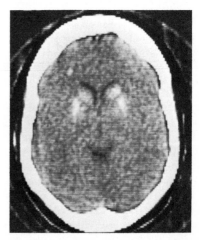

Figure 18–2. A 25-year-old woman had generalized seizures of nine years' duration, poorly controlled with medication. Neurological and general physical examinations were completely normal, including absence of Chvostek and Trousseau signs. CT scan showed multiple calcification in the frontal lobes, caudate nucleus and globus pallidus. This finding led to further laboratory studies, which demonstrated low calcium and elevated phosphorus.

density lesions that cause ventricular obstruction may be detected by CT.

Sturge-Weber Syndrome. Calcification may be detected in 50 to 60 percent of patients but is not usually seen radiographically in younger patients until the calcification becomes denser, and by the teens this is invariably present. The calcium is deposited in the underlying atrophic cortex in a characteristic "tram or railroad track" pattern and is not located

rare. In several cases the metabolic evaluation was initiated on the basis of a CT abnormality that suggested this diagnosis (Fig. 18–2). In other patients who have clinical disorders involving the basal ganglia, calcification of these structures may rarely be demonstrated by CT only. Detection of this abnormality is an important finding, since the movement disorders in these patients may be refractory to drug therapy.

Infectious-Inflammatory Conditions. Certain viral (cytomegalic inclusion-body disease), parasitic (toxoplasmosis, cysticercosis, schistosomiasis, paragonimiasis, echinococcosis) and tuberculous ·infections cause intracranial calcification. In toxoplasmosis, CT may detect multiple scattered periventricular high-density lesions, which may be associated with hydrocephalus (Fig. 18–3). Tuberculous granuloma shows solitary high-density nodules, which may be single or solitary, and CT may detect an enhancing lesion that may not be differentiated from other abscesses or neoplasms. Old healed lesions may show evidence of intraparenchymal calcification.

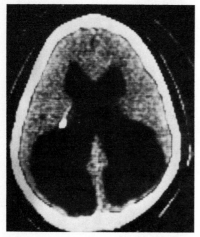

Figure 18–3. A four-year-old child with a history of congenital toxoplasmosis. CT findings: severe hydrocephalus, with a round area of calcification in the periventricular region on the left side, consistent with calcified nodules of toxoplasmosis.

Vascular Lesions. Aneurysms that show radiographically demonstrable calcification include those of basilar, middle cerebral and carotid origin. Plain skull radiogram shows a curvilinear or solitary ring if the diameter is less than 2 cm, whereas aneurysms exceeding 2 cm show dense egg-shaped calcification.[8] With CT it is possible to outline the calcification in the wall; it is deposited in fibrous tissue that has replaced the normal muscular and elastic component of the vessel wall. Dense clumps or lamellated rings of high-density material probably represent calcification in a thrombus in the sac of the aneurysm. CT evaluation may be important, as the sac of the aneurysm may be completely filled with clot, and angiography may not visualize the aneurysm. The plain skull radiographic evidence of calcification in angiomas is 10 to 25 percent, and appears as curvilinear, multiple flecks or dense clumps. Of 15 angiomas, plain CT showed high density calcification in seven cases and in only one was there radiographic evidence of calcification.

Neoplasms. The incidence of calcification in tumors is highest in the slow-growing and less malignant lesions.[9] Grade I astrocytoma, oligodendroglioma and meningioma are much more likely to show calcification on plain skull radiogram, and histological evidence of calcification may be even more frequent in these neoplasms. Glioblastoma, medulloblastoma and metastatic neoplasms are unlikely to demonstrate radiographic calcification because of their rapid growth despite the presence of foci of hemorrhage and necrosis. Glioblastoma and medulloblastoma show radiographic calcification in less than 1 percent of cases, whereas ependymomas calcify in 15 percent. Utilizing preinfusion CT study, the incidence of calcification in both medulloblastoma and glioblastoma has been approximately 5 to 10 percent; the appearance has varied from speckled areas to dense globular deposits. Oligodendroglioma invariably showed densely calcified regions, and in Grade I and II astrocytoma calcification is a prominent finding and is more frequent than the 25 percent reported with plain skull radiogram.

CT scan was entirely accurate in predicting the presence of macroscopic calcification, and in no pathologically verified case had CT not predicted its presence. Despite the presence of psammomatous bodies in meningiomas, radiographic evidence of calcification is not common although other bony changes are detected in 40 to 65 percent. In at least one half of meningiomas there was CT evidence of a mottled high-density region, which was believed to represent psammoma bodies. Of the sella tumors, craniopharyngioma may show a small dense clump of high-density material (60 to 80 units) although the actual tumor mass that is obstructing the intraventricular foramina may be isodense. Lipomas of the corpus callosum frequently calcify and in two cases CT showed a high-density mass on plain scan that had not been detected by radiography. Atypical teratoma and pinealoma may show calcification in the region of the anterior or posterior third ventricle, but this CT finding is not distinctive enough to permit definitive differential diagnosis from other lesions in this location. Both dermoid and epidermoid tumors may show nodular or curvilinear high-density areas associated with low-density well-marginated lesions, a pattern consistent with this diagnosis.

In several cases single or multiple discrete round high-density lesions (greater than 45 units) were detected by CT and were not associated with mass effect or any enhancement. In all cases a careful history excluded the possible etiologies of prior infection or vascular or metabolic disturbance. Isotope scan and EEG were

both normal, and skull radiogram did not visualize these calcifications. All patients had angiography and no underlying angioma or tumor was detected.

BONY ABNORMALITIES

Hyperostosis Frontalis Interna. There is thickening of the inner table, with sparing of the outer table, which tapers down toward the midline. It is not attached to the falx and this may help to differentiate from the bone change detected in meningioma. If the abnormal area is unila-

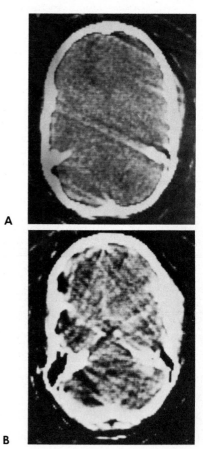

A

B

Figure 18–4. Skull radiography in a ten-year-old child showed evidence of fibrous dysplasia. CT findings: localized thickening of bone in the right temporal region (A), which shows striking enhancement (B). Angiography shows no evidence of tumor.

teral, tangential views and negative isotope scan usually exclude this diagnosis. With CT there may be high density and thickened bone, and there is no contrast enhancement or mass effect (Fig. 18–4).

Fibrous Dysplasia. Radiographically, there are hyperostotic lesions involving bones at the base of the skull and facial bones, with cystic lesions found in the diploic spaces. Patients with this condition may have nonelevated brown pigmented skin lesions and endrocrine dysfunction (precocious puberty). Pathologically, there is replacement of normal bone matrix by whorls of actively proliferating fibroblasts. Occasionally, localized radiographic changes may be consistent with meningioma, and isotope scan may show uptake by dysplastic bone. CT may demonstrate localized thickening of bone, and the presence of enhancement may also be detected, not always corresponding to cases with positive isotope scan (Fig. 18–5). Angiography may show no tumor.

Paget's Disease. In osteitis deformans there is an increase in density of bone with loss of normal architecture such that areas of bone destruction are filled with hyperplastic connective tissue. The diagnosis is established by skull radiograph with a characteristic pattern, and CT shows a thickened bone pattern.

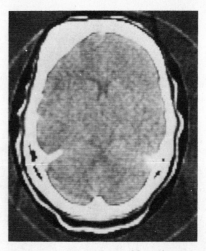

Figure 18–5. A 15-year-old girl presented with a generalized seizure disorder. Skull radiograph showed frontal hyperostosis and isotope scan was positive in the left frontal region. CT scan showed hyperostosis but no enhancement or parenchymal involvement, and subsequent angiography was negative.

Osteoma. Benign tumors may project externally from the other table or internally from the inner table. They have smooth contour with uniform density and CT shows localized high-density lesion.

Metastases. These osteolytic or blastic changes are defined by skull radiogram and sensitively detected by isotope bone scan. CT may show bone thickening with enhancement but this is less sensitive than conventional skull radiograph (Fig. 18–6).

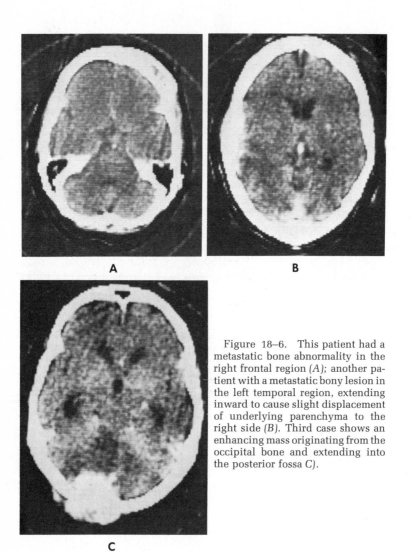

Figure 18–6. This patient had a metastatic bone abnormality in the right frontal region (A); another patient with a metastatic bony lesion in the left temporal region, extending inward to cause slight displacement of underlying parenchyma to the right side (B). Third case shows an enhancing mass originating from the occipital bone and extending into the posterior fossa C).

REFERENCES

1. Wagner JA, Slager UT: Incidence and composition of radiopaque deposits in basal ganglia of brain. Am J Roentgenol 74:232, 1955.
2. Goree JA, Wallace KK, Bean RL: The pineal tomogram: visualization of the faintly calcified pineal gland. Am J Roentgenol 89:1209, 1963.
3. Hahn FJY, Rim K, Schapiro RL: The normal range and position of the pineal gland on CT. Radiology 119:599, 1976.
4. Newton TH, Potts DG: Radiology of the Skull and Brain. CV Mosby, St. Louis. 1971. pp 823–830.
5. Bruyn GW: Calcification and ossification of the cerebral falx and superior longitudinal sinus. J Neurol Neurosurg Psychiatry 66:98, 1963.
6. DiChiro G: Pituitary stones. Ann Int Med 83:66, 1975.
7. Bennett JC, Maffy RH, Steinbach HL: The significance of bilateral basal ganglia calcification. Radiology 72:368, 1959.
8. Bull JWD: Massive aneurysms at the base of the brain. Brain 92:535, 1969.
9. Kalan C, Burrows EH: Calcification in intracranial gliomata. Br J Radiol 35:589, 1962.

Chapter 19 Children with Increasing Head Circumference

CT has become the initial diagnostic study in evaluating children with an enlarging head circumference. Prior to CT, if there were associated abnormalities, including an unusual head configuration (frontal bossing, lateral parietal prominence), an abnormal transillumination pattern, neurocutaneous lesions and abnormal neurological signs, air study and angiography were immediately initiated. Alternatively, if the child was neurologically intact but had several consecutive measurements that indicated progressive head enlargement, observation to follow serially the rate of head growth and pattern of neurological development was frequently done, although this approach may be potentially hazardous, as irreversible damage may occur during this period. In these latter cases, CT may be of the most benefit in early diagnosis, as the presence of severe hydrocephalus may now be detected in a noninvasive manner more sensitively than with echoencephalogram and before clinical signs develop and the cortical mantle is further compressed. CT may directly demonstrate ventricular size and, if increased, may accurately localize the anatomical level of obstruction and define distortion or displacement of the ventricular system. Because the scan provides only morphologic data, more precise information concerning the precise pattern of CSF obstruction is provided by air study or possibly by CT study utilizing cisternally injected Metrizamide. The information obtained by standard CT

study is usually adequate to determine the need for shunt; complementary information may determine the type of shunt to be performed; complementary air study is now infrequently performed.

In infancy hydrocephalus is the commonest cause of macrocephaly, but it may be due to other causes. If CT demonstrates that the lateral and third ventricles are dilated, aqueductal stenosis may be inferred indirectly, but CT cannot differentiate obstruction due to congenital stenosis with forking from that due to an acquired lesion in which the ependy-

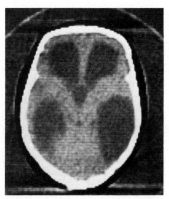

Figure 19–1. A four-month-old child was evaluated because of a rapidly enlarging head and failure to develop normal head control. There was a diffuse abnormal transillumination pattern, especially prominent in the occipital region. CT findings: marked lateral and third-ventricular dilatation, with small-sized fourth ventricle; convex shape of the third ventricle, which is directed posteriorly; no visualization of basilar cisterns, minimal rim of cortical mantle, and no change with contrast infusion. A shunt was inserted successfully without subsequent air study.

mal and subependymal layers are replaced by gliotic tissue resulting from hemorrhage or infection; this may sometimes be possible with air study.[1] The diagnosis of aqueductal stenosis may be established if the fourth ventricle is of small or normal size with dilatation of the remainder of the ventricular system; there is no visualization of the basilar cisterns, and the dilated posterior third ventricle has a convex shape that is directed posteriorly (Fig. 19–1). Because of the difficulty of accurately and completely visualizing the posterior fossa in infants, some children with this CT pattern are still found by air study to have communicating hydrocephalus.

With its small size and degree of angulation relative to the scanner, the dilated proximal portion of the aqueduct is only rarely seen (Fig. 19–2). The characteristic disproportional occipital horn enlargement may be visualized, and surrounding the frontal horns is a periventricular low-density rim that is confined to the white matter and may represent transventricular reabsorption of CSF (Fig. 19–3).[2, 3] Dilatation of the suprapineal recess with extension backward into the

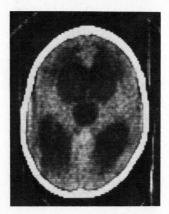

Figure 19–3. Symmetrical ventricular enlargement with semilunar low-density area surrounding the anterior frontal horn of the lateral ventricle. Ventriculogram confirmed the diagnosis of communicating hydrocephalus; pressure was high, consistent with an acute process.

quadrigeminal cistern may result from the effect of prolonged intraventricular pressure and may appear as an irregularly shaped low-density lesion in the region of the posterior

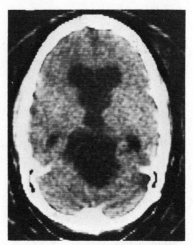

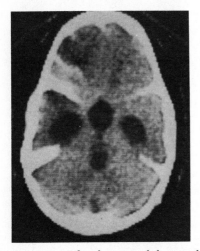

Figure 19–2. Dilated temporal horns, third ventricle, with unusual visualization of a dilated proximal portion of the aqueduct.

Figure 19–4. A child with a diagnosis of aqueductal stenosis, established by ventriculogram and shunted several years previously. CT findings: dilatation of lateral and third ventricle with sharply marginated, irregularly shaped, low-density lesion directly posterior to the third ventricle; the lesion truncates the third ventricle and extends backward into the quadrigeminal cistern. Ventriculogram showed this to be a dilated suprapineal recess.

third ventricle, but differentiation from other cystic lesions may require air study (Fig. 19–4).

Obstruction of CSF dynamics may be due to cystic dilatation of the fourth ventricle (Dandy-Walker malformation), which results in displacement and deformity of the fourth ventricle with associated absence of the inferior vermis, cerebellar dysplasia and other cerebral malformations, including agenesis of the corpus callosum. There may be a posterior prominence of the head, and lateral skull radiogram shows an elevated portion of the groove of the transverse sinus caused by the presence of a dilated

cyst, which prevents downward movement of the transverse sinus and torcular region. CT visualizes a posterior fossa midline cyst with no evidence of a normal fourth ventricle and elevation of the tentorial region; there may also be an associated hydrocephalus (Fig. 19–5). In other cases, there is a partially formed fourth ventricle and an absent inferior vermis; CT scan shows a CSF cyst extending posteriorly from the fourth ventricle with a prominent vallecula.

The presence of associated anomalies in patients with the Dandy-Walker syndrome, including agenesis of the corpus callosum, aqueductal stenosis and leptomeningeal cysts, may be well defined by CT without air study (Fig. 19–6).[4] Posterior fossa arachnoid cysts displace anteriorly and superiorly a normal fourth ventricle, which may also be compressed, and the tentorium may be elevated. An enlarged retrocerebellar space, as seen in communicating hydrocephalus, may simulate this posterior fossa cyst, but the fourth ventricle is enlarged and not

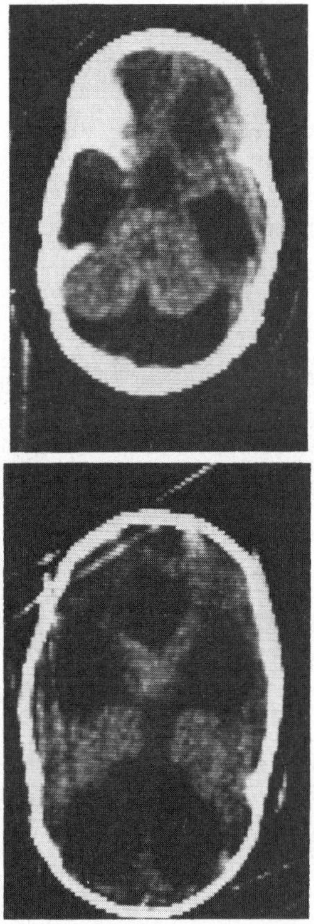

A

B

Figure 19–5. Scan shows lateral and third-ventricular enlargement, with reversal of normal convexity of the posterior third ventricle. Fourth ventricle is visualized (A) and there is a large cyst in the posterior fossa which is elevating the tentorium (B), consistent with Dandy-Walker syndrome.

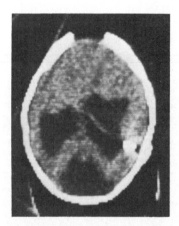

Figure 19–6. A six-month-old child, evaluated because of increasing head circumference, appeared normal neurologically. Air study showed Dandy-Walker cyst and shunt was inserted, but head continued to grow. CT findings: marked ventricular dilatation and small fourth ventricle with large retrocerebellar cyst. In addition, there is a high-riding third ventricle, with separation of lateral ventricles, consistent with agenesis of corpus callosum.

displaced in communicating hydroce-phalus.[5] Best definition of the intra- or extra-axial location of the posterior fossa cyst is achieved by air study or Metrizamide cisternal CT.

The Arnold-Chiari malformation, alone or in combination with other congenital or acquired abnormalities, may cause hydrocephalus by ob-structing the outlet foramina of the fourth ventricle with caudal elonga-tion and angulation of the fourth ven-tricle with obliteration of the sub-arachnoid spaces at the base of the brain. The diagnosis requires air

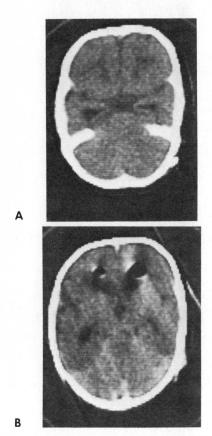

A

B

Figure 19–7. A nine-month-old child became lethargic and appeared unsteady while sitting up. CT findings: hydrocephalus with no visualization of the fourth ventricle and upward displacement of the posterior third ventricle (A) by nonenhanc-ing low-density mass in vermis (B). In addition shunt tube and air from previous ventriculogram are visualized. Pathological diagnosis was medul-loblastoma.

study but may be suspected from CT scan if there is an enlarged CSF-containing space representing the caudally elongated fourth ventricle, but a more frequent finding is a sym-metrical dilatation of all ventricular cavities, including the fourth ventri-cle. If an associated syringomyelia is present with Chiari malformation, CT may demonstrate the central lining within the spinal cord and medulla, as Pantopaque is present in the syrinx cavity after the myelogram.[6]

Tumors in the first year of life are rarely (1 to 4 percent) responsible for hydrocephalus, but increasing head size may be the only manifestation of the tumor. Present experience with CT is too limited to reach any conclu-sions concerning the indication for contrast enhancement in the child with hydrocephalus. A review of cases has shown that an isodense tumor may not be detected on prein-fusion study, although the presence of intraventricular obstruction and displacement or distortion of any por-tion of the ventricular or cisternal system raises suspicion of tumor, and contrast infusion must be performed in these cases (Fig. 19–7). The loca-tion of the majority of these tumors in children is midline and they have previously required ventriculography, but if these lesions are detected by CT, the necessity for air study may be further reduced (Fig. 19–8).[7] An-giography is required to define vascu-lar malformation, of which aneurys-mal dilatation of the vein of Galen is a rare but characteristic cause of this syndrome.

In neonates, congestive heart fail-ure is the most frequent clinical symptom of this malformation, whereas increased head size with in-traventricular obstruction is usually seen in infants. With CT a large dilat-ed vein appears as a midline high-density mass, which is consistent with circulating blood, and intravas-cular blood volume shows striking enhancement with contrast; there is associated obstruction of the posterior

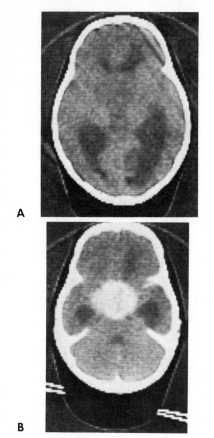

A

B

Figure 19–8. This one-year-old child had progressive head enlargement, lethargy, weight loss and impaired upward gaze. CT findings: plain scan shows lateral ventricular dilatation with obstruction of intraventricular foramina and visualization of round, slightly low-density lesion (A), which showed striking dense homogeneous enhancement (B). Air study and angiography demonstrated solid hypothalamic glioma without a cystic component.

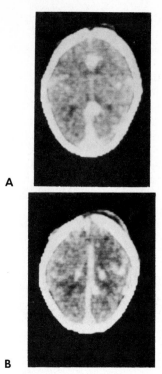

A

B

Figure 19–9. A five-day-old child was evaluated for congestive heart failure; isotope scan showed midline uptake. CT findings: marked dilatation of vein of Galen and anterior cerebral vein (A), with draining veins in both cerebral hemispheres, consistent with vascular malformation (B). This was verified by angiography.

third ventricle or aqueduct by the lesion.[5] In neonates the mass may be less prominent but the filling of the venous channels in midline may be very prominent (Fig. 19–9). In rare instances of infants who have clinical evidence of increased intracranial pressure there is no evidence of mass effect and the ventricles are normal in size and position on CT; subsequent pneumography has been normal in all cases, confirming the diagnosis of pseudotumor cerebri and obviating the need for ventriculography.

Following head trauma, increasing head circumference may be the only symptom of extradural hematoma, cyst formation or hydrocephalus. In some cases it is not possible to differentiate subdural hematoma, which is of low density and does not have an enhancing membrane, from leptomeningeal, subarachnoid or porencephalic cyst. This may require air study or angiography to determine the precise anatomical location of the fluid-filled space and to determine if there is actual communication with the ventricular system. If there has been a fracture it may continue to grow in the presence of an underlying leptomeningeal cyst. A porencephalic cyst is an expanding lesion

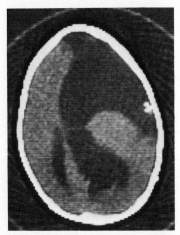

Figure 19–10. Scan shows large low-density lesion in the right frontoparietal region; it is dilating the ventricle and appears to communicate with the ventricle, and there is displacement of the ventricle to the left side. Air study confirmed the diagnosis of porencephalic cyst.

and may communicate with the ventricles to displace the ventricles and cause hydrocephalus (Fig. 19–10). CT may localize the position of the cyst and determine if it is single or multiple (porencephaly), but air study is necessary to define ventricle commu-

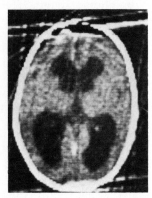

Figure 19–11. A four-month-old child without known history of trauma had increasing head size. Examination showed full and tense fontanelles, bilateral retinal hemorrhages and increased tone in legs. Subdural taps revealed 20 ml of bloody fluid on the left side and 10 ml on the right. CT scan performed five days later showed only symmetrical ventricular dilatation. Repeat taps performed within 24 hours after scan showed 15 to 20 ml of serosanguineous thick fluid on both sides; this had not been visualized by CT.

nication. Subarachnoid cysts are dilated and encysted spaces which are usually located in the middle and posterior fossa, and, if they are located over the hemisphere, may have features similar to those of porencephalic cysts.

The diagnosis of subdural hematoma and hygroma may usually be made with CT, but occasionally they are isodense and symmetrical, cause no ventricular displacement, distortion or compression and may have associated hydrocephalus; these may be detected only by subdural taps or angiography (Fig. 19–11). The differen-

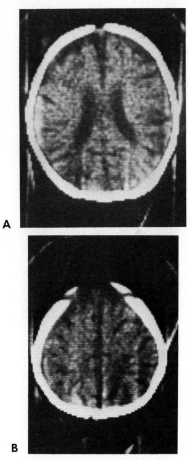

Figure 19–12. This child had normal head circumference but delayed developmental milestones. CT findings: enlarged ventricles with large bilateral extracerebral space, which extends into the interhemispheric fissue (A), and enlarged sulci (B), consistent with atrophic process.

tiation of subdural hematoma from enlarged extracerebral space with widened sulci and fissures due to an atrophic process is usually possible with CT (Fig. 19–12). In rare instances the head circumference continues to increase and subdural taps show 10 to 20 mm xanthochromic or normal CSF, but the scan shows enlarged extracerebral space and ventricular enlargement. In these cases, repeated subdural taps and shunt have been performed to arrest the enlargement of the head and prevent the fur-

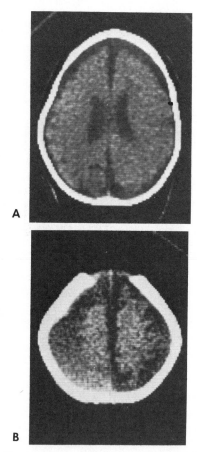

A

B

Figure 19–13. This ten-month-old child has had repeated subdural taps for bilateral subdural collections. The head size has continued to grow progressively and 15 to 25 ml of high-protein fluid has been removed. CT findings: extracerebral fluid collection bilaterally (A), extending into the anterior interhemispheric fissure, with prominence bilaterally of the cortical sulci (B).

ther compression of the underlying cortex. Further experience with this group of patients, some of whom are neurologically intact, and correlation with air study and isotope cisternography may demonstrate the mechanism of the fluid collection and ventricular enlargement.[8] In addition, serial studies in the neurologically intact children may document if there is progressive head enlargement or possibly spontaneous remission (Fig. 19–13). These cases may alter our concept of the development of hydrocephalus, as previous air study findings have indicated that the presence of widened extracerebral spaces and cortical sulci is indicative of an atrophic process that does not respond to shunt; this concept may now have to be re-examined.

Extraventricular obstructive hydrocephalus or obstruction of the outlet of the fourth ventricle due to adhesions causes symmetrical dilatation of the entire ventricular system, either with or without visualization of the basal cisterns. This may result from adhesions that thicken and obliterate reabsorptive space of the arachnoid villi and may be caused by infection, trauma or hemorrhage. The scan usually shows dilatation of the fourth ventricle but this need not always be present; dilatation of the basal cistern suggests the diagnosis of communicating hydrocephalus (Fig. 19–14). Hydrocephalus frequently develops in children who were premature and had subependymal germinal matrix hemorrhage. This usually causes severe neurological deficit in the neonatal period as a result of intraventricular hemorrhage.[9] Prior to CT, this diagnosis was made clinically and by finding blood in the CSF. Occasionally the patient may be clinically asymptomatic and lumbar puncture is not performed; therefore the etiology of the hydrocephalus is never established, but with CT these hemorrhages are well visualized.

Following shunt procedure, CT may be used to assess ventricular size

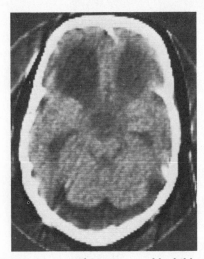

Figure 19–14. This six-year-old child with hydrocephalus had multiple shunt procedures. CT findings: lateral and third ventricular dilatation with normal size and position of fourth ventricle and huge cisterna magna or retrocerebellar cyst. Air study demonstrated communicating hydrocephalus with enlarged basilar cisterns.

and to evaluate the potential complications of shunt therapy. Following the insertion of a shunt, there may be a rapid decrease in ventricular size, and this may lead to the development of subdural hematoma, which may be detected by CT (Fig. 19–15). The hydrocephalus may arrest so that ventricular and head size are no longer increasing and CSF pressure is normal following the insertion of a shunt. This may lead to shunt dependency in which CSF circulation is impaired because the frontal horns have become small owing to subependymal fibrosis, which prevents their re-expansion, and CT scan shows either ventricular collapse on the shunted side or small frontal horns with enlarged occipital horns.[3, 5] Other complications of the shunt include intracerebral hematoma, porencephalic cysts, and perforation of brain parenchyma by the shunt tube, and these may be visualized with CT. In some children, the hydrocephalus arrests spontaneously; this is believed to result from the in-creased capacity of the ventricular ependymal surface to reabsorb CSF or from decreased production of CSF.

Serial CT may permit determination of any change in the ventricular size or the thickness of the cortical mantle and perhaps increase the latitude of the decison to delay shunt in asymptomatic patients, as CT is more accurate than indices of ventricular size determined by echoencephalography. If the ventricular size continues to increase there is reduction in size of the cortical mantle, with the majority of changes occurring in the white matter. There may be diffusion of CSF into the periventricular white matter, with stretching of the walls of the lateral ventricles, especially in the posterior occipital region, with subsequent thinning of the cortical ribbon and infarction (atrophy, cyst) due to marked compression of the superficial arteries. The thickness of the cortical mantle may be assessed by CT although the outcome of shunt has not been correlated with this measurement, but normal intelligence frequently correlates with a cortical mantle of greater than 2.8 cm thickness and early shunt.[10]

Less commonly, increase in head size is not related to impaired CSF circulation, but megalencephaly is related to an increase in brain substance. Such increase may be caused by accumulation or abnormal storage of metabolic products or an abnormal cellular proliferation of fluid collection resulting from a congenital or acquired insult with consequent destruction or poor development of the cerebral hemispheres. If structural damage has occurred, it may be visualized by CT, but definitive diagnosis may require air study or angiography, as the CT findings in hydranencephaly, hydrocephalus, holoprosencephaly and bilateral subdural effusion may be quite similar.[5, 11]

In hydranencephaly the cerebral hemispheres fail to develop owing to prenatal hypoplasia or occlusion of the internal carotid arteries, and only

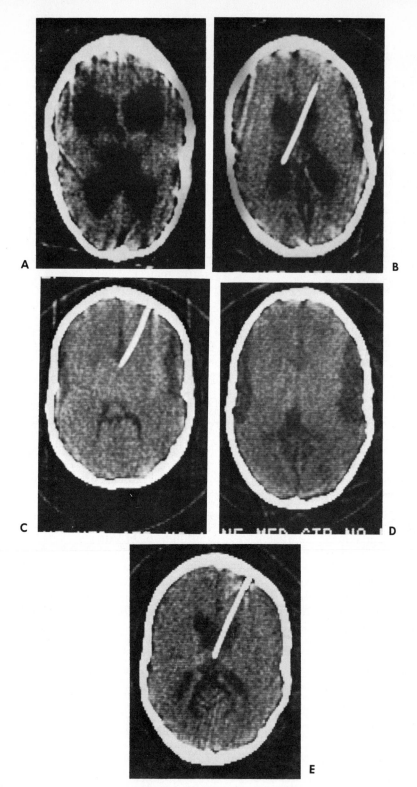

Figure 19–15. A child with marked hydrocephalus (A), who underwent ventriculo-peritoneal shunt. Two weeks later there was a dramatic decrease in ventricular size, but a small, subdural collection developed on the right side (B). This became bilateral on the next scan, which also shows compression of the ventricle (C and D). Following evacuation of the collections, the ventricles re-expanded to the initial postshunt size (E).

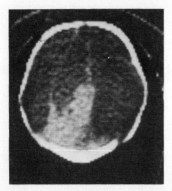

Figure 19–16. Low-density appearance indicates presence of CSF throughout both hemispheres, with sparing of left occipital region, basal ganglia, brain stem and cerebellum. In addition, there is a faint midline septum, and this is consistent with hydranencephaly.

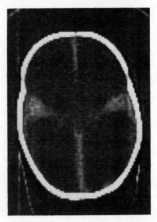

Figure 19–17. A child with meningitis developed seizures, focal neurological signs and increasing head size despite treatment. CT findings: huge ventricles with no cortical rim but midline small region of tissue. This pattern is consistent with severe hydrocephalus.

a remnant of the occipital region, brain stem, cerebellum and ganglionic mass may be identified without any discrete ventricular cavities or rim of cortical mantle (Fig. 19–16). Isotope scan flow study may suggest this diagnosis, but angiography is necessary to define the absence of the middle and anterior cerebral vessels.

In severe hydrocephalus, there may be no appreciable rim of cortical tissue adjacent to the enlarged ventricles, but the ventricular structure is preserved and usually there is an identifiable rim of preserved cortex, and midline septum persists (Fig. 19–17). Angiography may show severe compression and stretching of the middle and anterior cerebral vessels, but they are clearly visible. Large bilateral subdural hygromas may collapse the entire ventricular system and extend to the midline, but the fourth ventricle and posterior fossa should be preserved, and angiography shows that the cortical vessels are intact and markedly compressed inward and downward.

In holoprosencephaly, there is only a thin remnant of cerebral parenchyma. This may be divided into two forms: (1) alobar form in which there is no cerebral hemisphere but only a thin rim of primitive cortex that sur-

rounds a single ventricular cavity or two cavities; (2) lobar form in which there is partial separation into separate developed hemispherics but the frontal horns are fused and CT shows a batwing appearance (Fig. 19–18).

In other cases, CT may clearly define the specific abnormality. Agenesis of the corpus callosum is defined by the presence of a high-riding elevated third ventricle with separation of the lateral ventricles, and evidence

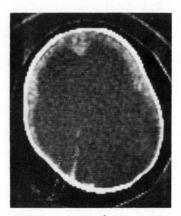

Figure 19–18. Scan shows monoventricle surrounded by rim of primitive cerebral tissue. At necropsy, diagnosis of holoprosencephaly was made.

of a midline cyst separating the lateral ventricles; this may represent the dilated third ventricle (Fig. 19–19). This abnormality may be associated with lipoma of the corpus callosum, which appears as a midline low-density lesion that frequently calcifies and is easily detected by CT. With CT, it may be possible to suggest the presence of lissencephaly from the finding of enlarged ventricles and subarachnoid spaces, with a smooth cortical pattern; this may be confirmed by angiogram showing a wavy pattern of the superficial cortical vessels that occurs in the absence of cortical sulci.

Other disorders, including polymicrogyria, schizencephaly and heterotopias, show no characteristic patterns. In septo-optic dysplasia, the absence of the septum pellucidum results in a flattened arterial appearance of the frontal horn.[11] The characteristic CT findings in tuberous sclerosis (periventricular calcification) and Sturge-Weber vascular malformation have been previously discussed.[2, 12] The characteristic low-density lesion in the white matter region is characteristic of the leukodystrophies including Schilder's disease.[13] CT is important in defining the presence of associated anomalies. If one is present, there is a markedly increased incidence of finding an associated abnormality, as in Dandy-

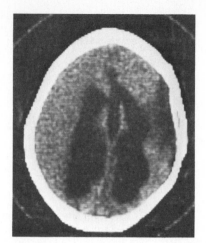

Figure 19–19. A high-riding and dilated third ventricle, with splayed lateral ventricles and a porencephalic cyst in the right hemisphere.

Walker disease with agenesis of the corpus callosum or aqueductal stenosis, tuberous sclerosis with subependymal astrocytoma, or neurofibromatosis with tumors including optic glioma.

In other cases of neonatal intraventricular hemorrhage, in cranioschisis (meningomyelocele, encephalocele) and in cases of microencephaly, CT may provide enough diagnostic information to assess the prognosis without invasive contrast studies, but it should be stressed that complete evaluation of many of these abnormalities still requires complementary air study and angiography.[5]

REFERENCES

1. Taveras JM, Wood EH: Diagnostic Neuroradiology. Williams and Wilkins, Baltimore, 1964. pp 1348–1356.
2. Gomez MR, Reese DF: CT of the head in infants and children. Pediat Clin N Am 23:473, 1976.
3. Naidich TP, Epstein F, Liu JP, Kricheff I, et al: Evaluation of pediatric hydrocephalus by CT. Radiology 119:337, 1976.
4. Ostertag C, Hemmer R, Mundinger F: Observations on the differentiation of hydrocephalus occlusus in infancy and early childhood using CAT. Neuropediatric 7:322, 1976.
5. Harwood-Nash DC, Fitz CR: Neuroradiology in Infants and Children. CV Mosby, St. Louis, 1976. pp 461–504.
6. DiChiro G, Axelbaum SP, Schellinger D, et al: CT in syringomyelia. N Engl J Med 292:13, 1975.
7. Kazner E, Lanksch W, Steinhoff H: Cranial CT in the diagnosis of brain disorders in infants and children. Neuropediatric 7:136, 1976.

8. Robertson WC, Gomez MR: External hydrocephalus in communicating hydrocephalus. Abstract presented at Child Neurology Society, Carmel, California, October, 1976.
9. Krishnamoorthy KS, Fernandez RA, Momose KJ, et al: Evaluation of neonatal intracranial hemorrhage by CT. Pediatrics 59:165, 1977.
10. Young HF, Nulsen FE, Weiss MH, et al: The relationship of intelligence and cerebral mantle in treated infantile hydrocephalus. Pediatrics 52:38, 1973.
11. Harwood-Nash DC: Congenital craniocerebral abnormalities and CT. Semin Roentgenol 12:39, 1977.
12. Gomez MR, Mellinger JF, Reese DF: The use of CT in the diagnosis of tuberous sclerosis. Mayo Clin Proc 50:553, 1975.
13. Duda EE, Huttenlocher PR: CT in adrenal-leuko dystrophy. Radiology 120:349, 1976.
14. McCullough DC, Kufta C, Axelbaum SP, et al: CT in clinical pediatrics. Pediatrics 59:173, 1977.

Chapter 20 CT in Evaluation of Treatment Modalities

CT is the most reliable diagnostic study to evaluate the results of surgery, radiotherapy, corticosteroids and chemotherapy including antineoplastic agents. This is due to its ability to distinguish directly varying pathological changes within the lesion and the surrounding parenchyma with greater accuracy and specificity than is possible with EEG, isotope scan, angiography or air study.

Following surgery or radiotherapy, EEG findings do not always correlate with the patient's clinical status, as the electrical potential generated from the area of the lesion does not always accurately reflect the pathological changes that are evolving within the lesion. For example, the development of a focal spike pattern in EEG after treatment may be indicative of multiple pathological processes, including hemorrhage, edema, necrosis, tumor recurrence or the development of a cerebral scarring process. There have been reports of decrease in the extent of the EEG abnormal pattern as the tumor actually was increasing in size, and the converse situation is also true.

Isotope scan may be difficult to interpret in the postoperative period because there may be uptake in the more superficial tissues owing to the effect of the craniotomy, and this may persist for up to six months.[1] Furthermore, an isotope scan may be negative despite the presence of substantial tumor recurrence, especially if the tumor is cystic; and alternatively radiotherapy and antineoplastic drugs may induce damage within the region of the tumor that may make the ab-

normality seem more conspicuous on isotope scan despite good clinical response. Even if tumors decrease in size with treatment, no change may be detected in the isotope scan for six to eight weeks because this study demonstrates only marked differences in radionuclide concentration, and a large degree of tumor shrinkage must occur before it is detectable with isotope scan.[2] Also, isotope scan cannot accurately differentiate tumor from edema.

Angiography has been utilized as the most reliable postoperative study but it is usually employed only if there is a sudden and definite worsening in the patient's clinical status. It is not a feasible procedure to evaluate serially the response to therapy. In the postsurgical patient angiography is less sensitive because of the absence of vessels that have been previously utilized to define mass effect and tumor stain. Although angiography usually detects evidence of mass effect or hydrocephalus in those patients who develop recurrent symptoms, it is not always accurate in defining the mechanism of this mass effect, which may include edema, necrosis, hematoma or tumor recurrence.

The most reliable indicator of the recurrence or persistence of the pathological process is the clinical course, but not infrequently there may be certain changes in the clinical condition that may suggest tumor recurrence but may also represent spontaneous and intermittent fluctuations in the clinical course, an unrelated neurological disorder or a complication of therapy. In these cases, prior to CT, accurate differentiation was not always possible without angiography or it sometimes required surgical exploration.[3] Specific clinical problems relating to treatment investigated by CT include the following:

Deterioration in the Immediate Postoperative Period. Some patients fail to regain consciousness and do not show improvement in neurological function. This is most usually due to persistent mass effect resulting from edema, necrosis or hematoma of

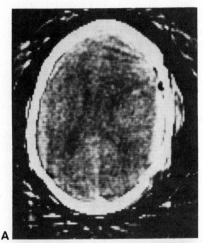

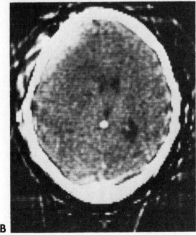

Figure 20–1. Following right temporal craniotomy, this patient's level of consciousness failed to improve. CT findings: displacement and distortion of the right lateral ventricles by an acute subdural hematoma (A). This is contrasted with evidence of blood under the bone flap and slight left hemispheric edema, which resolved in several days, but no definite evidence of extracerebral hematoma, confirmed by angiography (B).

intra- or extracerebral origin; CT is the most sensitive study to differentiate these conditions. Intracerebral hematoma is visualized as a round high-density lesion in the region of the surgery; it may be single or multiple, is associated with mass effect and does not enhance, but confusion may occur if a hematoma and residual enhancing high-density tumor are both present. Postoperative acute epidural or subdural hematomas have a characteristic high-density pattern and shape, but these lesions must be differentiated from a small amount of blood under the bone flap, which may have a similar appearance and usually resolves in several days (Fig. 20–1). Postoperative edema, residual tumor, necrosis or encephalomalacia may be visualized as low-density or isodense lesions that cause ventricular displacement and distortion with no enhancement; this latter feature distinguishes them from recurrent or residual neoplasm, which usually enhances. Occasionally with necrotic tissue there may be a peripheral rim of enhancement, which is due to a surrounding area of neovascularity and does not represent capsule formation or residual tumor. This enhancing high-density rim is not seen with postoperative edema (Fig. 20–2). Less frequently, immediate postoperative clinical deterioration is due to hydrocephalus rather than to mass effect, and this assessment of the ventricular size and the location of obstruction are established by CT, which also affords a reliable baseline for further studies.

Evaluation of Completeness of Surgical Resection of Neoplasm, Abscess or Hematoma. CT findings usually correlate directly with the clinical condition; worsening of neurological function is usually associated with CT demonstration of an increase in tumor size, extent, mass effect, central lucent region, and intensity of enhancement pattern. In tumors that have been completely extirpated the CT scan may be normal or show evidence of a well-marginated low-density area consistent with CSF caused by porencephalic

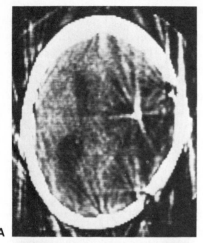

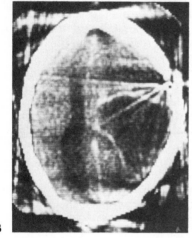

Figure 20–2.   Following surgical removal of a right hemispheric vascular angioma, this patient remained obtunded with worsening of left hemiparesis. CT findings: compression of the right lateral ventricle, with bowing and stretching of falx cerebri by a low-density lesion (A) in right hemisphere, with peripheral rim of enhancement (B).

cyst. Regression of the neoplasm is usually visualized as decrease in tumor and edema size, reduction of the mass effect and frequently diminution of the intensity of the contrast enhancement, although the latter is a less consistent finding.[3a] In 10 to 15 percent of cases clinical and CT findings do not correlate, and this is similar to the results obtained in previous studies of isotope scan; but CT was able to define more precisely the pathophysiological mechanism underlying the clinical deterioration, including hemorrhage or cyst formation, a determination not

previously possible.[2,4] Following surgical removal in inflammatory disorders, CT may define the presence of residual contiguous satellite or distant abscesses not detected by isotope scan or angiography. Completeness of removal and normalization of cerebral structures visualized by CT usually correlate with clinical recovery, but in several cases the CT scan failed to provide any possible explanation for poor clinical response. After surgical removal of an intracerebral hematoma, the scan usually demonstrates a low-density cystic space, but there have been necropsy reports that substantial remnants of hematoma or neoplasm may persist without a corresponding high-density CT scan pattern. Following surgical removal of extracerebral lesions, the mass effect and size of fluid in these spaces are diminished. A recent report showed that in epidural hematoma the scan is negative if clinical recovery occurs, but in subdural hematoma there may be surprisingly little reduction in the mass effect or extracerebral space size despite clinical improvement.[5]

Effect of Radiation Therapy. Immediately following the initiation of irradiation, there may be edema and tumor necrosis, which increase mass effect and result in clinical worsening. Administration of corticosteroids may prevent this complication or may be used to treat it if it occurs. This may be especially important in the treatment of pituitary adenomas, as surgical intervention may be necessary if visual function worsens significantly and does not respond to corticosteroids. The production of this inflammatory response in the tumor and surrounding brain occurs in all primary and metastatic neoplasms. It is infrequently responsible for clinical worsening in supratentorial tumors, but its presence is visualized by CT. With primary brain tumors there was CT evidence of regression in the size of the tumor in one to three months following initiation of radiation therapy, and this may continue for up to nine months after completion of the course of treatment.[3a] In rare instances, irradiation may precipitate hemorrhage within the tumor, which may be demonstrated by comparison of pre- and post-treatment nonconstrast CT scans. Delayed radiation necrosis may occur several months to years after treatment and, because it may be associated with progressive neurological deterioration consistent with the presence of a mass lesion, differentiation from recurrent neoplasm or edema may be quite difficult. In radiation necrosis angiographic findings include demonstration of an avascular intracerebral mass without evidence of tumor stain or abnormal vascularity, and, rarely, irregular narrowing of arteries similar to the vessel abnormality seen in collagen disease may be visualized.[6] The CT findings in radiation necrosis, in which pathological findings have verified the absence of recurrent tumor, have been varied, including irregularly shaped, mottled, low-density lesions causing significant mass effect with minimal evidence of enhancement and mass effect with a ring enhancement pattern; others have shown evidence of white matter degeneration. Differentiation from recurrent neoplasm has usually been based upon the paucity of enhancement, but this is not entirely reliable, and definitive diagnosis is based upon the findings of surgical exploration and biopsy.[7]

Previous pneumographic studies have demonstrated cerebral hemispheric atrophic changes following radiation therapy, and this may coexist with evidence of tumor recurrence. Wilson reported symmetrical enlargement of the lateral ventricles three to six months after irradiation in one half of patients who had received 3000 to 6000 rads to the head, and Robertson demonstrated atrophic changes in the posterior fossa following irradiation of brain stem gliomas.[8, 9] These radiation-induced effects are believed due to changes in the glial cells, especially the oligodendrocytes, which produce demyelination and white matter degenera-

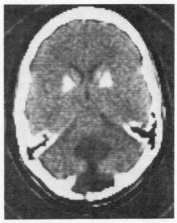

Figure 20–3. A 20-year-old man who underwent posterior fossa exploration and biopsy 12 years previously for brain stem glioma has now developed progressive gait unsteadiness. CT findings: marked enlargement of the fourth ventricle, vallecula cisterna magna and basilar cisterns, consistent with atrophic process. In addition, there is dense calcification in both basal ganglia.

tion. These previous pneumographic findings have been confirmed by serial CT studies. In addition, bilateral calcification of the basal ganglia has been detected several years following irradiation of brain stem gliomas (Fig. 20–3).

Delayed Clinical Deterioration in Neoplasms Following Surgical or Ir-

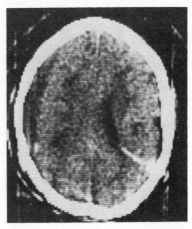

Figure 20–4. A 60-year-old man with dementia, urinary incontinence and gait disturbance had a right-sided ventriculo-peritoneal shunt for communicating hydrocephalus. Postoperatively, he began falling to the right side. CT scan showed a left-sided chronic subdural hematoma.

radiation Therapy. Patients with metastatic tumors and gliomas frequently develop recurrent symptoms several years following surgical resection despite the surgical evidence that tumor removal was complete. This may be due to tumor recurrence, cyst formation or radiation necrosis, but may also be due to scar formation or vascular damage. Norman showed that CT may reveal recurrence or progression of the tumor several months prior to clinical worsening, but the experience of others, as well as our own, with patients with neoplasms who were clinically stable has not confirmed this finding.[3a] CT is a most reliable study to define the exact patho-

physiology underlying the clinical deterioration and determining if it is related directly to the neoplasm, in which case further treatment may be necessary. In all cases of clinical deterioration due to recurrent neoplasm, CT clearly demonstrated the tumor, especially in identifying those conditions that do not require further treatment, and in these cases only a contrast infusion study without preceding plain scan is necessary.

Drug Treatment. Corticosteroids act to decrease cerebral edema by stabilizing the capillary basement, and CT scan may show evidence of decreased mass effect and a less intense enhancement pattern. Certain

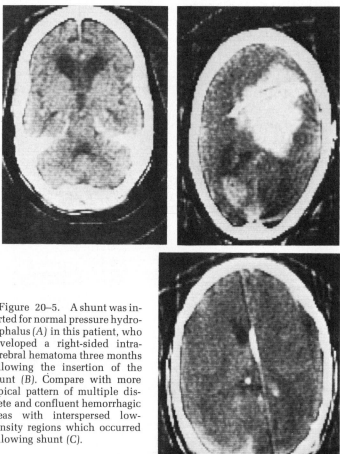

Figure 20–5. A shunt was inserted for normal pressure hydrocephalus (A) in this patient, who developed a right-sided intracerebral hematoma three months following the insertion of the shunt (B). Compare with more typical pattern of multiple discrete and confluent hemorrhagic areas with interspersed low-density regions which occurred following shunt (C).

immunosuppressive and antineoplastic agents, including methotrexate, may cause a necrotizing leukoencephalopathy that has CT features similar to abscess, neoplasm or hematoma. In this disorder, the most extensive damage occurs in the periventricular white matter, and in the more chronic stage calcification has been detected by CT.[10, 11] It may not be possible to differentiate necrotic change in white matter from edema by CT.

Shunting Procedures. Following insertion of a diversionary shunt, CT may be used to assess changes in ventricular size and to indirectly assess shunt function. Usually there is a dramatic decrease in ventricular size several days after shunt placement. If there is too rapid decrease in size, subdural hematomas may develop, and this occurrence is defined by CT (Fig. 20–4). Another unusual complication is the development of an intracerebral hematoma one to three months after insertion, and it is always located ipsilateral to the shunt (Fig. 20–5). Less commonly, clinical improvement occurs after shunt placement, but this is not associated with significant reduction in ventricular size, whereas in other cases there is collapse of the ventricles on the shunted side. CT is invaluable to determine the position of the shunt tube and to follow the development of cystic spaces.

REFERENCES

1. Waxman AD, Siemsen JK, Wolfstein RS: Evaluation of postcraniotomy patients by radionuclide scan. J Neurosurg 43:471, 1975.
2. Handel SF, Malcolm MR, Wilson CB: Scintiphotographic evaluation of response of brain neoplasms to systemic chemotherapy. J Nucl Med 12:292, 1971.
3. Lin JP, Payn N, Naidich TP, et al. CT in the post-operative core of neurosurgical patients. Neuroradiology 12:185, 1977.
3a. Marks JE, Gado M: Serial CT of primary brain tumors following surgery, irradiation and chemotherapy. Radiology 125:119, 1977.
4. Norman D, Enzmann DR, Levin V, et al: CT in the evaluation of malignant glioma before and after therapy. Radiology 121:85, 1977.
5. Dolinskas C, Zimmerman RA, Bilaniuk LT, et al: The course of mass effect following surgical evacuation of an extracerebral hematoma. Abstract presented at American Society of Neuroradiology, Bermuda, April, 1977.
6. Rottenberg DA, Chernik NL, Deck MDF, et al: Cerebral necrosis following radiotherapy of extracranial neoplasms. Ann Neurol 1:339, 1977.
7. Pay NT, Carella RJ, Lin JR, et al: The usefulness of CT during and after radiation therapy in patients with brain tumors. Radiology 121:79, 1976.
8. Wilson GH, Byfield J, Hanafee WN: Atrophy following radiation therapy for CNS neoplasms. Acta Raidol (Ther) 11:361, 1972.
9. Robertson EG: Pneumoencephalography. CC Thomas, Springfield, Illinois, 1967. p 377.
10. 10. Mueller S, Bell W, Siebert J: Cerebral calcification associated with methotrexate therapy in acute lymphocytic leukemia. J Pediat 88:650, 1976.
11. Bjorgen JE, Gold LHA: CT appearance of methotrexate induced necrotizing leukoencephalopathy. Radiology 122:377, 1977.

Index

Note: Page numbers in bold refer to illustrations.